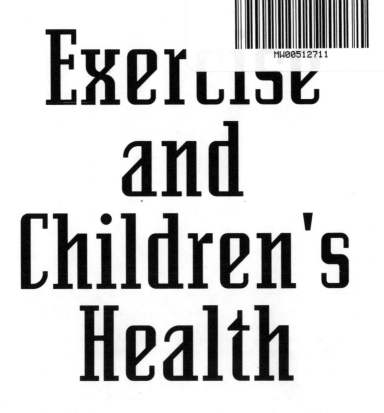

Exercise and Children's Health

Thomas W. Rowland, MD
Baystate Medical Center
Springfield, Massachusetts

Human Kinetics Books
Champaign, Illinois

Library of Congress Cataloging-in-Publication Data

Rowland, Thomas W.
    Exercise and children's health / by Thomas W. Rowland.
      p.   cm.
    Includes bibliographical references.
    ISBN 0-87322-282-2
    1. Exercise for children--Health aspects. 2. Physical fitness for
children. I. Title.
    [DNLM: 1. Exercise--in infancy & childhood. 2. Health.
3. Physical Fitness. QT 255 R883e]
    RJ133.R68 1990
    618.92--dc20
    DNLM/DLC
    for Library of Congress   89-71708
                                              CIP

ISBN: 0-87322-282-2 (case)
      0-87322-810-3 (paper)

Photos on pages 2, 215, and 275 by Kimberlie Henris. Photos on pages 11, 47, 129, 161, and 283 © CLEO Photography. Photos on pages 21 and 181 courtesy of University of Illinois Physical Fitness Research Laboratory. Photo on page 101 by Gary Reiss, Champaign, Illinois, courtesy of Champaign Park District. Photo on page 235 by Mark Robbins, courtesy of *Daily Illini*, University of Illinois at Urbana-Champaign. Photo on the back cover by Carl Bartels.

Developmental Editors: Holly Gilly, Marie Roy; **Copyeditor:** Wendy Nelson; **Assistant Editors:** Robert King, Timothy Ryan; **Proofreader:** Pam Johnson; **Production Director:** Ernie Noa; **Typesetter:** Sandra Meier; **Text Design:** Keith Blomberg; **Text Layout:** Kimberlie Henris; **Cover Design:** Jack Davis; **Illustrations:** Kimberlie Henris, Barbara Cook; **Photo Acquisition:** Valerie Hall, Margaret A. Gates-Wieneke, Amy Hurd; **Printer:** Braun-Brumfield

Printed in the United States of America   10 9 8 7 6 5 4 3 2 1

Human Kinetics Books
A Division of Human Kinetics
P.O. Box 5076, Champaign, IL 61825-5076
1-800-747-4457

Canada: Human Kinetics, Box 24040, Windsor, ON N8Y 4Y9
1-800-465-7301 (in Canada only)

Europe: Human Kinetics, P.O. Box IW14, Leeds LS16 6TR, England
0532-781708
Australia: Human Kinetics, Unit 5, 32 Raglan Avenue, Edwardstown 5039, South Australia
(08) 371 3755

New Zealand: Human Kinetics, P.O. Box 105-231, Auckland 1
(09) 309-2259

Contents

Preface

Every book needs to tell a story, and this one is very, very old (the story, not the book). It begins some 2 billion years ago, when the earth was covered by scant vegetation that was long accustomed to inspiring an atmosphere of nitrogen, carbon dioxide, water vapor, and hydrogen. A new gas, oxygen, was making its appearance in the air, the work of a group of blue-green algae that had "discovered" photosynthesis, combining the sun's rays with carbon dioxide to create a carbohydrate food source, and were now excreting oxygen as a by-product.

To most primitive organisms this new gas was a lethal poison, but for a few it unlocked the way for providing new and more abundant energy sources. These innovative survivors learned how to use oxygen in more efficient oxidative metabolic pathways, and, making good use of their newfound energy source, they began to *move*. Slowly at first, about a centimeter a day, they crawled about, invaginating and altering the shapes of their outer cell membranes.

Little controversy arose surrounding the health benefits of this new mobility. Here was a means of improving the odds on securing food, escaping enemies, and assuring sexual reproduction. It wasn't long (a few hundred million years or so) before the earth's animals were flopping, winging, slithering, and hopping their ways in this classic Darwinian saga.

Early *Homo sapiens* were no exceptions. They combined developing intellect with mobility to permit survival of the fittest hunters, farmers, and warriors. The ancient civilizations thrived with this symbiosis of mental and physical prowess, and the survival of nations at war was often held in balance by the physical capabilities of their soldiers. It is not surprising, then, that the quality of physical fitness has been revered throughout human history.

The role of physical activity in our modern society is, of course, vastly different. No longer do we rely on physical prowess for survival. One can earn a living, enjoy leisure time, obtain food, avoid enemies, and procreate with little or no physical effort whatsoever. Is there a price to be paid for this ease of modern living? Many are concerned that the "wholeness" of the individual is threatened—perhaps even destroyed—by the technological conveniences that surround us.

The irony is striking, then, that regular physical activity can play an important role in preventing and treating the ills produced by our contemporary lifestyles. Darwinism, alas, is alive and well, but the venue has shifted from the stagnant pools of prehistoric swamps to the proximity of the high school track. It's survival of the fittest all over again, but this time it's obesity, coronary artery disease, hypertension, smoking, diabetes, mental illness, and just plain boredom that have provided a new importance for physical activity in our daily lives. A sedentary lifestyle is dangerous to your health, a fact that would not have been any surprise to our prehistoric ancestors.

The major causes of morbidity and mortality in developed nations—and those most influenced by physical activity—are largely diseases that are both heavily influenced by lifestyle and have their roots in childhood and adolescence. It follows that individuals responsible for the health care and education of children should have key roles in public health strategies to reduce the incidence of these diseases. The promotion of physical activity thus joins the list of childhood interventions (along with proper diet, avoidance of obesity, early detection of hypertension, smoking cessation, and so on) designed to prevent diseases that will surface clinically only in the later years of life.

One rationale for advocating and guiding children in physical activities is based on studies that link these chronic diseases with sedentary lifestyle. But the current interest in children's exercise has been stimulated by other concerns as well. These are outlined in the introduction that follows, and all bear importantly on health. To the physician falls the responsibility as well as the opportunity to guide these young patients into safe and healthful forms of physical activity. It is for these health care providers that this book was written.

Young subjects differ from adults in many facets of exercise physiology. Part I of this book is designed to provide basic information regarding children's physiological responses to exercise, emphasizing developmental changes that occur during the growing years. Practitioners need to possess a basic understanding of these concepts, both for interpreting the results and meaning of children's fitness tests and for designing therapeutic exercise programs.

Part II reviews the scientific grounds for promoting exercise as a beneficial health measure. The importance of physical activity in preventive medicine is emphasized as well as the use of exercise as a therapeutic intervention in specific disease states. Clearly the days of simply recommending that the patient "get more exercise" are gone. Part III provides specific strategies for increasing physical activity in children by both structured and unsupervised programs; its practical guidelines give physicians and other professionals useful materials for "prescribing" exercise programs for young patients.

This book endeavors to paint a broad picture of the role of exercise in children's health. Because each aspect cannot be examined in all its depth, efforts have been made to include review-type references for readers in search of more comprehensive discussions.

A great deal more needs to be learned regarding exercise in children and the implications of physical activity and fitness for good health. But the information reviewed in this book provides persuasive evidence that the promotion of physical activity in young individuals is a valuable effort that can pay significant long-term health dividends.

Thomas Rowland, M.D.

Acknowledgments

I wish to express my appreciation for the support and encouragement I have received from Dr. Oded Bar-Or, whose contributions to the field of exercise in children have laid much of the foundation for this book. The following individuals deserve thanks for their helpful suggestions in the preparation of various chapters: Dr. Alan Morris, Dr. William Kraemer, Dr. Thomas Manfredi, Dr. Lorraine Bloomquist, Coleen Walsh, Dr. Judy Siegel, James Robertson, Dr. Russell Pate, and Dr. Paul Dyment. Ms. Lily Peng and her staff of the Health Sciences Library at the Baystate Medical Center provided invaluable assistance in securing reference material. Rainer Martens, Marie Roy, and Holly Gilly at Human Kinetics Publishers were encouraging mentors in keeping the book moving to completion. A special thanks goes to Barbara Sheldon, whose devoted and tireless secretarial efforts made it all possible. And, finally, I am grateful to my wife, Margot, and children, Todd, Geoffrey, and Elizabeth, without whose patience and support this book would not have been written.

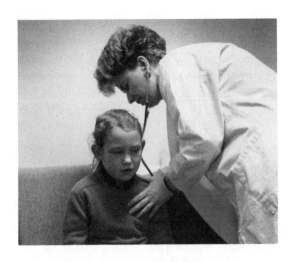

INTRODUCTION

The Role of the Physician in Pediatric Exercise Medicine

In 1978 Pate and Blair challenged primary health care providers to take up the role of "lifestyle counselor" for children, contending that "physicians must expand their traditional role of healer and begin truly to embrace the concept of preventive medicine" (p. 273). Theirs was a cogent argument. A sedentary life during the pediatric years creates a lifelong hazard to health, and pediatricians and family practice physicians are in the best positions to improve children's exercise habits. Others have subsequently underscored the role that primary care physicians can play in effecting changes in their young patients' fitness levels (Bar-Or, 1983; Rowland, 1981; Strong, 1987).

Advocating a healthy lifestyle during the growing years was not a foreign concept to these physicians. The promotion of a diet low in fats and salt, early detection of hypertension, avoidance of obesity, and smoking cessation had become as much a part of preventive medicine for children as immunizations, fluoride, and accident prevention. But seeing that their patients exercised sufficiently was a novel role for those whose previous involvement with sports medicine was limited to ritualistic preparticipation exams and management of minor injuries. Sports medicine, after all, was an orthopedic subspecialty.

The ensuing decade has witnessed dramatic changes in perceptions of exercise and its relationship to health, particularly with respect to growing children. The recognition of the health benefits of regular physical activity was only the first of many social and scientific forces that have reshaped the role of the primary care physician in sports medicine and the promotion of exercise. These trends have created both new responsibilities and new opportunities for physicians that can enhance the quality of their practices while helping ensure the safety and health of their patients:

• **Concern over the fitness of American children.** The results of mass exercise testing of children in the United States have been interpreted as indicating that our youth are in seriously poor physical condition (Safrit, 1986). Although the validity of these conclusions has been challenged (Murphy, 1986; Simmons, 1986), the wide dispersal of this information by the scientific and lay media has stimulated efforts to improve the physical fitness of American youth (Bailey, 1973). This movement has coincided with—and has been fueled by—two additional considerations that add immediacy to the promotion of exercise in children.

First, scientific evidence has become compelling that a sedentary lifestyle carries a risk for the development of coronary artery disease, obesity, hypertension, diabetes mellitus, and other chronic diseases of adulthood. Although these problems become clinically manifest during adulthood, they are lifelong processes with origins in the pediatric years (Berenson, 1986). The importance of promoting exercise for children, as Pate and Blair (1978) emphasize, lies in instilling physical activity as a habit that may help forestall these chronic illnesses over a lifetime.

The physician must play a key role in this effort. The need and justification exist for assessment, prescription, and support of physical activities for all children. Evidence in adults suggests that the health benefits of exercise may be related as much to regular physical activity as to physical fitness or athletic capabilities. If so, the impetus from physicians may be best placed on preventing a sedentary lifestyle in their patients rather than on specifically improving fitness levels.

The perceived lack of fitness in the pediatric population has also prompted a close look at America's physical education programs, which are considered a logical focus of action for improving children's physical capacities. That close look has produced, in turn, genuine concern. The National Children and Youth Fitness Study released in 1984 indicated that elementary school children in the United States attend physical education class only once or twice a week, and that just 50 percent of high school juniors and seniors participate in physical education at all. The same study indicated that physical education classes "appear to have little effect on the current physical fitness levels of children and, furthermore, have little impact on developing life-long physical activity skills" (Iverson, Fielding, Crow, & Christenson, 1985, p. 212).

Improving America's physical education efforts will be impeded by widespread disagreement over the goals of these classes. Fitness training, formal exercise education, and simply providing restless students a 45-min release of physical energy have all characterized contemporary physical education programs. Moreover, in an age of fiscal restraint, embattled school administrators often view physical education as an expendable portion of the curriculum.

Physical educators clearly should direct efforts to improve these programs, but the importance of increasing physical activity as a positive health measure signals an important role for physicians as well. As credible spokespersons for children's health, physicians can initiate community action to support innovative, health-related physical education programs in the schools (American Academy of Pediatrics, 1987).

• **The development of the "new sports medicine."** The days are gone when health care for young athletes was limited to the management of sport injuries. The physiological and psychological impacts of athletic competition during childhood and adolescence have created health concerns that encompass broad areas of medical practice. As a result, sports medicine has become well-suited to the comprehensive perspective of the primary care physician. Athletes need to know about dietary habits that both safely and effectively maximize performance. They deserve guidance into proper selection of sports and screening for fitness, strength, and flexibility that should help reduce the incidence and severity of injuries. Competitive athletes need to understand the psychological implications of participation and how to avoid "burnout." They should know the physiological bases of training, the facts regarding risks and benefits of ergogenic aids, and the prevention of heat injury.

These broader health aspects of sport competition—the "new sports medicine"—call for an equally new involvement by medical care providers. Sport participation for most young athletes is an enjoyable activity that improves fitness and offers the opportunity for emotional growth. In the role as spokesperson for the health safety of these athletes, the physician is in a vital position to assure that the experience from sport participation is a positive one (Shaffer, 1983).

The task of supervising the health needs of adolescent athletes is not a small one. In the 1986-87 school year, over 5 million boys and girls participated on high school sports teams in the United States. That represented a 25 percent rise since 1970, an increase due largely to a greater participation by girls (Figure I.1). Statistics from the National Federation of High School Associations indicate, for instance, that the number of girls on high school teams rose from approximately 300,000 in 1970 to just over 2 million in 1978. It is estimated that one half of boys and one fourth of girls between 14 and 17 years old are involved in organized competitive sports (Shaffer, 1979). In Canada, 84 percent of 14-year-old children participate in one or more sports, the most popular being swimming and ice skating (Shephard, 1982). The health implications of this volume of participation are enormous, and the need for physician input is clear-cut.

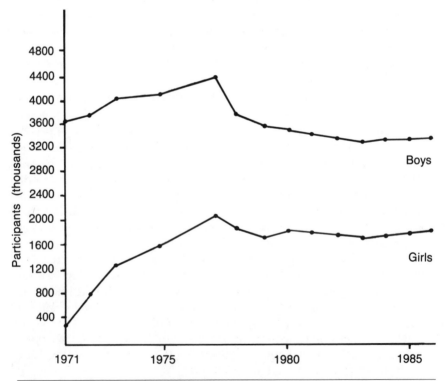

Figure I.1 High school sports participation in boys and girls. *Note.* Data from the National Federation of State High School Associations.

• **The replacement of free play by organized sports.** Despite the concerns of educators and lamentations by sentimentalists over the demise of sand-lot play, adult-directed organized sports programs for preadolescents have burgeoned (Berryman, 1982). Between 2 and 5 million children are play-ing soccer, more than 2 million (between 8 and 18 years old) participate in Little League baseball, and approximately 1 million compete on com-munity tackle-football teams. Altogether, at least 8 million girls and boys are involved in out-of-school organized sports (Goldberg, Veras, & Nicholas, 1978).

Strong arguments have been made for both the advantages and the risks of this downward age-trend of the free-play–structured sports transition (Martens, 1978). Good or bad, the rise of organized sport for youngsters does offer an opportunity for the physician to provide input into safe pro-gram design, matching of athletes, coach education, and other health-related measures that were previously lacking in the free-play setting.

The philosophy of these programs needs to be safeguarded by physi-cians as well. The era has ended when sport participation was enjoyed only by those few talented boys in football and basketball while the rest watched. *All* children should be involved in regular exercise, and sport organizations need to provide opportunities for every youngster to reach his or her potential for physical activity. For the most part, sport pro-grams for preadolescents have fostered the goals of enjoyment and par-ticipation over those of competition and victory, so they can provide social, physical, and emotional benefits to a large population of children rather than only to the highly talented. To this end they deserve support and involvement by the primary care physician.

• **The emergence of the elite prepubertal athlete.** Although there is little documentation of this trend, highly talented children have been increas-ingly obvious in many areas of sport participation. By their mid-teens many elite gymnasts, swimmers, skaters, and divers have been involved in intensive training regimens for nearly a decade (Feigley, 1984). The health risks incurred from the physical and psychological stresses on these immature athletes are uncertain and worrisome. Of particular concern is the observation that heavy training and competition during childhood may produce burnout during the teen years and withdrawal from sport participation altogether (Feigley, 1984).

Nutritional, psychological, and training counseling, in addition to treat-ment and prevention of injuries, is particularly important for this high-risk group of athletes. Unfortunately, however, many questions regard-ing the safety of high-level sport participation during the growing years remain unanswered. In addition, some evidence suggests that these child athletes do not often turn to physicians for advice and support on health- and performance-related issues. In a questionnaire study, 40 competitive distance runners under age 14 years were asked to indicate factors that motivated them to run (Rowland & Walsh, 1985). They ranked encourage-ment from a parent, friend, or coach first; not a single runner felt that a doctor's support was a motivational factor. And among the seven runners who reported having experienced a significant running-related injury (preventing full-time participation), only one sought advice from his physician.

• **The use of exercise as a therapeutic modality.** The ability to perform physical activity is reduced by the effects of many chronic diseases of childhood (Bar-Or, 1986). Patients with congenital heart disease, asthma, cystic fibrosis, and muscle disorders may be limited both by the physiological hindrances imposed by their disease and by the effects of secondary hypoactivity (Bar-Or, 1983). Growing experience with structured exercise programs for these children indicates that improvements in physical and psychological well-being can be achieved with regular physical activity. In some cases, as well, exercise training may serve to ameliorate the basic disease process.

Physical exercise thus provides a valuable therapeutic option for physicians in managing these patients. Physicians can play a valuable role in organizing community resources to provide structured exercise programs for children with chronic illnesses. The physician's guidance can be particularly vital, as well, in enabling athletes with diabetes, asthma, and seizure disorders to participate safely and effectively in competitive sport.

If physicians are to accomplish these growing tasks, they must be adequately prepared. Unfortunately, exposure of medical students and residents to health-related aspects of exercise during their training has been minimal. Knowledge in these areas has instead been gained principally through publications and continuing medical education programs (Hage, 1983). In these areas a great deal of progress has been made. In 1978 Goldberg, Veras, and Nicholas noted that in the previous 3 years not a single original article on the effect of sport participation during childhood had appeared in the two major pediatric journals. From 1985 through 1987 there were 12, and a new journal, *Pediatric Exercise Science*, was created in 1989 devoted specifically to exercise in children. Numerous national and regional symposia have addressed the unique aspects of exercise in the pediatric age group. The newly formed North American Society of Pediatric Exercise Medicine has dedicated itself to gathering and disseminating research information on exercise as it affects children's health and fitness. Clearly, continued efforts to improve the education of physicians regarding health-related aspects of exercise in children are essential.

Given the real needs of children and the growing expertise and interest of physicians, is there evidence that doctors can effectively change exercise behaviors in their patients? No information is available in the pediatric age group, but the question has been addressed regarding adults, with a mixed answer (Dishman, Sallis, & Orenstein, 1985). Almost half of sedentary individuals in one study indicated that a recommendation by a physician would stimulate them to increase their physical activity, and in another report 23 percent of adults stated that their doctor's orders to be active were an important reason for exercising. But in yet another survey only 3 percent indicated that they exercised because of a physician's advice (Clarke, 1973).

In summary, the role of the physician in supervising and encouraging exercise in young patients has expanded. The medical profession can fulfill these new responsibilities through a greater awareness of the risks and benefits of physical activity in the pediatric age group.

PART I

Developmental Exercise Physiology: The Physiological Basis of Physical Fitness in Children

An understanding of developmental exercise physiology—how the body changes in its response to physical activity with growth—enables physicians to more effectively guide their patients into both a healthy lifestyle and safe sport participation. Physical fitness, or the ability to perform physical exercise, is affected by physiological, anatomical, biochemical, and psychological alterations that parallel both growth and biological maturation. Adding to that complexity, there are various forms of physical fitness (endurance, strength, speed, agility), each with its own physiological mechanisms, training responses, and implications for health.

Why is it important to examine exercise responses in young subjects and decipher the meaning of differences between children and adults? Perhaps foremost, an understanding of developmental physiology promises insights into the determinants of exercise capacity at all ages. Changes that occur with biological maturation in children mimic many of the physiological effects observed after physical training in adults (see chapter 4).

Research data in adults indicate a connection between habitual physical activity and fitness and favorable changes in blood lipids, body fat, blood pressure, and blood coagulability. Comparable information in children is limited. The identification of similar relationships during childhood would provide grounds for improving physical education programs and exercise activities for children.

Certain markers of physiological fitness (such as maximum oxygen consumption, anaerobic threshold, submaximal economy) have been utilized to guide training regimens of adult athletes. Whether these are applicable to children is unknown. There is a clear need for physiological training markers in prepubertal athletes that could help avoid the risks of overtraining and injuries.

As noted previously, regular exercise may prove beneficial to children with chronic illness, particularly illness involving disturbances in cardiac or pulmonary function. If improvements in cardiopulmonary efficiency with physical training can be demonstrated in these patients, a sound rationale is created for developing pediatric exercise rehabilitation programs.

Physicians need to know about exercise physiology in children for the same reasons. Exercise recommendations need to be based on sound physiological principles. The ability to interpret new information such as the results of mass fitness testing is enhanced by an understanding of normal exercise responses in children. An increasingly knowledgeable group of children, coaches, and parents deserve counseling from equally informed medical care providers.

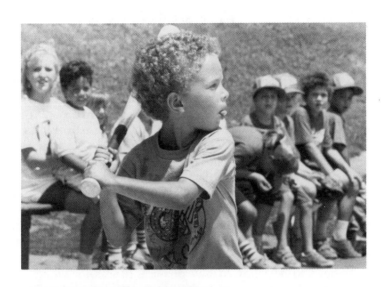

CHAPTER 1

A Primer of Exercise Physiology

An understanding of exercise physiology in children is best gained against a backdrop of the much greater body of information available regarding adults. This chapter provides a review of exercise basics, which will help readers unfamiliar with the subject to interpret subsequent chapters devoted to children's exercise responses. The information is, by necessity, brief and in summary form. Those desiring more comprehensive reviews of exercise physiology should consult standard sources (Åstrand & Rodahl, 1986; Fox, 1984; McArdle, Katch, & Katch, 1981).

TYPES OF FITNESS

Not many years ago the popular image of physical fitness consisted of virile men with bulging muscles, posing powerfully in comic book advertisements. For a fee, these titans would gladly send you their weight-training secrets. This was indeed a genuine opportunity, for these exercises, besides building muscle, would make a "real man" out of you and prevent you from having sand kicked in your face by bullies at the beach. Thousands of boys and young men, anxious to "get in shape," apparently took advantage of the opportunity.

But clearly physical fitness means more than being a "muscle man." Contrast the football linebacker's "pumping iron" with the speed of the sprinter, the agility and reflexes of the table tennis champion, or the endurance of the cross-country skier. All are examples of physical fitness, but clearly the neuromuscular skills, training regimens, and health-related benefits differ dramatically. The lesson: Questions regarding physical fitness need to be followed by "physical fitness for what?"

There is a great deal of specificity in training responses, both within and among types of fitness. Sprint training will not make an athlete a stronger jumper. Weight training will not improve coordination in figure-skating competition. The selection of exercises for a fitness program therefore depends on the program's goals. If improved performance is to be expected, athletes must train with those physiological mechanisms relevant to their sports. The mechanisms include the following:

- Strength
- Flexibility
- Speed
- Aerobic fitness

Strength

The wrestler, weight lifter, and water skier all engage in resistance, or isotonic, exercise, contracting their muscles with large force against loads with little motion. Resistance training improves strength, which results from enhanced protein synthesis and increased muscle mass. Strength may keep you safe on the beach, but most evidence indicates that weight training does little to improve cardiovascular fitness.

Isotonic exercise results in a relatively high escalation of blood pressure with a small rise in heart rate; the result is increased left-ventricular pressure work and myocardial oxygen requirements. Cardiovascular efficiency is not increased with training, and in patients with diminished left-ventricular function isotonic exercises may be hazardous. Caloric expenditure during weight training is overly brief to make these exercises useful in controlling excessive body fat. Resistance training with weights or mechanical devices is advocated primarily for improving strength and preventing injuries in sport competitions.

Flexibility

Expertise in certain forms of physical activity, like gymnastics and ballet dancing, calls for a wide range of joint motion, or flexibility. The ability to stretch connective tissue surrounding muscles and joints may be more important than simply improving athletic performance, however. Lack of flexibility may predispose to sport injuries, a major reason that athletes perform stretching exercises before training sessions and competition. Poor flexibility has also been associated with lower-back disease. Excessive flexibility, on the other hand, can be responsible for joint instability and a tendency for sprains and dislocations.

Speed

Fitness in running sprints or carrying a football is largely dependent on moving quickly. Speed in these events involves more than the neuromuscular capacity of rapid limb movement; strength, coordination, agility, and short-term muscle endurance all are important components of rapid body motion. Performance in sports that involve high-intensity bursts of speed, such as basketball, track sprints, and baseball, uses anaerobic sources of energy that do not rely on the cardiovascular system for oxygen delivery.

Aerobic Fitness

Improved cardiovascular efficiency, high caloric output, and decreased risk of coronary artery disease are associated with regular endurance exercise. Such sports involve repetitive, low-tension contractions of large muscle groups and are termed "aerobic" because they rely on a supply of oxygen for energy release. Running, swimming, bicycling, walking, and cross-country skiing all fit into this category. Repeated bouts of aerobic exercise, or training, improve the body's ability to use oxygen and increase cardiac efficiency. The result is greater endurance performance, associated with a sustained caloric expenditure. No gains are observed, however, in muscle strength or flexibility.

Maintaining fitness of all varieties is an important goal, but most health benefits of exercise have been related to aerobic activities. An understanding of aerobic fitness is thus particularly important for those advocating exercise as a means to good health.

WHAT DETERMINES AEROBIC FITNESS?

Aerobic fitness is a matter of the performance of muscle, the motor unit. This motor unit's functioning is dependent on many variables—biochemical, mechanical, neurological, physiological, and psychological. Although great emphasis has been placed on cardiovascular function in endurance activities, it is important to remember that these many other factors contribute to—and can limit—performance as well (Figure 1.1). Therefore, another lesson: Beware of oversimplification in the measurement of physical fitness. For example, consider the performance of a runner in a 10K road race. Certainly the functional capacity of lungs, heart, and circulatory system to deliver oxygen to the exercising muscles will be crucial in determining her or his finish time. But so will the runner's coordination and economy of gait. How much extra baggage she or he is carrying as body fat will be a major influence, too. Likewise, consider the importance of the runner's motivation to finish well and the skills and tactics of pace employed during the race.

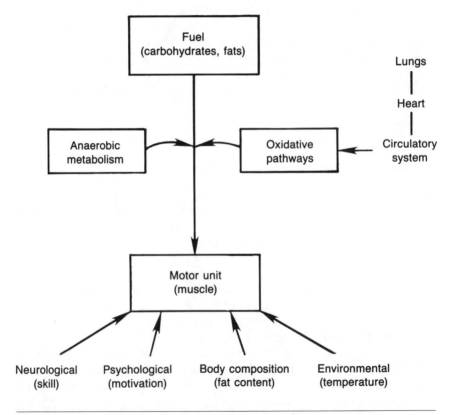

Figure 1.1 Components of endurance exercise performance.

Like any other motor, an exercising muscle needs fuel, in this case glucose and fatty acids, as well as a means of releasing energy. The preferred mechanism is oxidative metabolism, made possible through the intricate cooperation of lungs, heart, and circulatory system. When the limits of this oxygen-delivery chain are exceeded during high-intensity exercise, increasing utilization of glycolytic, or anaerobic, pathways is triggered. Anaerobic metabolism is only 1/13 as effective as aerobic means of providing energy and produces lactic acid as a by-product. Starved for energy and poisoned by falling intracellular pH, the muscle rapidly fatigues.

Oxygen Uptake

A subject running on a treadmill with increasing speeds or grade experiences a progressive rise in the energy demands of muscular contraction. These are met by a parallel increase in the supply of oxygen provided by the cardiovascular system. The amount of oxygen utilized by the exercising muscle is defined as the oxygen consumption, or uptake ($\dot{V}O_2$), expressed in liters per minute. Oxygen uptake is easily determined by measuring the oxygen content and volume of expired air; the oxygen content of inspired air is known, and $\dot{V}O_2$ is calculated as the difference. Oxygen uptake serves as a reliable marker of muscular activity as well as of the functional capacity of the pulmonary and cardiovascular systems to deliver oxygen to exercising muscle.

Oxygen uptake measured during a progressive treadmill test increases linearly up to high work loads but then typically levels to a plateau (Figure 1.2). The point where $\dot{V}O_2$ does not rise despite increasing treadmill speeds or grade is termed the "maximum oxygen consumption" ($\dot{V}O_2$max), or "maximal aerobic power." This value presumably indicates the limits of the oxygen delivery capacities of the combined pulmonary and cardiovascular systems. Once $\dot{V}O_2$max is reached, exhaustion rapidly sets in, as energy for increasing work must be obtained through glycolytic metabolic pathways. The average sedentary adult can increase $\dot{V}O_2$ tenfold over resting values, and in elite athletes $\dot{V}O_2$max may reach 18 times that of preexercise levels.

Maximal oxygen uptake reflects peak cardiovascular function during exercise and is a numerical marker of aerobic fitness. High $\dot{V}O_2$max values indicate a superior capacity for oxygen delivery and uptake by exercising muscle and the potential for excellence in endurance sports. As expected, $\dot{V}O_2$max values measured relative to body weight are greatest in competitors in cross-country skiing, marathon running, and distance cycling. Male athletes in these sports typically demonstrate $\dot{V}O_2$max levels of 70 to 80 ml kg^{-1} min^{-1} compared with values of 40 to 50 seen in untrained young men.

Adult women have lower $\dot{V}O_2$max values than men when adjusted for body weight. Several factors appear involved in this difference. Females

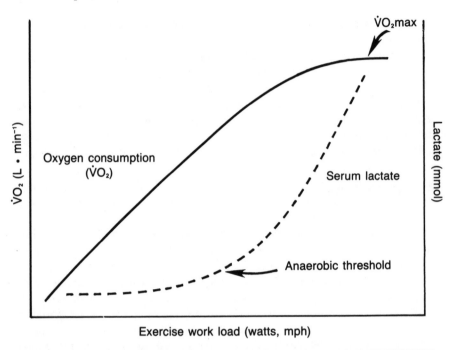

Figure 1.2 Rise in oxygen uptake and serum lactate with progressive exercise.

have less muscle mass (the tissue most responsible for oxygen uptake) than men, with a higher percent body fat. They also have lower blood-hemoglobin concentrations, which reduces oxygen delivery. Social factors impeding vigorous physical activities by women have also been implicated in gender-related differences in aerobic capacity.

Components of Oxygen Delivery

With increasing work loads the cardiac output parallels the rise in oxygen uptake. The heart augments its minute output from a resting value of 5 L to a maximum of 20 to 30 L in young men. During upright exercise, stroke volume reaches maximal values early in the course of a progressive test, rising little after a level of 40 percent $\dot{V}O_2$max has been reached. Beyond this intensity, cardiac output is generated solely by heart rate.

Hematological factors affect oxygen uptake as well. Not unexpectedly, there is a direct correlation between $\dot{V}O_2$max and hemoglobin concentration, and anemic individuals do not perform well in endurance events. Conversely, polycythemia should improve oxygen delivery and aerobic exercise performance (at least below those hemoglobin concentrations where increased blood viscosity might restrict blood flow). Limited studies with red cell transfusions ("blood doping") indicate this is probably true.

Oxygen supply to muscles during exercise is also increased by the redistribution of peripheral blood flow. Circulation to the skeletal musculature increases from 15 percent of blood flow at rest to 80 percent during vigorous exercise. This flow is generated at the expense of renal and gastrointestinal perfusion. Blood flow to the brain remains essentially unchanged, and coronary circulation is related to increases in myocardial work. Blood is also shunted to the skin for removal of the heat burden incurred with muscle activity.

During maximal exercise, the rate of oxygen extraction from the blood by the exercising muscle increases threefold. Factors at the receiving end of the oxygen supply chain, such as mitochondrial density, myoglobin concentration, and activity of aerobic enzymes, may be responsible for limiting oxygen uptake.

The population of muscle fiber types also determines exercise performance. There are two separate fiber types, with differing oxidative capabilities, in human skeletal muscle. Slow-twitch red fibers are rich in myoglobin and mitochondria and have a high capacity for oxidative metabolism. Fast-twitch white fibers have low myoglobin levels and few mitochondria but possess a high capacity for glycolytic metabolism. These anaerobic pathways provide energy for intensive activities of short duration. Athletes with a greater percentage of fast-twitch fibers are therefore more likely to excel in short-burst sports that do not rely on aerobic metabolism (e.g., sprints) than in endurance events. The ratio of slow-twitch to fast-twitch fibers varies greatly among individuals and is probably genetically determined.

The Training Effect

If the oxygen supply system is repeatedly stressed by endurance exercise training, it becomes more efficient. This, of course, is simply another way of stating that athletic training creates a state of improved fitness. This effect is particularly evident in previously sedentary subjects. The physiological correlates of this increased performance are listed in the box on the next page. The amount of exercise necessary to achieve this fitness effect in adults has been defined by type (endurance sports), duration (approximately 30 min per session), frequency (at least three times per week), and intensity (exercise at a heart rate 60 to 90 percent of maximum).

Anaerobic Threshold

Finally, it should be noted that the measurement of serum lactate (as a marker of intracellular anaerobic metabolism) during exercise testing may be a useful marker of endurance fitness (Figure 1.2). During a progressive cycle or treadmill exercise test, serum lactate levels rise slowly until an intensity equivalent to 50 to 70 percent of $\dot{V}O_2max$ is reached. The

---

The "Fitness Effect" From Endurance Training

Endurance training decreases . . .
. . . resting heart rate.
. . . resting blood pressure.
. . . percent body fat.
. . . submaximal heart rate.

Endurance training increases . . .
. . . submaximal stroke volume.
. . . maximal cardiac output.
. . . maximal oxygen consumption.
. . . maximal stroke volume.
. . . maximal serum lactate.
. . . maximal arteriovenous oxygen uptake.

---

typical acceleration in lactate at this point may reflect the onset of oxygen deprivation in the exercising muscle. The timing of lactate rise can be estimated by ventilatory parameters as well, because the buffering of lactate produces excessive carbon dioxide production, which in turn stimulates a nonlinear acceleration in minute ventilation.

The metabolic significance of this anaerobic threshold has been vigorously debated, but regardless of its biochemical basis, measurement of the anaerobic threshold appears to have clinical utility. Expressed as either absolute $\dot{V}O_2$ or percent $\dot{V}O_2max$, this point has been reported to correlate well with endurance exercise performance. Conceptually this makes sense, because it implies that subjects with high anaerobic thresholds are able to sustain greater exercise intensities (e.g., higher running or cycling speeds) without anaerobic metabolism, lactate accumulation, and fatigue.

SUMMARY

Most attention in this chapter has been focused on endurance activities for the following reasons:

- Endurance forms of exercise that rely on aerobic metabolism are most often linked to health benefits.
- Fitness in these activities (measured as the maximal oxygen uptake) is the reflection of the capacity of heart, lungs, and vascular tree to deliver oxygen to exercising muscle.
- Endurance fitness can be improved through exercise training of specific duration, frequency, and intensity.

However, physical fitness is not limited only to endurance. In addition to how long one can run, physical fitness is how fast one can swim, and how much weight one can lift. In table tennis, fitness is defined as agility; in gymnastics, it is strength and flexibility. These are all forms of fitness, each calling on particular neuromuscular mechanisms and energy substrates. Each responds in a specific fashion to training, and each has its unique benefits to health. It is important to realize, then, that physical fitness needs to be defined in terms of distinct forms of exercise, and when physical fitness is promoted as a means of improving well-being, health goals need to match the benefits offered by particular forms of exercise.

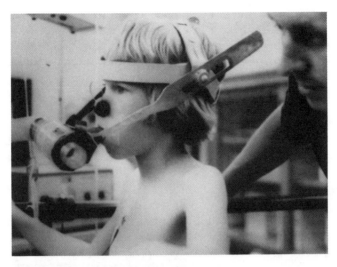

CHAPTER 2

The Special Problems of Pediatric Exercise Research

Understanding children's responses to exercise calls for valid testing of young subjects in both laboratory and field settings. This chapter focuses on the unique difficulties confronting the researcher studying the growing pediatric subject.

ETHICAL AND METHODOLOGICAL LIMITATIONS

We have fewer insights into children's responses to exercise than into the responses of adults, because technical and ethical constraints are involved in studying young subjects (Bar-Or, 1984b). It would be valuable, for instance, to compare serial quadriceps-muscle biopsies during exercise training in children and adults to examine differences in substrate utilization and aerobic enzyme activities. Cardiac radionuclide scans would help tell whether children really have depressed myocardial contractile responses with exercise compared to adults. The favorable impact of propranolol on the cardiac function of children with Marfan syndrome could be more easily assessed if echocardiographic evaluation of normal youngsters on this drug were possible. Adults might be convinced to volunteer for these procedures, but for children the procedures are clearly inappropriate. Testing methods that are painful or that might adversely affect growing subjects are unjustified on ethical, legal, and humanitarian grounds. Children often cannot truly give informed consent for participation in research projects, and their well-being needs to be protected by parents and researchers alike (Clarke, 1986).

This obstacle has created many gaps in the knowledge of pediatric exercise science, resulting in a surfeit of descriptive studies of exercise responses in children but little understanding of the underlying mechanisms or relationships to growth. Newer, noninvasive technologies such as bioimpedance, ultrasound, and magnetic resonance imaging may provide better means of learning more about children and exercise without placing young subjects at risk.

Testing modalities that are useful for adult subjects may not always prove adaptable to children. Little maximal data is available on preschool children, who are often unable (or unwilling) to maintain their balance on a rapidly moving or steep treadmill belt. The effect of low ventilation rates, mouthpiece deadspace, tubing diameter, and mixing-chamber size during measurement of gas exchange parameters in small subjects has not been evaluated. Body-fat determinations by underwater weighing techniques are unreliable in children because of uncertainties regarding growth-related variability in body tissue density (Lohman, Boileau, & Slaughter, 1984).

Most exercise-related research in children has involved older prepubertal boys who are lean and athletically inclined, because these subjects are more likely to volunteer for research projects and are capable of performing on routine exercise tests (e.g., maximal treadmill studies). Consequently a broad picture of the exercise capacities of both boys and girls across a wide range of ages, body habitus, and habitual physical activity is not yet available. Newer means of assessing physiological responses to exercise will be necessary before this can be accomplished.

INFLUENCES OF GROWTH

The list of unique difficulties faced by the pediatric exercise physiologist is long, but no factor is more confounding than the growth process itself. Consider these problems:

- How are exercise variables best compared between the immature prepubertal boy and the muscular 25-year-old college student?
- How can the physiological effects of exercise training be separated from those of normal biological development?
- How can two parameters of exercise function be related causally if both are changing in a parallel fashion with growth?

Compounding the problem, growth rates are not linear during childhood and adolescence. Also, although the many physiological components that determine exercise performance clearly change with growth, no evidence indicates they necessarily all do so at the same rate, and it is unclear whether the development of exercise parameters relates best to chronological, skeletal, sexual, or physical maturation (Janos, Janos, Tamas, & Ivan, 1985).

Measures of Maturity

Chronological age serves poorly as a marker of biological maturity, because at a given age children may differ significantly in work capacity and motor proficiency purely on a developmental basis. Height and weight have been used extensively as indices of physical performance because they are easily measured, but these are affected by changes in body proportion and composition with growth. Skeletal age, as indicated by bone X rays, is considered the most valid measure of biological maturity (Hebbelinck, 1978). Cumming, Garand, and Borysyk (1972) demonstrated that, among a large group of boys and girls at a track and field camp, bone age predicted performance better than chronological age, height, or weight for nearly all events. This technique is not often readily applicable in either the clinical or the research setting, however.

Consider the plight of the researcher attempting to predict future distance-running abilities in a group of 10-year-old boys. A maximal treadmill test is administered, and based upon measurements of $\dot{V}O_2$max and treadmill endurance time, the future running potential of each child is rated compared to his peers. The conclusions, however, may be highly inaccurate. During biological development the factors that contribute to physical fitness mature, and performance in exercise tests (strength, speed, and endurance) steadily improves (Bar-Or, 1983). But the *rate* of this exercise-related maturation does not necessarily parallel chronological age and may demonstrate significant intersubject variability (Mirwald & Bailey, 1986). Those 10-year-old boys are likely to be at very different places on their exercise developmental curves, and a cross-sectional fitness test may have little ability to discriminate those who will become superior athletes in later adolescence (Figure 2.1). How much a child will maintain her ranking in athletic performance measures compared to her peers as she grows is unknown. More information regarding the ''tracking'' of exercise development with age is necessary before these tests in growing children can be used to predict future athletic capabilities.

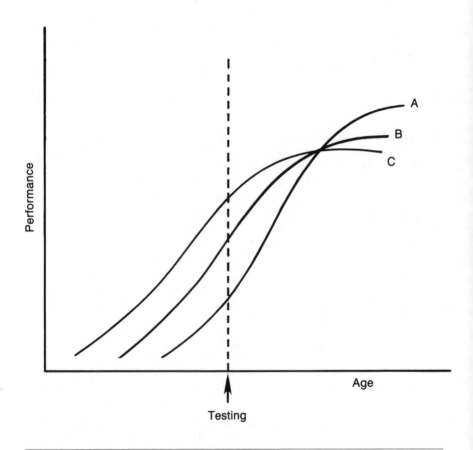

Figure 2.1 Results of exercise testing at a given chronological age may not be predictive of ultimate performance capabilities.

It is important for the physical educator to recognize this pitfall as well. A child's poor test result on a mile run might have several explanations. For example:

- The child may possess a limited genetic capability for endurance activities.
- The child may be overly sedentary, obese, unmotivated, or for some other reason not fulfilling physical potential.
- The child may simply be at an early stage of normal exercise development.

Each of these options might call for a different intervention by the physical education teacher. Unfortunately, there is no good way to pinpoint the relative contributions of each of these factors.

The same dilemma is faced by the investigator who studies cross-sectional differences in the exercise responses of prepubertal athletes and sedentary children. During normal development, for instance, sub-maximal running economy (oxygen cost at a given running speed) progressively improves, assumedly an advantage for endurance-event performance. A comparison of athletic and nonathletic children of the same age that indicates that athletic children have superior running economy could be explained by the effects of training or by the selection of sport participation by those who are genetically gifted with excellent running economy. The influence of biological development creates an equally tenable third possibility: The athletic group may simply be the children who have matured early in the factors responsible for energy requirements during submaximal running compared to sedentary subjects.

The "Denominator Problem"

Comparisons of exercise capacities between children and adults must include a consideration of differences in body dimensions. The same caveat applies when changes in fitness with training programs are assessed during the growing years. The young adult male has a higher absolute maximal oxygen uptake when running on a treadmill than does the average prepubertal boy. Does the adult possess greater aerobic fitness? Not necessarily. The child has less muscle mass, a smaller cardiovascular system, and—importantly—less body mass to move. Considering his smaller dimensions, the child could have aerobic machinery just as efficient as the older subject's.

Suppose a child is placed in a program of regular bicycle exercise, four times a week, at age 10, and maintains his training for 2 years. Measurements of absolute $\dot{V}O_2$max taken at 6-month intervals demonstrate a progressive rise in maximal aerobic power. Was the training program successful in improving cardiovascular function, producing a "fitness effect"? Maybe. But during the testing period, normal growth of heart, lungs, and muscle tissue also improved oxygen delivery, and absolute $\dot{V}O_2$max would have been expected to improve even if the exercise sessions had been replaced by television viewing.

How can all these factors be taken into account so that exercise performance in individuals of different ages and sizes can be compared in a meaningful way? How can changes with training be related to those expected with normal growth? Clearly, a denominator is needed to "equalize" exercise measurements across age and size groups. But which one? Age, body weight, height, surface area, or lean muscle mass?

There is no simple answer. When physiological data is collected during an exercise test, the investigator seeks to compare values recorded for the determinants of that exercise with those expected at the biological developmental level of the subject. What is needed is an easily measured marker of those expected normal values. In other words, the proper denominator should be directly related to the normal development of the exercise parameter being measured.

The determinant most thoroughly assessed in this regard is maximal oxygen uptake. When longitudinal measurements of absolute $\dot{V}O_2$max were studied in boys over an 8-year period, maximal aerobic power correlated best with (height)$^{2.46}$ (Bailey, Ross, Mirwald, & Weese, 1978). Other longitudinal studies have related the rise of $\dot{V}O_2$max to height exponents ranging from 1.51 to 3.21 (Bar-Or, 1983). Additional suggested denominators, based on geometrical considerations and animal studies, include (height)^3 (Asmussen & Heeboll-Nielsen, 1955), lean body mass (Von Dobeln & Eriksson, 1972), and (height)$^{2.25}$ (McMahon, 1973). The choice of these indices may have important—and contradictory—effects on testing results. When using (height)^3 or body weight, $\dot{V}O_2$max remains relatively constant during childhood but then declines at older ages. The use of (height)^2, conversely, results in an *increase* in $\dot{V}O_2$max with age (Bailey, Ross, Mirwald, & Weese, 1978; Bar-Or, 1983). Little longitudinal data is available on the relationship of other exercise parameters such as cardiopulmonary function and muscle endurance to body dimensions, chronological age, and other markers of biological maturity.

Dimensionality Theory

The means of relating geometrically similar objects of varying size has intrigued mathematicians, engineers, and biologists for centuries (Schmidt-Nielsen, 1984). Based on Euclidean geometry, areas of objects of different sizes but similar proportions can be related to each other by the square of their linear dimensions. Likewise, volumes are comparable by (length)³. This *dimensionality principle* holds true for animals, explaining, for instance, why the leg bones of elephants are proportionally thicker and heavier than those of the mouse. The increased mass of larger animals is a cube function of body length, but the cross-sectional area of most bones is related to the length squared; because as an animal increases in size, the strength of bone must increase to support the animal's weight, the cross-sectional area of the leg bones must increase by the cube rather than the square of the length.

According to dimensionality theory, physiological functions can be compared among animals of different sizes in the same way. Those that involve cross-sectional or surface area (e.g., muscle strength, heat loss) can be related by (length)², whereas body volumes (e.g., stroke volume) are comparable with (length)³ as a denominator. Because time is expressed as a linear function of length, oxygen consumption (liters per minute) should be related to L^3/L or L^2. This contrasts to the previously mentioned experimental studies that have identified exponents of L ranging from 1.51 to 3.21 (Bar-Or, 1983). From these data, Bar-Or (1983) concluded that dimensionality theory had not been confirmed experimentally and offered no practical advantage over the use of body weight for growth-related comparisons.

Body Weight

In most research studies, exercise parameters have been related to body weight because this is a readily obtained value that correlates with measures of most cardiopulmonary functions in normal individuals. It is important, however, to recognize that expressing factors such as oxygen uptake "per kilogram" may have several different implications in the following areas:

• **Body mass and the oxygen supply chain.** Body mass is, in general, directly related to the functional dimensions of the oxygen supply chain. $\dot{V}O_2$/kg at a given work stage may therefore be interpreted as "actual oxygen delivery compared to the potential for maximum O_2 delivery." In this case, submaximal $\dot{V}O_2$/kg is also a measure of exercise intensity. It follows that at maximal exercise $\dot{V}O_2$/kg is indicative of peak cardiopulmonary function, a value that can be used to compare individuals of different sizes. This will be true only, of course, if non-oxygen delivery mechanisms (such as motivation and muscle function) are not limiting exercise performance.

• **Absolute oxygen consumption and muscle mass.** Absolute oxygen consumption during physical activity is related to mass of muscle employed during that particular exercise; i.e., $\dot{V}O_2$max during arm work is less than during leg exercise. An ideal denominator for comparing $\dot{V}O_2$ between individuals, then, is the lean body mass actually performing the exercise.

Usually this measurement is not feasible, so body weight is used as a substitute. This should prove acceptable, providing the exercising muscle represents the same proportion of body weight in each of the subjects being studied. The obvious conclusion is that differences in body composition, particularly in body fat, influence the appropriateness of body mass as a "normalizing" denominator for comparing exercise test results among individuals.

• **Oxygen consumption and load measure.** When oxygen consumption is measured during weight-bearing exercise (e.g., treadmill running), "per kilogram" becomes—in addition to the above considerations—a measure of the load the muscles are required to move. On a cycle ergometer the work load is produced by resistance applied to the wheel, but during running the burden is created by body mass. $\dot{V}O_2$/kg, then, is how much metabolic work must be done to move 1 kg of body mass at a given speed and elevation. The mode of exercise is therefore important in evaluating exercise parameters related to body weight.

CONFUSIONS IN CAUSALITY

Because most exercise parameters change with the child's growth and development, strong correlations demonstrated between these markers do not necessarily imply a cause-and-effect relationship (Figure 2.2).

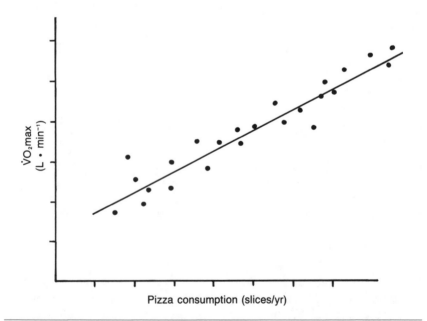

Pizza consumption (slices/yr)

Figure 2.2 Hypothetical relationship between maximal oxygen uptake and pizza consumption during the childhood years, illustrating that apparent causal relationships can be observed between independent factors that are both related to age.

Decreasing stride frequency and improved running economy are closely related in children as they grow, but based on this information alone one cannot conclude (though it is tempting to do so) that children utilize more energy than adults when running at a given speed because they take more steps. These could be independent variables correlated with biological development by separate mechanisms.

SUMMARY

This chapter has outlined the ethical and methodological constraints currently limiting research into developmental exercise physiology.

- Procedures that might entail any significant risk are taboo in pediatric subjects.
- Testing methods that are appropriate for adults may not be so for children.
- The ability to perform certain exercise tests (e.g., treadmill running) may define the results obtained; that is, testing fit children will produce results limited to fit children.
- The factors determining exercise performance change with biological development, which may not necessarily parallel chronological age. It is unclear how to best factor out this effect in training studies. Currently, relating exercise parameters to body weight is common practice, using appropriate control groups of nontrained subjects.

Given these problems, it is not surprising that current understanding of exercise physiology in children is far from complete. Newer technology will be necessary to overcome many of the ethical and methodological barriers to studying young subjects. There is a clear-cut need for valid, easily measurable markers of normal biological development as it relates to exercise performance; these would permit comparisons between individuals of different ages and allow investigators to sort out the effects of physical training from those of normal growth. Longitudinal studies will be essential for establishing normal developmental curves for the determinants of exercise performance, which is not an easy task in either young or older populations (Rutenfranz, 1986).

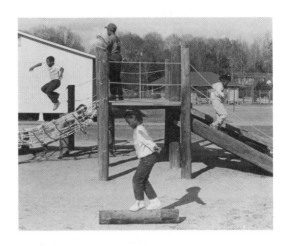

CHAPTER 3

Physical Fitness and Habitual Physical Activity

Whether health benefits from exercise stem from the amount of daily physical activity or from one's abilities to perform in exercise tasks (physical fitness) is controversial. This chapter considers that question in relation to children, examining the trends of daily activity as the child grows, reviewing the means of measuring activity, considering the evidence linking health-related outcomes to habitual activity and/or fitness, and finally, addressing the question of current levels of fitness in children living in developed countries.

THE HEALTH–EXERCISE LINK

There is little doubt that regular exercise is an important part of a healthy lifestyle, but the mechanisms by which muscular activity contributes to wellness are not well understood (Haskell, Montoye, & Orenstein, 1985). Certainly they are diverse:

- Biochemical (rise in HDL-cholesterol levels)
- Physical (increased strength, flexibility)
- Physiological (decreased resting blood pressure)
- Anatomical (increased bone strength)
- Psychological (improved self-esteem)

These adaptations are all outcomes that have been observed following exercise training programs. Given these varied responses it could be predicted that multiple mechanisms link exercise with improved health.

Most epidemiological data in adults associates health gains from exercise with the extent of an individual's daily physical activity (Haskell, 1985; LaPorte, Dearwater, Cauley, Slemenda, & Cook, 1985). The contribution of physical fitness (as measured by the ability to perform on specific exercise tasks) per se to health is an unsettled issue. Despite a great deal of attention paid to fitness levels in children, it is not at all clear whether performance capabilities in any exercise event can be directly related to health outcomes (Cureton, 1987). In this respect it is important to realize that there are many forms of fitness, some which may have more influence on health than others (Caspersen, Powell, & Christenson, 1985).

DAILY PHYSICAL ACTIVITY OF CHILDREN

No parents of a normal 3-year-old need to be counseled to increase their child's physical activity. These youngsters are supercharged dynamos who deserve gold medals for emptying supermarket shelves and escaping through backyard fences. With increasing years this intense level of spontaneous activity declines as children enter the confines of the classroom and come under the influence of television, computers, and car pools. (These environmental factors are not fully responsible, though. It is clear that the decrease in habitual activity with age is a primary biological trend, observed in other animals as well.) Finally, as teenagers they reach the other end of the spectrum, closing themselves in their rooms where they are not heard from for weeks, being nourished only by pizzas slipped beneath closed doors (Bombeck, 1971).

This rate of decline of habitual exercise during childhood is both dramatic and disturbing. Many of the health-related benefits of exercise relate to the amount of daily exercise, and it is assumed that exercise habits during childhood predict adult patterns of physical activities. By understanding the factors that control daily exercise, appropriate strategies might be devised to moderate the age-related decline in regular activity. To this end more information is needed on the natural course of physical activity during childhood and how it relates to health.

Measuring Physical Activity

Measuring physical activity is difficult, particularly in children. Over 30 different techniques have been tried, none fully satisfactory (LaPorte, Montoye, & Caspersen, 1985). Daily physical activities involve a multitude of actions that are difficult to quantitate without interfering with the subject's normal patterns of exercise. As a rule, the easier and more convenient the technique for assessing these activities, the less valid it is likely to be. Methodology for measuring routine physical activity has been the subject of several extensive reviews (Bar-Or, 1983; Freedson, in press; Saris, 1986; Shephard, 1982).

The best means of quantitating physical activity is by measuring the energy expended during the exercise. This calls for measuring oxygen consumption, a procedure entailing mouthpiece, tubing, gas analyzers, ventilometers, and recording devices. Clearly this is not a practical technique for establishing activity levels in large groups of children. Durnin and Passmore (1967) described a method of establishing $\dot{V}O_2$ for certain activities, which could be related to activities recorded by subjects on an exercise diary. This method requires not only that laboratory-established $\dot{V}O_2$ activities match those of daily living but also, impractically for children, that subjects reliably record their physical activities.

At the other extreme, questionnaires or diaries completed by parent, teacher, or child are easy to administer but of variable reliability. Saris (1986) notes that children below the age of 10 or 12 can provide only limited information about their patterns of physical activity. Parents do not often observe their children in play activities away from the home, and teachers' views are limited to the classroom setting.

The development of small, portable, unobtrusive heart-rate monitors that record pulse rates over extended periods has greatly aided efforts to measure habitual physical activity. Individual regression equations relating heart rate to $\dot{V}O_2$, established during laboratory exercise testing, can be utilized to estimate daily energy expenditure (Saris, Elvers, van't Hof, & Binkhorst, 1986; Verschuur & Kemper, 1985). This technique offers the advantage of measuring exercise intensity without interfering with normal activity patterns. Klausen, Rasmussen, and Schibye (1986) noted, however, that the heart rate–$\dot{V}O_2$ relationship depends on the muscle mass being utilized during exercise as well as the type of physical activity (intermittent versus continuous). Likewise, emotional stress affects heart rate without parallel changes in oxygen uptake (Saris, 1986).

Earlier mechanical devices provided a very limited perspective on regular activity. The pedometer, a device to measure vertical movements at the waist, does not measure exercise intensity, and in some activities, such as cycling, does not record at all (Saris & Binkhorst, 1977). The actometer is worn like a wristwatch and measures both amount and intensity of movement by motion of a rotor. This device and newer electronic counters may provide more reliable activity information (Klesges & Klesges, 1987; Saris, 1986).

Decline of Physical Activity With Age

Cross-sectional and longitudinal studies of habitual physical activity during childhood and adolescence confirm the subjective impression that regular exercise diminishes with age. Saris et al. (1986) described the longitudinal changes in daily physical activity in boys and girls aged 6 to 12 years using 24-hr heart rate–$\dot{V}O_2$ correlations. Energy expenditure per kilogram body weight decreased progressively during the 6-year study, as did the percentage of time spent in vigorous physical activity (defined as a heart rate above 50 percent $\dot{V}O_2$max).

A longitudinal study of Dutch teenagers using comparable methods produced similar results (Verschuur & Kemper, 1985). Energy expenditure fell from age 12 to age 18 years, but at a slower rate than reported at younger ages (Saris et al., 1986). Combining the two studies provides a picture of the habitual activity pattern across much of the growing years (Figure 3.1). It is interesting to note that the shape of this exercise energy curve simulates that of the decrease in resting basal metabolism with increasing age (compare with Figure 4.10 on page 67).

The fall of the age–activity curve may be tempered by the fact that older children require less $\dot{V}O_2$ per kilogram than younger subjects performing the same exercise (Bar-Or, 1983). However, data from other studies that did not use measures of energy expenditure describe the same downward trend of regular exercise with age (Kucera, 1986; Sunnegardh, Bratteby, Sjolin, Hagman, & Hoffstedt, 1985). Based on studies utilizing parents' ratings of physical activity, this decline begins no later than the third year of life (Routh, Schroeder, & O'Tuama, 1974).

In these studies, boys were consistently more active than girls. A meta-analysis of 90 studies examining activity levels in children confirmed that males are generally more active than females at all ages, although the differences were smaller in early infancy (Eaton & Enns, 1986). Maccoby

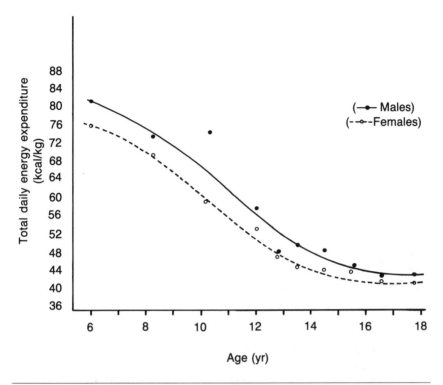

Figure 3.1 Daily physical activity as indicated by energy expenditure during childhood and adolescence. *Note.* From "Changes in Physical Activity of Children Aged 6 to 12 Years" by W.H.M. Saris, J.W.H. Elvers, M.A. van't Hof, and R.A. Binkhorst. In *Children and Exercise XII* (pp. 121-130) by J. Rutenfranz, R. Mocellin, and F. Klimt (Eds.), 1986, Champaign, IL: Human Kinetics. Copyright 1986 by Human Kinetics. Adapted by permission. And from "Habitual Physical Activity in Dutch Teenagers Measured by Heart Rate" by R. Verschuur and H.C.G. Kemper. In *Children and Exercise XI* (pp. 194-202) by R.A. Binkhorst, H.C.G. Kemper, and W.H.M. Saris (Eds.), Champaign, IL: Human Kinetics. Copyright 1985 by Human Kinetics. Adapted by permission.

and Jacklin (1974) had concluded earlier that there was no evidence for sex differences in physical activity under age 1 year.

The evidence affirming the downhill curve of physical activity with age invokes a flurry of questions for which there are not yet adequate answers.

- How much of the decline in physical activity with age is an inevitable part of normal maturation (as suggested by its striking parallel course with basal metabolic rate)?

- To what extent can the curve be manipulated by external influences?
- What are the key ages for intervention?
- What constitutes inadequate physical activity for children?
- Can normal curves be established, and would it be possible for physicians to identify children at risk by a standardized means of assessing physical activity?
- How does the shape of the curve predict exercise levels during adulthood?

Clearly a large group of extrinsic and intrinsic influences can alter the shape of the activity curve. Anthropometric, social, psychological, physiological, and geographical factors all potentially play a role in determining regular levels of exercise. These will be addressed in the last section of this book when motivational factors for exercise are considered. An intriguing concept is that there is an intrinsic, central-neurological regulator of habitual activity underlying these influences. Anand (1961) reviewed data indicating that animals with lesions in the medial hypothalamus exhibit hypoactivity, whereas removal or lesions of the rostral hypothalamus, basal ganglia, or ungulate gyrus of the cerebrum produces hyperkinetic behavior. Selective chemical inhibition of dopamine metabolism in young animals has repeatedly been shown to increase levels of physical activity (Shaywitz, Gordon, Klopper, & Zelterman, 1977). A similar mechanism of dopamine depletion has been postulated in children with attention-deficit disorder ("hyperactive children") (Raskin, Shaywitz, Shaywitz, Anderson, & Cohen, 1984). It would be valuable to understand the extent to which any such "activity center" determines the age-related curve of habitual exercise or can be altered through external influences.

Studies assessing the routine physical exercise of children have recently been reviewed (Simons-Morton, O'Hara, Simons-Morton, & Parcel, 1987). Although the amount of daily vigorous activity by children has been described as "shockingly low" (Sallis, 1987), this information is difficult to interpret because the threshold amounts of physical activity to achieve health effects are unknown, and no comparative data are available from the pretelevision era to establish that, in fact, children are becoming more sedentary. It is assumed, however, that in a society where getting to school, going upstairs, opening a can of tuna, or sharpening a pencil can all be achieved with zero extra energy expenditure, the age–activity curve must be shifted downward. The 20 hr of television time the average schoolchild watches per week alone cuts into approximately 50 percent of a youngster's "free time" (Schramm, Lyle, & Parker, 1961). But even before television, evidence suggested that children favored sedentary pastimes (Sullenger, Parke, & Wallin, 1953).

EXERCISE AND HEALTH:
PHYSICAL FITNESS OR HABITUAL ACTIVITY?

CASE: An obese adolescent with essential hypertension enters a 3-month jogging program, 30 min a day, three times per week. Two outcomes might be predicted:

- An improvement in endurance fitness associated with increased maximal aerobic power and cardiopulmonary function
- A fall in resting blood pressure, decreased body fat, favorable alteration in blood lipid profile, and enhanced self image

Questions: • Were the physiological changes associated with increased cardiovascular fitness responsible for the health benefits? Or were the positive health effects a direct result of physical activity itself?
- Were the same mechanisms operating for improvements in fitness and health effects following the increase in physical activity? Or were they independent responses bearing no relationship to each other?

Answer: The answers are not clear (Figure 3.2).

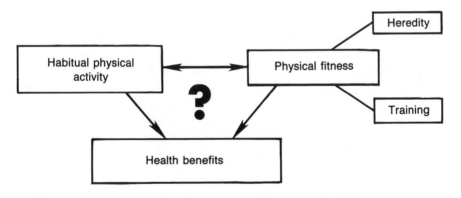

Figure 3.2 The pathways connecting exercise to physical and emotional well-being are unclear.

There is a growing sentiment that excessive emphasis has been placed on the importance of physical fitness and health outcomes, and that habitual physical activity may play a much greater role in the promotion of wellness (Simons-Morton et al., 1987). Epidemiological studies in adults that have correlated routine exercise levels with incidence of systemic hypertension, stroke, myocardial infarction, and sudden death have all utilized markers of daily physical activity. Specifically, cardiovascular morbidity and mortality have been related to these factors:

- Energy expenditure, in longshoremen (Paffenbarger, Laughlin, Gina, & Black, 1970)
- Stairs climbed, blocks walked, and daily sports, in college alumni (Paffenberger, Hyde, Wing, & Steinmetz, 1984)
- Occupational physical activity (Kannel & Sorlie, 1979)
- Weekend leisure activity (Morris et al., 1973)

Less information is presently available directly relating physical fitness with a lower incidence of mortality or morbidity from chronic diseases of adulthood (LaPorte, Dearwater, Cauley, Slemenda, & Cook, 1985). Ekelund et al. (1988) followed 4,276 men aged 30 to 69 years for an average of 8.5 years after initial treadmill testing and assessment for coronary artery disease risk factors. Using submaximal heart rate and treadmill endurance time as markers of physical fitness, they found that fitness levels were inversely related to subsequent death from coronary heart disease independent of other risk factors. Long-term health outcomes have not been studied with respect to either regular physical activity or fitness in children.

Clearly children can gain health advantages from regular exercise without concomitant increases in levels of fitness. Obese children who increased their low-intensity daily exercise levels demonstrated declines in body fat without parallel changes in cardiovascular fitness. At the same time subjects enrolled in a structured exercise training program improved their fitness levels but showed less effective weight loss than the low-intensity exercise group (Epstein, Wing, Koeske, Ossip, & Beck, 1982).

It has been suggested that the intensity of exercise involved in formalized programs designed to meet criteria for improving aerobic capacity may prove unacceptable to young children (Cureton, 1987). Exercise goals to improve fitness might then be counterproductive, creating a negative reaction to exercise that would inhibit rather than promote habits of regular physical activity. Simons-Morton et al. (1987, p. 301) concluded that "due to lack of evidence of substantial carry-over effects of youth fitness to adult health . . . and the likelihood of resistance by children . . . there is little reason to recommend [a cardiorespiratory training regimen] in structured physical activity programs."

Physical fitness cannot be dismissed entirely as a goal for health-related exercise, however (Blair, 1985). Favorable serum lipid changes with training have been demonstrated to correlate with maximal aerobic power in both adults and children (Savage et al., 1986). Improvements in functional fitness during rehabilitation exercise programs for children with chronic diseases helps these patients improve their ability to tolerate exercise during their daily lives (Bar-Or, 1983). Strength, muscle endurance, and flexibility may all contribute significantly to preventing athletic injuries as well as to averting degenerative neuromuscular disease. Even skill-related fitness such as throwing, sprinting, and jumping can play a beneficial role in exercise programs for children by adding to the enjoyment of physical activity (Seefeldt & Vogel, 1987).

It would appear that many forms of physical activity and physical fitness can serve to improve children's health. Specific exercise programs need to be devised relative to their desired outcomes (see boxed information). Regular low-grade activity to increase energy expenditure would seem most logical in the management of obesity. The same types of activities might be appropriate for maintaining bone strength and preventing osteoporosis. Resistance exercise for improving strength fitness is important for certain athletes. An increase in functional fitness will allow the child following heart surgery to more fully enjoy life.

Contributions of Physical Activity and Fitness to Health

Health concern		Effect of physical activity
Obesity	→	Increased caloric expenditure
Osteoporosis	→	Increased bone mineralization
Atherosclerosis	→	Improved blood lipid profile, reduction of other risk factors
Emotional disorders	→	Improved self-esteem, self-mastery
Health concern		Effect of physical fitness
Impaired exercise capacity	→	Improved aerobic capacity
Chronic back disease	→	Improved flexibility and strength
Athletic injuries	→	Increased muscle strength
Systemic hypertension	→	Decreased sympathetic tone

THE RELATIONSHIP BETWEEN FITNESS AND PHYSICAL ACTIVITY

Intuitively, individuals who are more active in their daily lives should also possess greater levels of physical fitness (as measured by $\dot{V}O_2$max or motor performance tests). We would make these assumptions:

- The child who is more fit will enjoy and participate in more regular physical activities.

OR

- The youngster with a high level of habitual physical activity might achieve improved fitness through a training effect.

Whether either assumption is true—or whether, in fact, there is any correlation at all between fitness levels and habitual activity—remains uncertain. Resolution of this question is an important goal for exercise scientists because the answer carries significant implications for both the understanding of pediatric exercise physiology as well as strategies for testing and promotion of health-related exercise.

Can Children Improve Fitness by Training?

Whether prepubertal children can improve aerobic fitness by endurance training is controversial (Rowland, 1986). Evidence related to this question will be addressed in chapter 4. Proponents of the view that $\dot{V}O_2max$ does not respond to aerobic training in children have suggested that the high daily activity levels of youngsters effectively act as training stimuli. According to this argument, children are already maximally trained by their own habitual exercise (Hamilton & Andrew, 1976). As summarized by the American Academy of Pediatrics (1976, p. 88), "the pre-school child who characteristically uses his large muscles during many hours of the day is continuing a self-improved program of physical fitness."

Will Fitness Result From Activity?

Do children in fact exercise vigorously enough during their daily lives to improve cardiovascular fitness? Comparisons of heart rate monitoring in prepubertal subjects with training criteria in adults indicate that the *total* time spent in high-intensity exercise (pulse rate over 160 bpm) might be enough to improve fitness but that vigorous activity typically comes in short bursts and is not sustained for a duration that would be expected to increase aerobic capacity (Gilliam, Freedson, Geenan, & Shahraray, 1981; Verschuur & Kemper, 1985). This analysis is complicated, however, by the absence of proof that standards of exercise intensity, duration, and frequency for aerobic training in adults can equally be applied to children. Certainly the contention that aerobic capacity is maximized by high levels of habitual activity during childhood would be weakened by a failure to demonstrate a positive correlation between $\dot{V}O_2max$ and amount of daily physical activity.

The activity–fitness relationship in children is an important question from the standpoint of preventive medicine as well. As noted earlier, many of the health benefits derived from regular exercise may relate to habitual activity rather than to physical fitness. This is good news for physicians, because it is presumably easier to alter exercise habits in patients than to change performance capabilities, which are strongly influenced and limited by genetic endowment. If fitness and activity are related, the task of detecting children at risk for hypoactivity is also simplified. Tests of fitness and means of assessing daily activities would then equally well identify those individuals who need intervention and counseling. If physical fitness does not adequately predict levels of physical activity, and if activity is the major health benefactor, fitness testing provides little guidance. Measurement of fitness levels would then primarily identify children who possess the hereditary capacity to perform well on physical tasks, which might have little bearing on health.

The lack of a precise tool to measure daily exercise activity is only one of several obstacles to clearly defining the relationship between fitness and physical activity. Body habitus and composition, extrinsic motivation, previous athletic experience, and other factors that influence fitness need to be carefully considered when studying correlates to activity levels in children. These issues may help explain the conflicting data regarding the fitness–activity association.

Ashton (1983) assessed fitness parameters in two groups of 9- to 10-year-old girls designated as high- and low-active based on questionnaire and interview. The high-active group scored better on all tests in a battery of $\dot{V}O_2$max, work expenditure, or physical work capacity at a heart rate of 170 bpm (PWC_{170}), step performance, strength, anaerobic capacity, and distance run in 9 min, but the differences were only statistically significant ($p < .05$) for $\dot{V}O_2$max and PWC_{170}. A considerable overlap was evident, however, as girls with high and low $\dot{V}O_2$max values were observed in each group.

Cunningham, Stapleton, MacDonald, and Paterson (1981) studied the relationship of daily energy expenditure (by heart rate–$\dot{V}O_2$ correlation) and $\dot{V}O_2$max on a treadmill test in 12-year-old boys. Multiple regression analysis indicated that body weight and fitness made the only significant contributions to the variance, with little addition by daily energy expenditure or time spent in vigorous activities. Seliger, Trefny, Bartunkova, and Pauer (1974) could find no correlation between $\dot{V}O_2$max and 24-hr activity by diary in prepubertal boys, but subjects were few in number (11) and particularly sedentary.

$\dot{V}O_2$max correlated ($r = .67$) with habitual activity determined by questionnaire in 25 children (mean age 12 years) studied by Schmucker, Rigauer, Hinrichs, and Trawinski (1984). Body composition apparently was not considered, however, in the statistical analysis. Bailey (1973) also reported a relationship between activity by questionnaire and $\dot{V}O_2$max during a longitudinal study of Canadian boys.

In their longitudinal study of active and inactive boys, Mirwald, Bailey, Cameron, and Rasmussen (1981) showed no influence of habitual activity on $\dot{V}O_2$max before adolescence. At the age of peak height velocity, however, the active group demonstrated a greater rate of increase in maximal aerobic power, suggesting that a sedentary lifestyle during adolescence may have long-term implications for adult fitness.

Two reports have examined the relationship of habitual activity with anaerobic threshold as a marker of fitness. Weymans, Reybrouck, Stijns, and Knops (1986) showed a significant influence of regular physical activity (by questionnaire) on anaerobic threshold (measured indirectly by gas exchange parameters) in males 5 to 18 years old. Another study indicated that the amount of daily time spent in vigorous exercise by 9- to 10-year-old boys correlated significantly with $\dot{V}O_2$max but not with anaerobic threshold (Atomi, Iwaoka, Hatta, Miyashita, & Yamamoto, 1986).

FITNESS LEVELS OF AMERICAN CHILDREN

A series of mass fitness tests performed over the past 20 years has generated concern about the fitness levels of American children (Safrit, 1986). These tests purportedly indicate that physical fitness is a major problem during childhood that might be remedied by remodeling the country's physical education programs. The conclusions have drawn considerable public notice. Media attention to these reports has been matched, as well, by vigorous controversy among scientists and educators regarding the content and interpretation of these tests (Murphy, 1986; Simmons, 1986).

Fitness Tests

Large-scale assessment of childhood fitness began in 1957, when the American Alliance for Health, Physical Education, and Recreation (AAHPER) established national norms using a seven-item test. This Youth Fitness Test battery included pull-ups (arm and shoulder girdle strength), sit-ups (strength of abdominal and hip flexors), shuttle run (speed and agility), standing long jump (explosive leg muscle power), 50-yd dash (speed), 600-yd run/walk (cardiovascular efficiency), and softball throw for distance (sport skills). The "dismaying test results" stimulated efforts to upgrade the quality of physical education programs, and when the test was repeated in 1965 significant improvements were observed in most test items. A modified AAHPER test conducted in 1975 did not show many changes from 1965, however (Hunsicker & Reiff, 1976).

The AAHPER test was changed in 1980 in response to criticisms that testing items were not associated with scientifically documented health outcomes. This Health-Related Physical Fitness Test (HRPFT) consisted of a distance run, bent-knee timed sit-ups, sit-and-reach test, and sum of skinfolds. Five years later, the U.S. Department of Health and Human Services published results of the National Children and Youth Fitness Study (NCYFS) that contained the same test items (plus chin-ups). Comparison of the 1980 and 1985 results indicated that children performed better in almost all age groups in the earlier study. Safrit (1986) has noted that this apparent fall-off in fitness may relate to different sampling methods. The HRPFT used physical education students whose teachers volunteered to participate, whereas the NCYFS was based on a probability sample that included subjects who may or may not have been enrolled in physical education classes.

Testing Conclusions

The conclusion drawn from these tests, that there is a serious physical fitness deficit among American children, has been questioned (Corbin, 1987; Murphy, 1986; Simmons, 1986; Simons-Morton et al., 1987). Importantly, no information is available to link performance level on test items with specific health outcomes. The youngster who finishes in the lowest 10th percentile of her class on a distance run cannot necessarily be assumed to be at increased health risk, because the relationship between her performance and any health effect has not been quantified; what truly constitutes an acceptable finish time from a health standpoint is unknown, and the child's performance simply describes her field performance relative to that of her peers.

Performance items may be strongly influencd by factors other than the determinant they are designed to measure. A prominent example is the distance run, performance on which may be dramatically affected by differences in body-fat content, motivation, and pacing experience as well as by cardiovascular efficiency. This may help explain why laboratory-derived $\dot{V}O_2$max correlates only moderately well with field endurance tests in children. Moreover, the technical difficulties of test standardization in large studies involving many schools weakens comparisons made between tests spaced 10 years apart. Other problems of cross-sectional fitness testing have been previously discussed:

- At any given age the developmental level of biological factors related to physical performance may vary widely.
- It is impossible from field fitness testing to distinguish the physical "underachiever" from the child with genetic-based limitations of exercise capability.
- The tendency for testing results to "track" in a given individual with increasing age is unknown.

The health-related fitness levels of American youth may be low, and with improved physical education programs the situation may be remediable. But it is difficult to confidently justify these conclusions based on the results of mass fitness testing results alone (Shephard, 1982).

Is there any evidence that children's aerobic fitness levels have diminished as an effect of sedentary modern living? Little information is available. Maximum oxygen consumption values in boys reported 50 years ago by Robinson (1938) are comparable to those observed in present-day studies. Shephard (1982) noted that if the childhood population had sustained major declines in fitness, large gains in $\dot{V}O_2max$ would be expected in training studies; this has not been the general experience (see chapter 4). Based on this scant evidence, Pate and Blair (1978) concluded that "while there can be no question that a truly sedentary life-style leads to low cardiorespiratory fitness, evidence does not yet exist to indicate that this principle has expressed itself on the bulk of American children" (p. 269).

FUTURE DIRECTIONS

The story of fitness and physical activity and their influence on children's health is largely incomplete. Interpretation of testing results, implications connecting activity and health, and therapeutic interventions are being based on assumptions that do not always bear up to close scientific scrutiny. Present information suggests an important role for exercise in children's health, but effectively guiding youngsters into active lifestyles will require a much greater scientific foundation than is currently available.

The following list specifies areas where additional information would be helpful.

• **Normal physical activity levels.** More information is needed regarding "normal" levels of physical activity in children. How much is adequate? Are certain ages vulnerable periods for hypoactivity? Extrinsic factors influencing activity need to be delineated and the extent to which physical activity can be modified needs to be more completely understood.

• **Daily physical activity assessment.** An improved means of easily and accurately assessing daily physical activity is needed. With this information clinicians could more precisely identify hypoactive patients and examine responses to exercise interventions. A reliable tool for quantitating daily exercise would also provide researchers with a more effective means of testing relationships among physical activity and physical fitness, health outcomes, and factors influencing habitual levels of exercise.

• **Exercise thresholds.** The forms and thresholds of exercise necessary to achieve positive health outcomes need to be established. Interventional studies examining the relationships between increased exercise activities and health effects will provide more useful information than the current set of descriptive reports. Given these insights, the results of fitness testing will become more meaningful and exercise prescriptions more relevant to wellness.

• **Relationship of physical activity to fitness.** The relationship between physical fitness and activity in children remains clouded. More comprehensive studies carefully considering confounding variables will provide a better answer to whether physicians need to differentiate between the two in testing and therapeutic interventions.

• **Habitual physical activity.** The tendency for both physical fitness and physical activity to be sustained from childhood through the adult years has not been evaluated, yet the basic tenet of promoting exercise for children—that patterns of regular physical activity need to be instilled early in life—is based on the premise that such habits persist. Specific early interventions by physicians, parents, or teachers may be important in assuring continuity of a healthy lifestyle, but these are currently unknown.

SUMMARY

This chapter discussed how physical fitness is linked to habitual physical activity.

- Both physical activity and physical fitness may be important to health, depending on the outcome goals.
- An accurate assessment of daily physical activity is difficult. Studies on large populations of children are best performed using questionnaire or diary information; more accurate data on smaller numbers can be obtained by direct observation or heart rate determination. Newer mechanical devices show promise of providing better means of measuring activity levels.
- Levels of habitual energy expenditure relative to body size decline during childhood and adolescence. Although this appears to be a normal maturational change, the rate of activity decline may be strongly influenced by modifiable environmental factors.
- Studies examining children's physical activity and fitness have not provided a clear picture of the relationship between the two. Even if they are associated, it is difficult to determine whether fit individuals exercise more or whether greater levels of activity improve physical fitness.
- The ability to draw conclusions about the results of mass fitness testing of school children is hampered by a lack of research data linking physical performance with health-related outcomes.

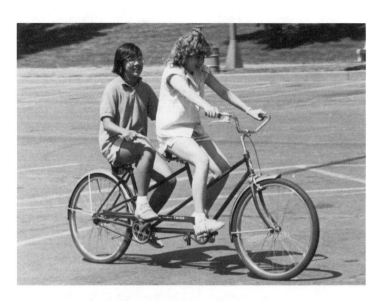

CHAPTER 4

Endurance Exercise Fitness

This chapter addresses the development of children's abilities to perform in endurance exercise (running, swimming, cycling, and so on) as they grow. More specifically, the discussion will consider the physiological mechanisms that account for improved performance in these activities during biological maturation. Long-term longitudinal investigations describing this developmental sequence are lacking, and most information has been derived from shorter serial studies and cross-sectional analyses comparing pre- and postpubertal subjects. In presenting this information, these three enigmas that continue to challenge developmental exercise physiologists will be addressed:

- In adults, maximum oxygen uptake (measured per kilogram body mass) is considered a marker of both cardiovascular functional reserve and endurance exercise capability. Yet in children $\dot{V}O_2max/kg$ does not increase during the growing years. By what physiological means, then, do the child's abilities in endurance events develop?
- A period of endurance training in previously sedentary adults is associated with anatomical and physiological adaptations (the "fitness effect") that include improvements in $\dot{V}O_2max$. Does the child respond similarly to training? If not, why not?
- Boys tend to exhibit greater levels of endurance fitness than girls, although not to the extent observed following puberty. What is responsible for gender-related differences in fitness in the childhood years?

Children by their nature do not typically engage in sustained forms of exercise (Gilliam et al., 1981). Yet endurance sports such as cycling, running, and swimming are those most frequently associated with the health benefits of exercise—and for a number of good reasons. These activities are not restricted to those few individuals with high athletic skill but can be enjoyed by all children. They are lifetime sports (it is difficult, on the other hand, to round up 21 of your 45-year-old friends for a tackle football game on Sunday afternoons), and, importantly, they improve the working efficiency of the cardiovascular system because of the exercising muscles' demands for oxygen delivery. It is tempting to link these improvements in heart function to a diminished risk for cardiovascular disease during adulthood. However, although regular exercise of sufficient degree to improve fitness may reduce that risk, there is little to suggest that the effects of improved cardiac efficiency itself are responsible (LaPorte, Dearwater, Cauley, Slemenda, & Cook, 1985).

It is important to realize that there is a considerable overlap in physical fitness between pediatric and adult populations. Certainly an active 25-year-old graduate student will demonstrate greater levels of functional and physiological fitness than an obese 10-year-old, and a slender 12-year-old who has been playing on a recreational soccer team will perform better on treadmill exercise testing than a sedentary 30-year-old office worker. Therefore it is very difficult to match groups of pre- and postpubertal subjects by levels of regular activity and body composition when examining differences in exercise physiology by cross-sectional studies. The comparisons cited in this chapter address *mean values* between sets of children and adults; they appear to demonstrate real age-group differences principally on the grounds of the consistency by which these differences are reported by different investigators. Also, it should be noted that the studies reviewed in this chapter have involved principally active, healthy, older, prepubertal boys, sometimes in comparison with young adult subjects. These observations cannot be assumed to be representative of "children" because females, children under age 8, and sedentary and obese youngsters are often ignored.

AGE AND ENDURANCE PERFORMANCE

Endurance exercise fitness can be described in three ways: First, in its purist sense, endurance fitness is defined by the time a subject can persevere before exhaustion limits exercise involving rhythmic motions of large muscle groups (e.g., as in running, swimming, and cycling). Obviously, the ability to persist on such a test is determined by the speed or intensity at which the exercise is performed; that is, a subject can last longer while running on a 5-mph rather than an 8-mph treadmill. Second, the definition of endurance capacity is altered in the competition setting, when the speed/endurance relationship is applied to a set distance: The marathoner with greater endurance fitness who can complete 26 mi at a pace of 5:05 per mile will defeat the runner who can maintain only a speed of 5:15 per mile for the same distance. Third, in the exercise laboratory, exercise fitness could be described as the maximal time sustained on a progressive treadmill test of increasing speed and/or slope. Treadmill endurance time represents somewhat of an anomaly, because this type of progressive exercise intensity to exhaustion is not duplicated in any sporting event. Still, endurance times during treadmill testing have been correlated with distance running performance (Kemper & Verschuur, 1985).

Considering these three ways of defining endurance performance, is there evidence that children possess more or less endurance fitness than adults? Procedural difficulties make field testing impractical for comparing functional endurance capacities between groups. For instance, if adults and children were to be tested for maximal distance run before exhaustion, what should be the starting pace? Subjects who start too fast will quickly tire and drop out, and slow starters will continue for longer periods (Katch, Pechar, McArdle, & Weltman, 1973). Endurance performance in the laboratory has been assessed by the pattern of fall-off in pedaling work on a high-resistance cycle protocol (Katch & Katch, 1972; Sady & Katch, 1981). In this test, all subjects begin at the same high work rate (approximately 100 percent $\dot{V}O_2$max) and pedal for the same length of time. A subject who maintains the same work rate for the duration of the test is considered to have 100 percent endurance. Those who decline in pedal rate as they fatigue have less endurance fitness, and this percentage decrement provides a useful means of making interindividual comparisons.

A study comparing prepubertal boys and adult men (mean ages 10.2 and 30.0 years, respectively), employing this technique, showed no difference in relative endurance fitness (Sady & Katch, 1981). The mean work load was 543 and 1,607 kgm • min^{-1} at $\dot{V}O_2$max for the boys and men, respectively, so absolute endurance fitness on this high-resistance cycle test was clearly greater in the adult subjects.

No significant differences have been observed in the physiological adaptations to prolonged low-intensity exercise in children and adults (Máček, Vávra, & Novosadova, 1976). Asano and Hirakoba (1984) measured exercise parameters in 10- to 12-year-old boys and 20- to 34-year-old men who cycled for 1 hr at a constant work load of 60 percent $\dot{V}O_2$max. Patterns of change in $\dot{V}O_2$, heart rate, respiratory rate, ventilation, respiratory exchange ratio, cardiac output, and blood pressure were similar in the two groups. These studies again measured responses at the same relative metabolic intensity rather than absolute work load.

Studies assessing performance by children of different ages on distance running events consistently demonstrate a progressive improvement in finishing times until at least early adolescence (Hunsicker & Reiff, 1976; Krahenbuhl, Pangrazi, Petersen, Burkett, & Schneider, 1978; Shephard, 1982) (Figure 4.1). A similar trend is observed in treadmill endurance times (Cumming, Everatt, & Hastman, 1978; Houlsby, 1986). Cumming et al. (1978) combined their own data with that of Bruce, Kusumi, and Hosmer (1973) to create an age–performance curve for endurance time on a standard treadmill protocol (Figure 4.2). Endurance rose to a peak at ages 16 to 18 in males and then declined through the adult years. A similar trend was observed in females, except the curve peaked earlier (at about age 12 years); at all ages values for females were lower than for males. Interestingly, the average endurance time for boys at age 8 years was equal to that for men at age 35. Among the females, a 5-year-old would be expected to perform better than a 35-year-old woman. A significant influence of body habitus and fat on these comparative treadmill times was emphasized by the authors (Cumming & Hnatiuk, 1980).

Based on these limited data it is reasonable to conclude that endurance fitness improves progressively throughout childhood and adolescence, at least in males. Information from treadmill running data as well as performance on standard step tests (Master & Oppenheimer, 1929) suggests that endurance performance peaks between the ages of 16 and 25 years in the average untrained male and then declines thereafter. The age–performance curve in females appears to be shifted downward and to the left compared to males. The conclusion, then, that prepubertal subjects possess greater cardiovascular fitness than other age groups based

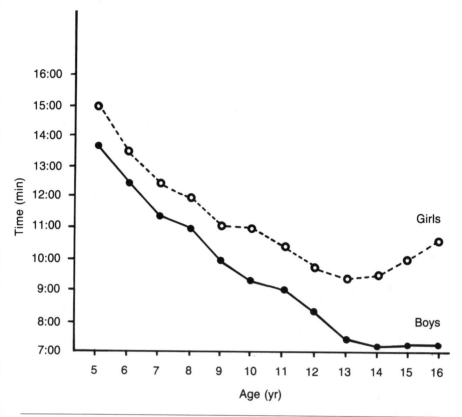

Figure 4.1 One-mile run times in children and adolescents (mean values for over 12,000 subjects). *Note.* Data from the American Alliance for Health, Physical Education, Recreation and Dance (1980).

on their high levels of maximal aerobic power (per body weight) therefore appears to be erroneous from a functional standpoint.

What factors are responsible for the progressive improvement in endurance performance during the growing years? Considerable research in adult subjects has indicated that maximum oxygen uptake and the ability to minimize oxygen uptake requirements at submaximal work loads (exercise economy) are strong predictors of endurance fitness. These determinants could be anticipated to play important roles in the development of endurance capacity in the pediatric age group as well. The following sections examine current knowledge of maximum oxygen uptake and exercise economy in children and how these factors might (or might not) relate to improvements in endurance performance with growth.

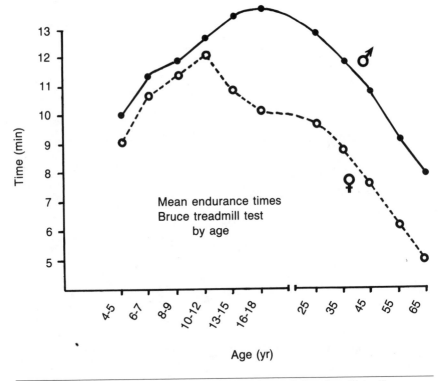

Figure 4.2 Treadmill endurance times in males and females. *Note*. From "Bruce Treadmill Tests in Children: Normal Values in a Clinic Population" by G.R. Cumming, D. Everatt, and L. Hastman, 1978, *American Journal of Cardiology*, **41**, p. 70. Copyright 1978 by Reed Publishing USA. Reprinted by permission.

MAXIMAL OXYGEN UPTAKE IN CHILDREN

The cardiovascular delivery and muscular uptake of oxygen are among the major physiological determinants of endurance fitness in adults (Snell & Mitchell, 1984). However, the validity of $\dot{V}O_2$max as a reliable marker of cardiovascular function or endurance capacity in children is open to question.

The Development of $\dot{V}O_2$max

Cross-sectional and longitudinal studies, in combination, have provided a reasonably clear picture of the development of maximal oxygen uptake during the childhood and adolescent years (Bar-Or, 1983; Krahenbuhl,

Skinner, & Kohrt, 1985). Prior to puberty, absolute $\dot{V}O_2$max levels, measured with either treadmill or cycle testing, improve steadily with growth of pulmonary, cardiovascular, and musculoskeletal systems (Figure 4.3). In most studies, values in males slightly but consistently exceed those in females at all ages. Pubertal influences then cause these curves to diverge during adolescence. Absolute $\dot{V}O_2$max accelerates at puberty in males, reflecting increases in muscle mass, whereas $\dot{V}O_2$max in females remains virtually unchanged after the early teen years.

The problem of how best to relate $\dot{V}O_2$ to the normal growth of body dimensions was discussed in chapter 2. Arguments for using body mass, height, various power functions of height and mass, lean body mass, lean

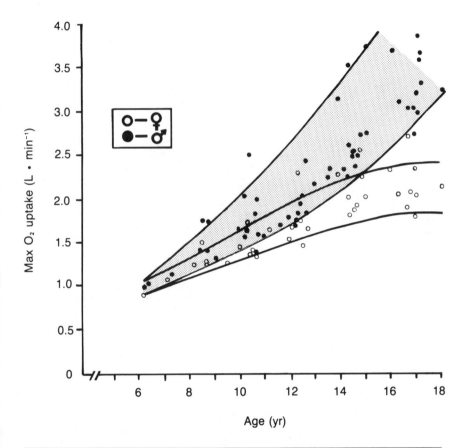

Figure 4.3 Changes in absolute maximal oxygen uptake with age. *Note.* From *Pediatric Sports Medicine for the Practitioner* (p. 4) by O. Bar-Or, 1983, New York: Springer. Copyright 1983 by Springer Verlag. Reprinted by permission.

leg volume, or skeletal age as the denominator to "factor out" the influence of growth on oxygen uptake have all been presented from both theoretical and empirical perspectives.

The ideal index, unfortunately, remains unknown. It has generally been concluded that body mass relates closely to $\dot{V}O_2$ in almost all studies and remains the most practical denominator for interindividual comparison of aerobic capacity (Krahenbuhl et al., 1985). Whether body mass is an equally appropriate reference for weight-bearing (e.g., running) and non-weight-bearing (e.g., cycling) exercise, or for subject populations with variable ranges of body composition, remains problematic.

When $\dot{V}O_2$max is related to body mass, maximal aerobic power on treadmill testing remains essentially constant in males (50 to 55 ml $\cdot$ kg^{-1}min^{-1}) across the wide age-range of 6 to 16 years (Figure 4.4). Thereafter weight-related aerobic power progressively drops off with advancing age. In

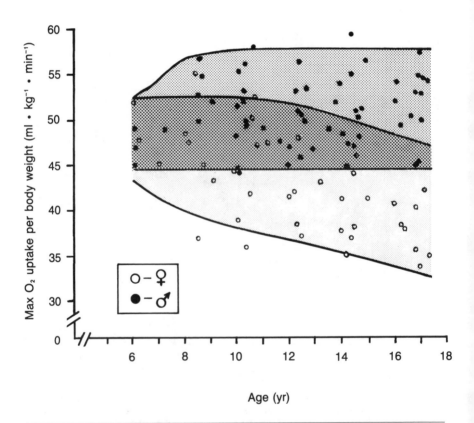

Figure 4.4 Changes in maximal oxygen uptake with age expressed per kg body weight. *Note.* From *Pediatric Sports Medicine for the Practitioner* (p. 5) by O. Bar-Or, 1983, New York: Springer. Copyright 1983 by Springer Verlag. Reprinted by permission.

females, on the other hand, a continuous decline in $\dot{V}O_2max/kg$ is observed from the midchildhood years, becomes exaggerated at puberty, and continues to fall throughout life (Åstrand & Rodahl, 1977).

$\dot{V}O_2max$ and Fitness in Children

When research efforts turned to understanding the growth of exercise capacity in children, much attention was focused on the development of $\dot{V}O_2$ and its determinants (Cunningham, Paterson, & Blimkie, 1984; Krahenbuhl et al., 1985; Shephard, 1982). These studies have somewhat surprisingly indicated that $\dot{V}O_2max$ is not so neatly related to endurance fitness in children as it is in older subjects (Davies, 1980; Day, 1981). The following lines of evidence suggest that high $\dot{V}O_2max/kg$ values are misleading and cannot be interpreted simply as indicative of superior fitness in children.

Evidence #1: Children's aerobic fitness components differ from adults'.
Analysis of the components of aerobic fitness in children suggests shortcomings compared with adults: Inferior ventilatory efficiency, possible impaired production of cardiac output and stroke volume, and low blood-oxygen carrying capacity are all characteristics of prepubertal subjects that improve as subjects grow.

Evidence #2: Moderate correlation in children's endurance performance exists when field and lab tests are compared.
Studies comparing field endurance performance with laboratory $\dot{V}O_2max/kg$ indicate only a moderate correlation in children as contrasted with the close relationship observed in adults (Burke, 1975). Massicotte, Gauthier, and Markon (1985) reviewed studies of $\dot{V}O_2max$ and distance-run performances in children and found typical correlation coefficients of .6 to .7.

Evidence #3: $\dot{V}O_2max/kg$ stabilizes or declines during growing years, but endurance improves.
During the growing years, endurance performance (defined as treadmill endurance time or by finishing times in distance runs) improves steadily, whereas $\dot{V}O_2max/kg$ remains stable or declines (Figure 4.5).

Evidence #4: Body composition factors may also account for $\dot{V}O_2max$ differences in children.
Evidence indicates that $\dot{V}O_2max$ differences in children are accounted for by factors other than cardiovascular function, particularly those involving body composition (e.g., lean body mass and percent body fat) (Day, 1981). $\dot{V}O_2max/kg$ thus represents an expression of the combined influences of anthropometric as well as physiological determinants of endurance performance. Mayhew and Gifford (1975) were able, for instance,

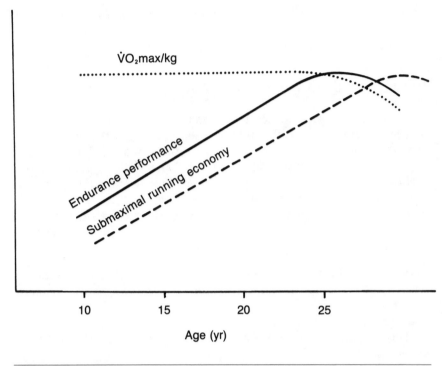

Figure 4.5 Changes in maximal oxygen uptake, running economy, and endurance performance with age.

to create a predictive formula in boys for $\dot{V}O_2$max based solely on anthropometric factors that gave a .85 correlation with directly measured $\dot{V}O_2$max.

Still, it is clear that maximal oxygen consumption plays an important role in determining children's performance in endurance activities, as it does in adults. Prepubertal endurance athletes demonstrate $\dot{V}O_2$max levels that are generally about 10 ml • kg^{-1} min^{-1} greater than nonathletic children (Mayers & Gutin, 1979) (Figure 4.6). Despite controversy, children can show improved $\dot{V}O_2$max with physical training (Krahenbuhl et al., 1985; Rowland, 1986), and in disease states where $\dot{V}O_2$ is curtailed, exercise performance declines (Bar-Or, 1986).

In longitudinal assessment of the individual child, however, $\dot{V}O_2$max/kg does not serve as a useful indicator of endurance fitness because, as noted earlier, maximal aerobic power does not increase over the years when endurance performance is dramatically improving. This discrepancy may be explained by the possibility that $\dot{V}O_2$max/kg does not provide an accurate assessment of ability to generate aerobic metabolism during exercise;

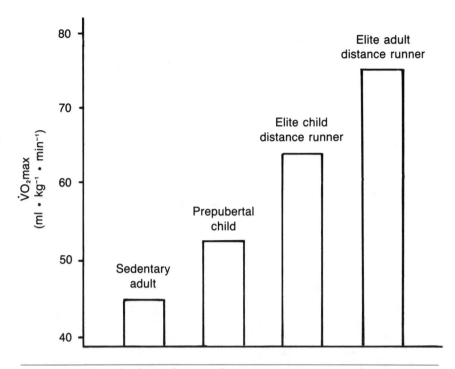

Figure 4.6 Typical values of maximal oxygen uptake in trained and athletic children and adults (males).

another possible explanation is that improvements in submaximal running economy during growth may enhance performance irrespective of maximal aerobic power.

Growth of Oxygen Delivery Systems

Although $\dot{V}O_2$max/kg does not increase during childhood, the maximal ability to deliver oxygen to exercising muscle—expressed as the multiple of resting levels of $\dot{V}O_2$, or the *metabolic scope*—progressively improves. This rise in the ratio of maximal to resting oxygen uptake occurs de facto, because $\dot{V}O_2$max/kg remains unchanged while the child grows and the resting metabolic rate per body mass declines. Metabolic scope should be expected to be independent of body size (Schmidt-Nielsen, 1984); the rise in this value with growth may thus indicate improvements in oxygen delivery above that accounted for by organ growth alone. If so, similar qualitative improvements should be observed in the components of the oxygen delivery chain. In fact, evidence does suggest that such changes occur.

Pulmonary

In adults, lung function has always been considered the strongest link in the oxygen delivery chain. Arterial pO_2 and pCO_2 in a healthy individual are maintained at normal levels throughout progressive exercise, and ventilation ($\dot{V}_E$) at peak effort does not tax maximal lung ventilatory capacity (Åstrand & Rodahl, 1977). Limited assessment of blood gases during exercise in children indicates similar findings (Godfrey, 1974).

Values for maximal ventilation with exercise throughout childhood and into the adult years parallel those for absolute $\dot{V}O_2$max. $\dot{V}_E$max progressively increases in males until 20 to 25 years of age, when values begin to decline. The peak in females is earlier, around the time of puberty (Åstrand, 1952; Åstrand, 1960). The age curve of $\dot{V}_E$max related to body weight also follows that of $\dot{V}O_2$max/kg. $\dot{V}_E$max/kg remains essentially stable during the childhood and adolescent years in boys, with values of 1.6 to 2.0 L • kg^{-1} (Åstrand, 1952) but decreases once early adulthood is reached. As with oxygen uptake, the ratio of maximal to resting ventilation improves during the growing years (Robinson, 1938).

Along with these high levels of lung work, children ventilate more to deliver a given amount of oxygen compared with adults. This high *ventilatory equivalent for oxygen* ($\dot{V}_E/\dot{V}O_2$) is evidence of inferior ventilatory efficiency in children and is observed at maximal as well as submaximal exercise (Åstrand, 1952; Rowland, Auchinachie, Keenan, & Green, 1987). There is a trend for $\dot{V}_E/\dot{V}O_2$ to decrease with age from childhood through young adult years, indicating that maturational factors influence breathing economy during exercise (Andersen, Seliger, Rutenfranz, & Messel, 1974). Why children should possess such reduced ventilatory efficiency is unknown. Prepubertal subjects may hyperventilate during exercise compared with older subjects, as limited data indicate lower end-tidal pCO_2 values in children (Andersen & Godfrey, 1971; Godfrey, Davies, Wozniak, & Barnes, 1971). This, in turn, may be a reflection of greater ventilatory sensitivity to pCO_2 levels in children (Cooper et al., 1987).

Because children have smaller lungs than adults, they would be expected to also demonstrate smaller tidal volumes with exercise. In fact, tidal volume (V_T) is even smaller than would be predicted for their size: V_T/kg is decreased in children compared to adults at both a given V_E and exercise intensity, and respiratory rates are correspondingly higher (Åstrand, 1952; Rowland & Green, 1988) (Figure 4.7). The relative contributions of breathing rate and V_T are normally adjusted to minimize ventilatory work (Godfrey, 1974). The wisdom of the shift in children to lower V_T and more rapid rates presumably lies in developmental aspects of lung mechanics that improve ventilatory efficiency with higher frequency: V_T ratios in this age group. The answer may lie in the relationship of falling airways resistance and rising compliance with age (Otis, Fenn, & Rahn, 1950). Increased lung-recoil forces observed in children compared to adults

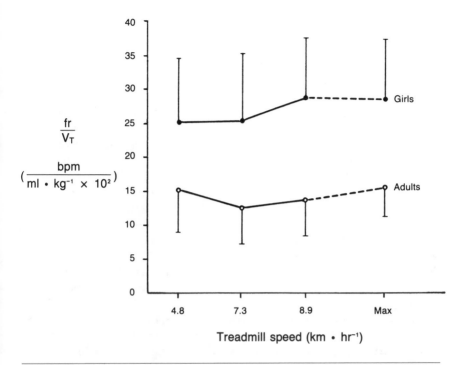

Figure 4.7 Ratio of respiratory frequency (*fr*) to tidal volume (V_T) in children and adults during treadmill exercise. *Note.* From "Physiological Responses to Treadmill Exercise in Females: Adult-Child Differences" by T.W. Rowland and G.M. Green, 1988, *Medicine and Science in Sports and Exercise*, **20**, p. 476. Copyright 1988 by the American College of Sports Medicine. Reprinted by permission.

may also play a role, because smaller tidal volumes in youngsters with increased pulmonary elastic fiber density would minimize ventilatory work (Zapletal, Misur, & Samanek, 1971).

The implications of these aspects of children's pulmonary function during exercise are unclear. Ventilation appears adequate for maximal exercise, but the added energy requirements created by greater $\dot{V}_E/\dot{V}O_2$ levels and perhaps higher breathing rates could potentially limit endurance capacity compared to older subjects (Åstrand & Rodahl, 1977).

Cardiac

In contrast to pulmonary function, methodological constraints have limited the understanding of cardiac responses to exercise during growth. It has long been proposed, though, that children's cardiovascular activity is different from adults'. In fact, as recently as 1967 these variations prompted concern that vigorous physical activity might pose a cardiac risk for children (Corbin, 1987). Subsequent data suggest that prepubertal subjects may have diminished cardiac function with exercise compared with young adults, but fortunately there is no evidence that exhaustive physical activity has any detrimental effect.

Heart Rate. Heart rates are high at rest and during submaximal exercise in small children and progressively fall throughout the pediatric years. The peak heart rate during progressive treadmill testing in children aged 9 to 13 years ranges from 195 to 215 bpm (Bar-Or, 1983); on cycle ergometer protocols the rate is usually about 5 bpm slower (Cumming & Langford, 1985). At puberty, peak rate begins to fall at a rate of 7 to 8 beats per decade (Robinson, 1938). The maximal heart rate attained depends on which exercise protocol is used as well as subject motivation. When children simply run at very high work loads (steady-state maximal exercise), the peak heart rate may be 10 to 15 beats higher than during a progressive test (Åstrand, 1952). On the other hand, short cycle tests with rapid increases in resistance (and thus shorter times at maximal work intensity) produce lower peak heart rates (Cumming & Langford, 1985).

As children grow, submaximal heart rates steadily decline at exercise at either equal intensity (percent $\dot{V}O_2$max) or work load. As outlined by Bar-Or (1983), these rates are influenced by multiple variables: Higher values are created by obesity, heat stress, anxiety, greater exercising muscle mass, poor cardiovascular fitness, and upright body position. Both maximal and submaximal heart rates are typically higher in girls than in boys (Godfrey, 1974).

Cardiac Output. It is even more difficult to measure children's cardiac output with exercise. The most precise techniques require vascular catheterization, and information on cardiac function from direct Fick, thermodilution, and dye-dilution methods in normal children is limited. These techniques are best performed under steady-state conditions, which make measurements difficult at maximal exercise; each involves assumptions and potential errors that limit accuracy and at best provide an estimate of cardiac output (Alpert, Bloom, Gilday, & Olley, 1979). Although safer and more acceptable for children, noninvasive methods of determining cardiac output (e.g., CO_2 rebreathing, Doppler flow, acetylene rebreathing, and thoracic bioimpedance) are subject to the same objections (Christie et al., 1987; Marks, Katch, Rocchini, Beekman, & Rosenthal, 1985).

Little difference is observed in resting cardiac index (cardiac output per square meter of body surface area) between children and adults (3 to 5 L/min per m²). During submaximal exercise, children demonstrate a lower absolute cardiac output at a given metabolic stress ($\dot{V}O_2$), the consequence of a dampened rise in stroke volume compared to that observed in adult subjects (Godfrey, 1974; Katsura, 1986; Rowland, Staab, Unnithan, & Siconolfi, 1988; Zeidifard, Godfrey, & Davies, 1976).

The results of cardiac output studies at maximal exercise in prepubertal boys are outlined in Table 4.1. Mean ratios of maximal to resting cardiac index of 2.5 and 3.1 have been reported in boys 10 to 12 years old, with an associated rise in stroke index by a factor of 1.1 to 1.35 (Eriksson, 1972; Rowland, Staab, Unnithan, & Siconolfi, 1988). In contrast, young adults typically increase their cardiac index to 4 to 6 times basal levels (depending on fitness level) while doubling stroke index (Fox, 1984; Karpman, 1987; McArdle et al., 1981; Miyamura & Honda, 1973). The limited comparative data thus suggest that young (about college-age) physically fit adults augment cardiac index significantly more than do active children during maximal exercise. If so, differences in stroke volume must be responsible, given that maximal heart rates are highest in prepubertal subjects. Studies of cardiac responses across pediatric age groups appear to indicate that these child–adult differences progress in a continuum during the growing years (Bar-Or, 1983; Cunningham, Paterson, Blimkie, & Donner, 1984; Gadhoke & Jones, 1969).

Why might children demonstrate decreased stroke index responses to exercise compared to adults? No age-related differences in cardiac preload or afterload have been identified, implying that changes in stroke volume are effected principally by increased cardiac contractility. Experimental

Table 4.1 Maximal Cardiac Output Studies in Prepubertal Boys

Reference	Method	Exercise	Subjects	Maximal cardiac index L/min/m²
Cumming (1977)	Dye dilution	Supine cycle	31	10.1
Eriksson (1972)	Dye dilution	Upright cycle	9	9.1
Yamaji & Miyashita (1977)	CO_2 rebreathing	Upright cycle	8	10.4
Gilliam, Sady, Thorland, & Weltman (1977)	CO_2 rebreathing	Upright cycle	36	10.4
Miyamura & Honda (1973)	CO_2 rebreathing	Upright cycle	16	11.7
Rowland, Staab, Unnithan, & Siconolfi (1988)	Bioimpedance	Upright cycle	15	9.2

evidence suggests several possible mechanisms for depressed myocardial contractile reserve in children. Decreased cardiac output, ejection fraction, and myocardial $\dot{V}O_2$ are reported in gonadectomized rats, and these markers of impaired myocardial function are reversed after testosterone administration (Schaible, Malhotra, Ciambrone, & Scheuer, 1984; Scheuer, Malhotra, Schaible, & Capasso, 1987). This suggests that adult–child differences in cardiac responses to exercise could relate to the effects of endogenous androgen stimulation occurring at puberty, at least in males.

The possibility of diminished sympathetic stimulation of the ventricular myocardium in children is suggested by studies indicating a positive correlation between age and mononuclear cell beta-adrenoreceptor density (Middeke, Remien, & Holzgrere, 1984; Roan & Galant, 1981). Also, newborn lambs studied by Romero and Friedman (1979) showed depressed left-ventricular stroke volume and contractility after an administered volume load compared to adult sheep. The authors attributed these findings to a lower ventricular compliance and failure to reduce peripheral resistance in the young animals.

Hematologic

The concentration of hemoglobin in the blood is a key determinant of oxygen delivery and aerobic fitness. Anemic individuals demonstrate diminished $\dot{V}O_2max$ levels and are impaired in their ability to exercise (Viteri & Torun, 1974); conversely, polycythemia (at least to the limits of increased blood viscosity) raises blood oxygen carrying capacity and may improve endurance fitness (Kanstrup & Ekblom, 1984).

The blood hemoglobin concentration and total hemoglobin per body weight increase steadily throughout childhood and adolescence (Åstrand, 1952). The normal hemoglobin concentration in a 10-year-old boy or girl is 13.0 g/100 ml compared to 16.0 and 14.0 g/100 ml in the adult male and female, respectively. The same child will possess a total hemoglobin mass per kilogram body weight of 72 percent of that of an adult male or 96 percent of an adult female.

Peripheral Uptake

Considering the possible cardiac and hematological limitations of oxygen delivery in children, prepubertal subjects would be expected to maintain sufficient $\dot{V}O_2$ for exercise by compensatory increase in peripheral oxygen extraction. When these calculations are made, children do demonstrate a higher arterial–venous oxygen difference at peak exercise than do older individuals (Rode, Bar-Or, & Shephard, 1973; Rowland et al., 1988). The physiological basis for augmented peripheral oxygen extraction in children is not, however, overtly obvious. The scant information available on mitochondrial density and cellular aerobic enzyme activity in children does not indicate significant differences from that in adults (Bell, MacDougall, Billeter, & Howald, 1980; Eriksson, 1980). There is some evidence, however, that muscle blood flow during exercise is greater in prepubertal subjects. Koch (1974) showed a greater muscle blood flow immediately after exercise in 12-year-old boys compared with adults, and follow-up studies 1 and 4 years later demonstrated a progressive decline with increasing age (Koch, 1978, 1980).

RUNNING ECONOMY

The previous section presented evidence indicating that improvements in oxygen delivery (beyond those expected by changes in body size) during growth could help explain the development of endurance performance in childhood. Another potential mechanism for performance changes—improved submaximal running economy—may occur without alterations in maximal oxygen delivery.

When a person begins to run on a treadmill, oxygen consumption rises from resting values to satisfy the energy requirements of contracting muscle. It is of interest to determine the oxygen requirements at submaximal exercise, because conservation of energy at these work loads might be expected to permit the subject to extend his or her performance to greater peak levels. Indeed, submaximal running economy has been related to endurance performance in both children and adults (Mayers & Gutin, 1979; Rowland, Auchinachie, Keenan, & Green, 1988).

Definition

Running economy is the metabolic cost (measured as oxygen uptake per kilogram body weight) for a given treadmill speed and slope. A *lower* oxygen uptake is therefore interpreted as *improved* economy. Examining the rise from preexercise $\dot{V}O_2$ to that at a given treadmill speed would give valuable information regarding running economy, but "resting" $\dot{V}O_2$ may be influenced by anxiety and anticipatory cardiovascular responses. Alternatively, the oxygen cost of increasing the treadmill a given unit of speed (or slope) during submaximal running offers another means of measuring exercise economy.

Adult–Child Comparisons

When the metabolic cost of treadmill running is compared between young adults and prepubertal subjects, the absolute $\dot{V}O_2$ is lower in the children at all speeds. This is expected, because the "work" of treadmill running is the propulsion of body mass, which is obviously less in the child.

The corollary, that when values of $\dot{V}O_2$ are related to body mass the child–adult economy differences should disappear, is, surprisingly, untrue. Both $\dot{V}O_2$/kg at a given speed and the oxygen cost of increasing treadmill speed 1 mph are greater for both boys and girls than for their adult counterparts (Figure 4.8) (Åstrand, 1952; Freedson, Katch, Gilliam, & MacConnie, 1981; Robinson, 1938; Rowland, Auchinachie, Keenan, & Green, 1987; Rowland & Green, 1988). Moreover, there is a continuum of improved running economy with growth during childhood and adolescence (Åstrand, 1952; MacDougall, Roche, Bar-Or, & Moroz, 1979).

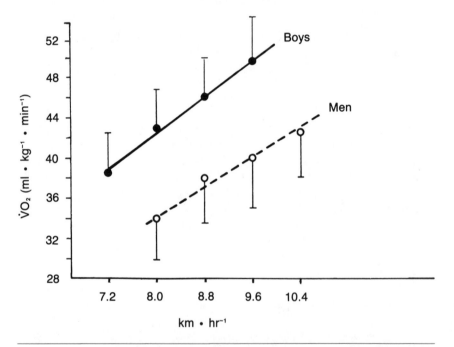

Figure 4.8 Submaximal treadmill running economy in prepubertal boys and adult males. *Note.* From "Responses to Treadmill Running in Adult and Prepubertal Males" by T.W. Rowland, J.A. Auchinachie, T.J. Keenan, and G.M. Green, 1987, *International Journal of Sports Medicine*, **8**, p. 295. Copyright 1987 by Thieme Medical Publishers, Inc. Reprinted by permission.

This increase in economy may contribute to the rise in endurance fitness during the pediatric years. As illustrated in Figure 4.9, $\dot{V}O_2$max/kg remains stable with increasing age while economy improves. This means that a child will run at a progressively lower percentage of $\dot{V}O_2$max, when tested at the same speed, as she or he grows. The older child should perform better in endurance events, because at a given speed the relative intensity of the exercise will be less as the subject ages. That is, compared to when she was 8 years old, the 12-year-old girl should be able to run a given distance at a faster pace, or run longer at a given speed. It should be noted that in this situation, better performance is related to improved economy, independent of aerobic power.

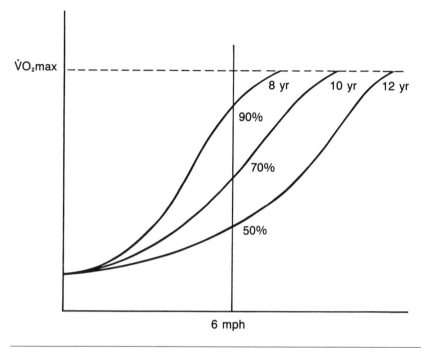

Figure 4.9 Improvements in running economy with age cause the older child to be exercising at a relatively lower intensity (percent $\dot{V}O_2$max) at the same speed. *Note.* From "Oxygen Uptake and Physical Fitness in Children" by T. Rowland, 1989, *Pediatric Exercise Science*, 1, p. 318. Copyright 1989 by Human Kinetics Publishers, Inc. Reprinted by permission.

Etiology of Economy Differences

Why should children exhibit such inferior running economy compared to adults? The answer lies somewhere in the myriad of determinants of treadmill work and their variability with age. In adult subjects, these factors of locomotion are important to energy economy (Cavanagh & Kram, 1985; Daniels, 1985):

- Vertical displacement
- Lateral motion
- Stride length

- Fuel utilization patterns
- Energy transfer between body segments
- Body composition
- Coordination
- Muscle strength and elasticity
- Muscle fiber types and vascularization
- Pacing
- Heat dispersion mechanisms
- Equipment (e.g., shoes)
- External factors such as wind resistance, temperature, humidity, and type of surface

The fact that running economy may also be altered by nonmuscular factors is vividly illustrated by experiments with exercising kangaroos (Dawson & Taylor, 1973). When a kangaroo begins to run on a treadmill using all four limbs, oxygen consumption, as expected, begins to rise. But at increasingly high speeds when the animal begins to hop only on hind legs, $\dot{V}O_2$ starts to *decrease*. This occurs presumably as energy is provided by the elastic recoil force of the kangaroo's large Achilles tendon.

Most of these factors have not been examined in prepubertal subjects, but the six that follow appear to be pertinent to explaining child–adult differences in running economy.

Ratio of Surface Area to Mass

This discussion has focused on improvements in running economy during childhood, but it is important to realize that children are less economical metabolically at *rest* as well. Basal metabolic rate related to body mass is maximal in early childhood and declines thereafter (Figure 4.10). In terms of oxygen uptake, the differences between a resting 10-year-old boy and a resting middle-aged man are small, usually no greater than 1 to 2 ml • kg^{-1} min^{-1}, but this amounts to an almost 25 to 35 percent greater metabolic rate in the child (MacDougall, Roche, Bar-Or, & Moroz, 1979). An understanding of the reasons behind this difference might have important bearing on explaining variations in economy with exercise.

Investigation of the metabolic activities of animals has provided insight into these child–adult differences (Schmidt-Nielsen, 1984). Since the mid-1800s biologists have recognized that smaller animals exhibit greater resting metabolic rates per unit body mass than larger animals (Figure 4.11). Much effort has since been expended searching for a way to match energy turnover among animals of varying size. The *surface law* states that the metabolic rates of animals of different size can be made similar when related to body surface area.

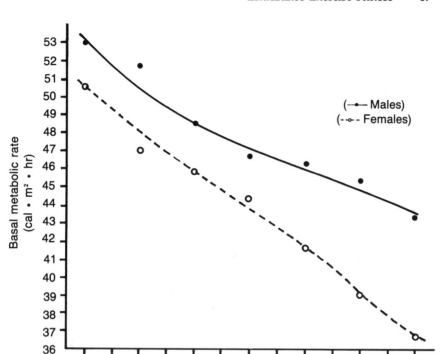

Figure 4.10 Changes in basal metabolic rate with age. *Note.* Data from Knoebel (1963).

Among the explanations offered for these metabolic differences among animals, the requirements for homeothermy appear to have the greatest validity. Warm-blooded animals maintain a constant body temperature by generating heat to match that lost through surface-related mechanisms (e.g., cutaneous vasodilatation and sweating). Energy production is therefore related to body surface area as a means for survival. Smaller animals (such as children) have a greater surface area:mass ratio and subsequently generate more energy per kilogram than large animals.

With exercise, metabolic processes geared to surface area might be expected to signal a need for greater $\dot{V}O_2$/kg in those with a higher surface area:body mass ratio. For smaller animals, a survival mechanism at rest then becomes an encumbrance with exercise, because physical activity calls for movement of body mass, not surface area.

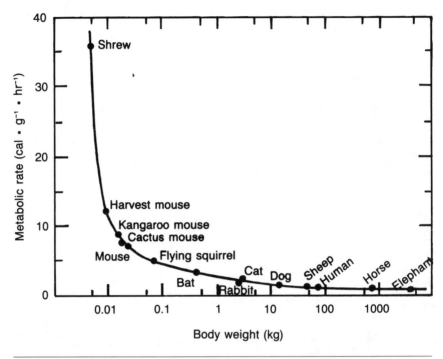

Figure 4.11 Smaller animals have a higher resting metabolic rate per kilogram body mass than larger animals. *Note.* Reprinted by permission from *Muscles, Reflexes, and Locomotion* (p. 281) by T.A. McMahon, 1984, Princeton, NJ: Princeton University Press. Copyright 1984 by T.A. McMahon, which was adapted from "Energy Metabolism, Body Size, and Problems of Scaling" by K. Schmidt-Nielsen, 1970, *Federation Proceedings, 29*, p. 1528.

It has also been suggested that body organs that are associated by size to body surface area will be relatively larger and consume more oxygen per kilogram of body weight in smaller animals. During growth, some of the organs with high rates of energy turnover (e.g., kidney, brain, and liver) do in fact decrease in size relative to body weight (Stahl, 1965). The extent of this decline is not sufficient, however, to explain the fall of weight-related metabolism (Schmidt-Nielsen, 1984).

The question of whether the metabolic rate of isolated tissues of children (and other small animals) is increased compared to larger individuals is not fully resolved (Kleiber, 1961). Early studies of tissue slices in animals indicated no differences in metabolic function *in vivo*. These findings suggested that the overall body metabolic rate is governed by a central factor that is operative only in the intact organism. More recently, rates of oxygen consumption for tissue slices in animals of different sizes have been shown to correlate well with body weight (Krebs, 1950). At the cellular level, mitochondrial density, cytochrome C content, and cytochrome oxidase activity have been demonstrated to relate closely with metabolic rate per kilogram across a broad range of animal sizes (Schmidt-Nielsen, 1984). These reports support the opposite notion; that is, the metabolic rates of different tissues vary with body size and in combination account for variations in total body metabolism.

Not surprisingly, there is little information surrounding this issue in children. Needle biopsy specimens of vastus lateralis muscle in 6-year-old youngsters have demonstrated a slightly higher mitochondrial density than in untrained adults 19 to 45 years old (Bell et al., 1980). Other reports, however, do not show increased biochemical markers of cellular aerobic metabolism in prepubertal subjects. No significant differences in succinate-dehydrogenase activity were observed in the muscle biopsy specimens of 11-year-old boys and adults reported by Eriksson (1980). Eriksson and Saltin (1974) showed increasing concentrations of creatine kinase with age in muscle biopsies of subjects 11 to 16 years old, and Webber, Byrnes, Rowland, and Foster (1988) elicited lower serum creatine kinase levels after downhill running in children than in college students.

Differences in body size do not totally explain the contrasts in metabolic rate between rats and elephants or between children and adults. Basal metabolic rate (BMR) in humans shows a persistent decline with age, most precipitously during the childhood years, even when related to body surface area, body weight, or (weight)$^{3/4}$ (Kleiber, 1961). These differences in metabolic rate independent of size have traditionally been attributed to anabolic activities associated with growth (Knoebel, 1963).

Stride Frequency

The higher metabolic rate at a given treadmill speed in children has often been attributed to children's obligatory greater stride frequency. This makes sense, because the oxygen cost of running is created by the muscle tension generated in repeatedly braking and accelerating the body's center of mass (McMahon, 1984).

Rowland, Auchinachie, Keenan, and Green (1987) studied stride length and frequency in boys and young adult males during a progressive submaximal treadmill test. The mean stride frequency of the prepubertal subjects remained approximately 90 per minute compared to 75 per minute in the adults, across a speed range of 4.5 to 6.5 mph. When oxygen consumption per stride was calculated at the various speeds, no significant differences were observed between the boys and the men (Table 4.2), implying that the increased stride frequency in the younger subjects was largely responsible for their inferior running economy.

In that study no correlation was observed between the stride length:frequency ratio and running economy within either child or adult groups. Assuming that homogeneity of performance capacity may have obscured such a relationship, Rowland and Green (1988) added the findings obtained with more athletic children to the prepubertal group. A significant

Table 4.2 Mean Oxygen Cost Per Stride in Boys and Men

Treadmill speed (mph)	Minute stride frequency		$\dot{V}O_2$ (ml • kg⁻¹min⁻¹)		$\dot{V}O_2$/kg per step	
	Boys	Men	Boys	Men	Boys	Men
5.0	90	74	43.0	34.0	.48	.46
5.5	90	75	46.0	38.0	.51	.51
6.0	91	75	49.5	39.9	.54	.53

Note. Data from Rowland, Auchinachie, Keenan, & Green (1987).

correlation was then observed in the pediatric subjects between stride frequency at 6 mph and economy defined as the $\dot{V}O_2$ cost of increasing treadmill speed by 1 mph (Rowland, Auchinachie, Keenan, & Green, 1988).

The differences in submaximal running economy observed between children and adults are also observed in animals of varying sizes (Figure 4.12). When 50 species were studied, from pygmy mice to horses, it became clear that the oxygen cost of running per kilogram body weight is greater in smaller animals at all speeds (McMahon, 1984). Schmidt-Nielsen (1984) pointed out that the metabolic cost of running is assumedly influenced by evolutionary forces, given that "we can expect animals live as economically as possible. For each animal the economy of moving about is as economical as its body size permits. The small animal must take more steps to move a given distance, and this costs more. If we related the cost of locomotion to one step we find animals to be equally economical, whether large or small" (p. 170).

If the dissimilarities in submaximal running economy between children and adults are related primarily to stride frequency, these differences should disappear during cycle exercise testing. They appear to. Work during submaximal cycle exercise is generally considered weight-independent (Adams, 1967); that is, the work load is created by the resistance provided by the cycle apparatus rather than by the movement of body mass. Submaximal $\dot{V}O_2$ during cycle testing can therefore be expressed in absolute terms rather than related to body weight for interindividual comparisons. Given small differences due to discrepancies in resting $\dot{V}O_2$, pedaling rate consistency, and relative work intensities, the absolute energy expenditure of children and adults is similar during submaximal cycle testing (Bentgsson, 1956; Girandola, Wiswell, Frisch, & Wood, 1981; Klausen, Rasmussen, Glensgaard, & Jensen, 1985).

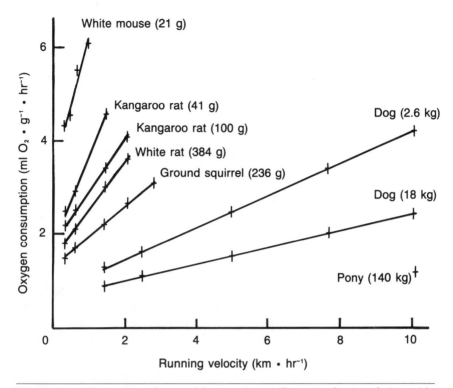

White mouse (21 g)

Kangaroo rat (41 g)

Dog (2.6 kg)

Kangaroo rat (100 g)

White rat (384 g)

Ground squirrel (236 g)

Dog (18 kg)

Pony (140 kg)

Oxygen consumption (ml O₂ • g⁻¹ • hr⁻¹)

Running velocity (km • hr⁻¹)

Figure 4.12 Oxygen uptake per kilogram in smaller animals rises faster with exercise than in large animals. *Note.* From "Scaling of Energetic Cost of Running to Body Size in Mammals" by C.R. Taylor, K. Schmidt-Nielsen, and J.L. Raab, 1970, *American Journal of Physiology*, **218**, p. 1105. Copyright 1970 by the American Physiological Society. Reprinted by permission.

The higher stride frequency of the child does appear to be important in increasing submaximal $\dot{V}O_2$ requirements during running. It should be pointed out, though, that purposefully lengthening a child's stride to decrease frequency and improve economy will be not only fruitless but also counterproductive. The natural stride length at a given speed is "selected" as the most economical, and either lengthening or shortening stride length will increase energy expenditure (Hogberg, 1952).

Immature Running Mechanics

The running styles of children differ from those of adults, progressing in a predictable sequence throughout the growing years (Wickstrom, 1983). Features typical of childhood running gait include greater vertical movement with each stride; increased hip, knee, and ankle extension at takeoff; increased time in the nonsupport phase of the stride; and decrease in the relative distance of the support foot ahead of the body's center of gravity at contact. Surprisingly high peak vertical ground forces have been described in 2- to 6-year-old children running at maximal speeds (Fortney, 1983). Cavagna, Franzetti, and Fuchimoto (1983) reported that for a 2-year-old child the muscle power per kilogram necessary to move the center of mass at a walking speed of 4.5 km/hr was more than twice that for an adult.

How much these age-related changes in running mechanics contribute to differences in submaximal economy between children and adults is unknown. Efforts to correlate running patterns in adults with submaximal oxygen requirements generally have not proven successful. In fact, these biomechanical studies have shown no clear-cut economy advantages to any particular running style (Williams, 1985).

Speed–Mass Mismatch

The speed at which a muscle contracts is inversely related to the force generated (Hill, 1939), and a proper balance between these two factors is important in the optimal conversion of energy into mechanical work (Wilkie, 1950). Davies (1980) suggested that this principle might help explain child–adult differences in running economy. In his study of 12-year-old boys and girls, greater $\dot{V}O_2$/kg values were—as expected—demonstrated at all treadmill speeds compared to those previously reported in adults. The children then ran the same protocol wearing weighted jackets equivalent to 5 to 10 percent of body weight. Oxygen cost per kilogram decreased, particularly at high running speeds, and economy values approached those of adults. Davies concluded that the light body weights of children may not be optimally matched with their obligatory faster leg movements during running compared with older subjects. He cautioned, though, that external loading of children may improve submaximal running economy but should not be expected to improve exercise performance.

In addition, Davies noted that the running economy of lightweight men is not significantly different from that of heavy men, and that light adult females are not less economical than men (Davies & Thompson, 1979). Further, studies of adult animals (running at relatively slower speeds) indicate that submaximal oxygen consumption *rises* in direct proportion to weight loading (Taylor, Heglund, McMahon, & Looney, 1980).

Differences in Anaerobic Energy

The oxygen supply to exercising muscle determines the extent of aerobic metabolic energy available for contraction. During the course of a progressive exercise test the limits of oxygen delivery are exceeded, and additional muscular work can be performed only by energy derived from anaerobic, or glycolytic, metabolism. The energy derived from these pathways is 1/13 that of aerobic metabolism, so fatigue rapidly sets in once the limits of oxygen delivery are met. It is difficult to quantitate the glycolytic contribution to high-intensity exercise because there are no good methods for measuring anaerobic energy yield (Åstrand & Rodahl, 1977).

Abundant evidence exists that children are unable to generate anaerobic energy as effectively as adults (see p. 80). The impact of these differences on endurance performance is unclear. It should be realized, however, that when submaximal running economy is measured as $\dot{V}O_2$ consumed at a given slope and speed, only the aerobic energy contribution is considered. Whether the anaerobic input is large enough to help account for child–adult differences in running economy (particularly at high work intensities) is uncertain. As treadmill speed increases, children do become progressively less economical than adults, while the older subjects demonstrate higher muscle lactate concentrations (and presumably greater anaerobic energy yield) (Eriksson, Karlsson, & Saltin, 1971). When the $\dot{V}O_2$ values of children and adults are compared at a given treadmill speed and slope, it is thus important that the two groups be exercising at similar intensities ($\dot{V}O_2$ as percent $\dot{V}O_2$max) to help minimize differences in anaerobic energy contribution.

Less Efficient Ventilation

Children need to ventilate more than adults for each liter of oxygen consumed, at all levels of exercise (Åstrand, 1952; Rowland, Auchinachie, Keenan, & Green, 1987). Why prepubertal subjects have a greater $\dot{V}_E/\dot{V}O_2$ (ventilatory equivalent for oxygen) is unclear. Children take relatively shallower, more rapid respirations than adults, which may result in larger dead-space ventilation (Cotes, 1979). Children also appear to hyperventilate during exercise compared to adults, with arterial pCO_2 values significantly lower in younger subjects (Bar-Or, 1983). This hyperventilation in children may be a manifestation of increased ventilatory responses to CO_2 production (Cooper et al., 1987). Differences in ventilatory equivalent for oxygen between children and adults relative to submaximal economy may be significant in considerations of exercise economy because at maximal work loads the oxygen cost of ventilation may reach 14 to 19 percent of total body $\dot{V}O_2$ (Pardy, Hussain, & MacKlem, 1984).

In summary, multiple factors may account for improvements in endurance-exercise capacity with growth. Despite the failure of $\dot{V}O_2$max/kg to rise, evidence does suggest that qualitative changes occur in oxygen delivery mechanisms. Running economy improves with age, permitting more exercise work to be done at equal intensity (percent $\dot{V}O_2$max) as the child grows. A progressive decrease in stride frequency at equal speeds and decline in surface area:mass ratio appear to contribute to the improvements observed in economy during childhood.

AEROBIC EXERCISE TRAINING IN CHILDREN

In adults, a regular endurance exercise program of sufficient intensity, frequency, and duration will produce a 6 to 25 percent improvement in $\dot{V}O_2$max as well as other cardiovascular adaptations collectively termed the "fitness effect." This includes lowered resting and submaximal heart rate as well as increased submaximal and maximal stroke volume. The ability to enhance peak stroke volume accounts for a greater maximal cardiac output observed following training, because few changes occur in maximal heart rate. Improved peak cardiac output is in turn responsible, along with increased peripheral oxygen extraction, for the rise in $\dot{V}O_2$max.

In the past, considerable doubt was cast on the ability of children to improve maximal aerobic power with physical training before puberty (Bar-Or, 1983; Katch, 1983). This has been explained as due to the inherently greater habitual activity levels of children, which place them closer to their maximal $\dot{V}O_2$ potential (Hamilton & Andrew, 1976). Studies indicating that children do not sustain high-intensity exercise for periods of time sufficient to improve fitness (by adult criteria) weaken this argument. Gilliam et al. (1981), for instance, showed that 6- to 7-year-old boys and girls produced heart rates over 160 bpm for 21 and 9 min per day, respectively, and these higher rates typically came in intermittent bursts. Extrapolation of adult standards suggests that sustained exercise to a heart rate of 160 to 170 bpm for 15 to 60 min at least three times a week would be necessary to increase $\dot{V}O_2$max in prepubertal subjects (American College of Sports Medicine, 1978).

Cross-Sectional Studies

Cross-sectional studies indicate that elite prepubertal athletes have superior cardiovascular function and higher $\dot{V}O_2$max values than their untrained peers. This, of course, does not answer the question of whether this greater aerobic fitness is a result of athletic training or whether their success in sports is due to an exceptional inherent cardiovascular capacity. Typical of these studies is the report by Mayers and Gutin (1979) of exercise testing in elite prepubertal cross-country runners. These highly-trained boys had a $\dot{V}O_2$max of 56.6 ml • kg^{-1} min^{-1} compared to an untrained control group with a $\dot{V}O_2$max of 46.0 ml • kg^{-1} min^{-1} The runners also demonstrated superior submaximal running economy, lower submaximal heart rates, and better anaerobic capacity.

Longitudinal Studies

Longitudinal studies examining the $\dot{V}O_2$max responses to exercise training in children have been extensively reviewed (Krahenbuhl et al., 1985; Sady, 1986; Vaccaro & Mahon, 1987). Whether children can truly improve aerobic capacity with training cannot easily be decided from these reports, because the results are conflicting. When only those that satisfy the training criteria for achievement of improved aerobic power in adults are considered, however, the picture is perhaps clearer (Vaccaro & Mahon, 1987). Rowland (1985) noted that none of five training studies of children that failed to show improved $\dot{V}O_2$max satisfied regimens expected to improve aerobic fitness in adults. In most of these cases, exercise was overly short and intense (short-distance interval running or high-intensity, brief, bicycle exercise). Nine other training studies appeared to follow adult fitness criteria (continuous activity of large muscle groups, 3 to 5 sessions per week for 15 to 60 min, at an intensity producing a heart rate 60 to 90 percent of maximum). Of these, six showed a rise in aerobic power after training, with a range of 7 to 26 percent, consistent with that observed in adult studies. Although this analysis appeared to indicate adult–child similarities in response to aerobic training, the author noted that these studies were marked by methodological flaws that tempered such a conclusion (small subject numbers, absence of controls, nonrepresentative samples, failure to document exercise intensity, and variable pretraining fitness).

Training Guidelines

These data appear to indicate that adult standards for improving $\dot{V}O_2$max with training are also applicable to children. Beyond this, few guidelines are available. Presumably if children are capable of improving $\dot{V}O_2$max, the training criteria differ according to factors such as age and previous level of physical activity. Massicotte and MacNab (1974) trained three groups of 11- to 13-year-old boys with cycle exercise at different heart rates over a 6-week period. Significant improvement in $\dot{V}O_2$max (11 percent) was observed in subjects cycling at a target heart rate of 170 to 180 bpm but not in those training at rates of 150 to 160 and 130 to 140 bpm. All three groups demonstrated decreases in submaximal heart rates following training, however.

The heart rate at anaerobic threshold (HR-AT) has been utilized as a target for endurance fitness training programs in adults, because this intensity presumably reflects a marker of stress on oxygen delivery systems (Dwyer & Bybee, 1983). In children, HR-AT has been reported between 165 to 170 bpm, which represents approximately 85 percent of maximal heart rate (Rowland & Green, 1989; Washington, van Gundy, Cohen, Sondheimer, & Wolfe, 1988). Attempts to utilize these rates as targets for aerobic training for children may be inappropriate, however, because of the wide range of AT-HR values (135 to 197 bpm).

Training Responses

Given the pitfalls of using $\dot{V}O_2$max/kg as an indicator of endurance fitness or cardiovascular capacity in children, it may be more instructional to examine the response of components of oxygen delivery to training in prepubertal subjects. The information here, however, is meager. Lowered submaximal heart rates in children following physical training has been reported in several studies (Vaccaro & Mahon, 1987). Only one study has examined maximal cardiac output changes with training. Eriksson (1972) showed an increase in maximal stroke volume from 67 to 80 ml and cardiac output from 12.5 to 14.6 L • min⁻¹ after 16 weeks of running and skiing training in 12-year-old boys. Rost (1987) described $\dot{V}O_2$max, radiologic measurement of heart volume, and echocardiographic findings in 8- to 10-year-old children engaged in competitive swimming training. In determinations 1 year apart, the swimmers showed a greater increase in $\dot{V}O_2$max and heart volume than did nonathletic controls. Small changes in left-ventricular end-diastolic dimensions were similar, however.

Eriksson, Gollnick, and Saltin (1973) studied the effects of exercise training on aerobic and anaerobic enzymes of 11- to 13-year-old boys with biopsies of vastus lateralis muscle. The concentrations of glycogen, creatine phosphate, and adenosine triphosphate (ATP) were greater at rest after a 4-month training program. Blood and muscle lactate levels rose 23 and 56 percent higher during maximal exercise testing after the training. In a second experiment, succinate dehydrogenase and phosphofructokinase activities were 30 and 83 percent greater, respectively, after a 6-week cycle training program.

Most authors now agree that given an appropriate exercise training stimulus, $\dot{V}O_2$max can be improved in children, and that increases in aerobic capacity can be most expected in subjects with lower pretraining fitness levels (Krahenbuhl et al., 1985; Shephard, 1982). Some studies have suggested that the training effect is greatest during the pubertal growth spurt (Kobayashi et al., 1978; Mirwald & Bailey, 1981). Other reports have failed to support these findings (Cunningham, Paterson, & Blimkie, 1984), and the concept of a critical period for enhancing cardiovascular function through exercise training remains controversial.

SEX DIFFERENCES IN ENDURANCE FITNESS

It is as difficult to compare endurance fitness between males and females as it is between adults and children: Such a large overlap exists between the sexes that there are more similarities than differences, and very few individuals possess characteristics of the "average" male or female. These considerations create major problems in selecting groups for comparative studies (Wells, 1985). One can conclude, however, that significant differences in *average* physiological and performance markers exist between the sexes, with males scoring higher in aerobic power and fitness tests based predominantly on their larger cardiopulmonary capacity and muscle mass. These trends are most prominent after puberty but in most cases are still visible during childhood as well. Although the physiological differences between boys and girls are small, the performance gap is often wider. Some have thereby concluded that females are less likely to fulfill their full potential for exercise fitness compared to males as a result largely of social rather than biological constraints (Raithel, 1987). For physicians who are promoting exercise during childhood for long-term health benefits, this gender gap has significant implications.

By almost any means of measuring endurance fitness, boys perform better than girls at all ages. The average 10-year-old boy can run a mile 2 min faster than a girl the same age (American Alliance for Health, Physical Education, Recreation and Dance, 1980). Treadmill endurance time on walking or running protocols is typically 10 to 20 percent longer in prepubertal males than in females (Cumming et al., 1978; Riopel, Taylor, & Hohn, 1979). However, Washington et al. (1988) could demonstrate no significant differences by gender in maximal work on progressive cycle ergometry testing of children aged 6 to 15 years. In a study better evaluating true endurance, Åstrand (1952) determined the maximal speed a subject could maintain for 5 min running on a treadmill. At most prepubertal ages, the boys exceeded the girls by only small speeds (i.e., 13.8 vs. 13.5 km/hr at ages 7 to 9 years).

Determinants of Sex Differences

Sex-related performance discrepancies stem at least partially from physiological differences that persist throughout childhood and become exaggerated at puberty. Even as boys, males have a lower percent body fat and greater relative muscle mass. Boys have relatively larger hearts on X rays, a corollary to their larger submaximal stroke volume and lower heart rates compared to girls (Shephard et al., 1969). In most studies maximal heart rates also tend to be slightly lower in males (Cumming et al., 1978; Riopel et al., 1979; Washington et al., 1988). Peak respiratory exchange ratio and lactate levels do not typically vary by sex, however (Åstrand, 1952; Shephard, 1982). Boys achieve greater maximal ventilation than girls, but ventilatory efficiency ($\dot{V}_E/\dot{V}O_2$) is similar. Blood volume, hemoglobin concentration, and amount of hemoglobin per body weight are essentially equal between the sexes before puberty. Thereafter, hemoglobin values are significantly greater in males (Åstrand, 1952).

The combined effects of these differences are manifest in $\dot{V}O_2$max levels (Bar-Or, 1983; Krahenbuhl et al., 1985). Until puberty absolute $\dot{V}O_2$max increases with age at the same rate in boys and girls, but mean values in males are always higher. Surrounding pubertal development $\dot{V}O_2$max accelerates in males as they gain in muscle mass; $\dot{V}O_2$max values plateau in females, who do not share this increased muscle bulk but gain body fat instead. When expressed per kilogram of body weight, $\dot{V}O_2$max remains stable in boys throughout the childhood and adolescent years but tends to decrease in earlier years in girls. Submaximal running economy is similar in prepubertal males and females (Åstrand, 1952), but in older age groups the data is conflicting (Wells, 1985). Girls appear to respond to an aerobic training stimulus as well as boys (Rowland, 1985).

Explanations for prepubertal male–female physiological differences have focused largely on body composition. Bar-Or (1983) concluded that sex differences in maximal aerobic power could be explained largely by the fact that $\dot{V}O_2$max is closely related to lean body mass, which is greater in males. Davies, Barnes, and Godfrey (1972) showed that $\dot{V}O_2$max differences between boys and girls during cycle testing disappeared when $\dot{V}O_2$ was related to leg volume. After puberty, too, little sex difference in $\dot{V}O_2$max is observed when expressed relative to lean body mass. As Wells (1985) points out, however, the explanation is academic; the female runner still has to carry the extra load of body fat and is thereby encumbered compared to the male.

Habitual Activity

Could females' lower habitual activity levels be limiting their endurance fitness? As pointed out earlier, virtually every pediatric study of routine physical activity has shown greater movement in boys. In their mega-analysis of sex differences in activity levels, Eaton and Enns (1986) reported that males scored higher even before the age of 1 year; the implications of this finding are unclear, they noted, because although "it lends credibility to the contention that [activity level] has congenital or genetic origins, . . . a complete disentangling of social influences from the child's endogenous characteristics is impossible even in the first postnatal days" (p. 20).

At later ages participation in sports continues to be dominated by males despite dramatic increases in the number of female athletes in the last decade. The number of women's sports being offered in United States high schools increased from 14 in 1971 to 33 in 1985. Over the same period, the number of participants increased from 293,345 to 1,757,884, with 1 of every 4.5 girls in the age group 14 to 17 years involved. This number is still only one half that of males. There is significant geographic variability to this participation: Iowa has nearly 8 times more female athletes per capita than Alabama or Mississippi (Ojala, 1987).

Just why girls should be less physically active and hold back from sport participation has sparked considerable discussion and concern. Limited opportunities for females continues to be an issue, as does the lack of appropriate role models (e.g., female coaches and officials). Girls' lack of interest in sport participation may be fueled by peer conduct (Eaton & Enns, 1986), and psychological barriers (such as sex role identity and perceived incompetence) may be critical in inhibiting females from physical activity.

GENETIC DETERMINANTS
OF PHYSICAL FITNESS

The current best advice to an individual wishing to become an elite marathon runner is to choose his or her parents carefully. Virtually all the factors affecting endurance performance are strongly influenced by genetic determinants, including not only anatomical, biochemical, and physiological components, but also psychological qualities such as competitiveness and motivation (Cowart, 1987).

Early studies of twins suggested that up to 90 percent of aerobic capacity is fixed by heredity (Klissouras, 1971). Although subsequent studies have tempered this estimate, current data indicate that the contribution of the genetic effect on $\dot{V}O_2$max is approximately 50 percent and for endurance performance up to 70 percent (Bouchard, 1986). Equally important, one's capacity for increasing $\dot{V}O_2$max with physical training is genetically influenced by a similar amount. An individual may then be a "high responder" or "low responder" to fitness training based on genetic endowment (Hamel, Simoneau, Lortie, Boulay, & Bouchard, 1986). The genetic contribution to the elite endurance athlete is therefore twofold: a high level of baseline aerobic fitness plus the inherent capacity to respond optimally to exercise training.

This prominent role of inheritance in influencing endurance capacity and response to training has several implications for the assessment of children's fitness. Although those with greater genetic fitness endowment might be expected to exercise more, this is not necessarily so. As a result, the amount of individual daily physical activity within a group of children might not correlate with results of fitness testing. Also, children who are genetically "low responders" might experience very limited improvements in endurance fitness with training compared to "high responders." Considering this genetic variability, the use of "untrained controls" in studies assessing the effect of physical training on children is open to question.

Any cross-sectional study of children that tests endurance exercise capacity is largely influenced by the genetic makeup of the group. The relative roles of habitual activity and heredity in determining the physiological, biochemical, anthropometric, and psychological contributions to exercise performance in children, and how these are influenced by biological maturation and training, remain to be clarified.

ANAEROBIC CAPACITY IN CHILDREN

Anaerobic metabolism (glycolysis) becomes important whenever oxygen delivery is inadequate to meet the energy needs of exercising muscle. This occurs in vigorous exercise of short duration (e.g., a 200-m run), briefly at the onset of longer exercise before muscle perfusion becomes established, and during endurance exercise when intensity exceeds 50 to 70 percent of $\dot{V}O_2$max. Anaerobic capacity is not typically associated with endurance fitness in adults, but, as alluded to several times earlier, the ability to draw on glycolytic pathways for energy may contribute to adult–child performance differences. Prepubertal subjects demonstrate increasing anaerobic capacity as they grow, paralleling improvement in speed, strength, and endurance capabilities. Just how much gains in energy from anaerobic sources contribute to these performance changes is unknown. Evidence for the development of anaerobic capacity with growth comes from several sources.

Lactate Production

The measurement of anaerobic metabolism during exercise is difficult, and only indirect means are available to determine glycolytic contributions. Because lactic acid is a by-product of anaerobic metabolism, the serum lactate level has been taken to be an indicator of glycolytic energy input. The pitfalls of this assumption are troublesome: Serum lactate levels may not reflect intramuscular anaerobic rate, and the blood level is a representation of the balance of production, metabolism, and elimination of lactate rather than simply a marker of intracellular anaerobic metabolism (Wasserman, Beaver, & Whipp, 1985).

These problems notwithstanding, prepubertal children demonstrate lower serum lactate levels than older subjects at all levels of exercise. Åstrand (1952) demonstrated a progressive increase in maximal blood lactate concentration throughout the childhood years, with a mean value in boys of 56 mg percent at age 6 years and 104 mg percent at age 17. Levels were similar in girls. Comparable trends have been reported by other authors (Máček & Vávra, 1985; Morse, Schultz, & Cassels, 1949; Robinson, 1938).

As Åstrand (1952) pointed out, these findings do not necessarily indicate an impaired anaerobic capacity. Children show a greater acceleration of oxygen uptake at the onset of exercise, almost twice the rate of adults (Máček, Vávra, Benesova, & Radvansky, 1984; Robinson, 1938).

This might result in lower initial lactate levels in prepubertal subjects but probably not during prolonged exercise (Máček, 1986). Máček (1986) suggested that the metabolic clearance of lactate might be greater in children. Sympathetic activity during maximal exercise is less in prepubertal subjects than in adults. Subsequently, lessened hepatic vasoconstriction in children might, for instance, allow more rapid liver metabolism of lactate.

Anaerobic Exercise Testing

Children perform less well on exercise tasks designed to measure anaerobic capacity. Results of the Margaria test, which records speed of ascending steps, and the Wingate test, which measures power output in a 30-sec all-out cycling bout, indicate that performance improves during the growing years (Bar-Or, 1983; diPrampero & Cerretelli, 1969; Inbar & Bar-Or, 1986). This improvement persists when related to body weight, implying that test results are not simply related to increased muscle mass.

Anaerobic Threshold

Although serum lactate accumulates from the early stages of a progressive exercise test, most individuals show accelerated lactate levels at an intensity of 50 to 70 percent of $\dot{V}O_2$max. Whether this anaerobic threshold truly reflects the point of aerobic starvation of muscles is controversial, but many have accepted this value as an indicator of aerobic capability. That is, the higher the anaerobic threshold, the greater the intensity or speed at which an individual can exercise with the benefit of aerobically derived energy. There is a second alternative interpretation. A high anaerobic threshold might indicate an inferior *ability* to generate energy anaerobically. Expressing the anaerobic threshold as a percentage of $\dot{V}O_2$max may be a better means of indicating this capacity (Weymans, Reybrouck, Stijns, & Knops, 1985).

Anaerobic threshold expressed as a percentage of $\dot{V}O_2$max decreases with age during childhood, consistent with the concept that anaerobic capacity improves with biological maturation (Paterson, McLellan, Stella, & Cunningham, 1987). Typically prepubertal children have values of approximately 65 percent, whereas the anaerobic threshold in older adolescents is 5 to 10 percent less. Girls have lower absolute anaerobic threshold levels than boys at the same age, but no sex differences are observed when threshold is expressed as a percentage of $\dot{V}O_2$max (Weymans et al., 1985).

Glycolytic Enzymes

Little is known about the biochemical basis for the apparent inferior anaerobic capacity in children. Activity of phosphofructokinase (PFK), a rate-limiting glycolytic enzyme, was one third of adult values in vastus lateralis muscle biopsies of 11- to 13-year-old boys (Eriksson et al., 1973).

Exercise training can improve anaerobic capacity in children. Eriksson (1972) reported increases in blood and muscle lactate levels after a 4-month training program in 11- to 13-year-old boys, and the muscle PFK activity increased 83 percent after 6 weeks of cycle training in the subjects studied by Eriksson et al. (1973). Rotstein, Dotan, Bar-Or, and Tenenbaum (1986) evaluated the effect of a 9-week training program of high-intensity exercise on 10- to 11-year-old boys. Anaerobic capacity improved 14 percent on the Wingate test, and $\dot{V}O_2max/kg$ increased 8 percent. Relative anaerobic threshold (percent $\dot{V}O_2max$) fell 4.4 percent. This decline may have reflected enhanced capability for anaerobic metabolism. In adults endurance training causes an *increase* in the anaerobic threshold expressed as percent $\dot{V}O_2max$, indicative of improved aerobic function (Ready & Quinney, 1982). Children undergoing a similar training program may show the same effect. Becker & Vaccaro (1983) demonstrated an increase in relative anaerobic threshold from 67 to 71 percent of $\dot{V}O_2max$ after 8 weeks of regular cycle exercise, 3 days a week for 40 min each session.

This combined evidence indicates that children are impaired in their ability to generate anaerobically derived energy, and that the effectiveness of glycolytic metabolic pathways increases with both age and training. These findings may help explain the improvements observed in both sprint and endurance exercise events during growth.

FUTURE DIRECTIONS

As children grow, the many factors determining endurance fitness develop in a progressive, predictable fashion. The curves describing these changes follow not only physical growth but functional maturation as well. Physicians are used to such developmental curves, routinely using them to follow the course of height, weight, head circumference, and neuromuscular development in children, knowing that disease states disrupt normal developmental patterns and cause these curves to deviate from expected norms. Could not the same means be used to create charts for a "cardiovascular developmental age" determined by exercise testing? Normal percentile grids for parameters such as submaximal heart rate, running economy, and $\dot{V}_E/\dot{V}O_2$ might be established for children during the growing years; factors like hypoactivity, obesity, anemia, and cardiac or pulmonary disease could then be expected to alter the curve of an individual compared to that established by age-related population norms. Such grids were created for endurance-run performances of 27,000 South African school children 50 years ago (see Jokl, 1978), a forerunner of today's mass fitness testing in youth. Grids for submaximal physiological parameters that do not rely on motivation might be created in the same way.

Before such charts are feasible, a great deal more information is necessary regarding the growth of physiological exercise parameters in children. Do they in fact "track" with chronological age (that is, remain at a similar percentile relative to the general pediatric population), or do the variabilities in onset and rate of physiological change prohibit the use of percentile grids for serial measurements? Does the level of habitual activity truly affect normal physiological growth? What are the triggers and controlling factors that determine the growth of exercise physiological function?

Another aspect of exercise fitness in children bearing further investigation is the intriguing set of similarities between the changes due to normal physiological growth and those observed following physical training (the "fitness effect") (Wells, 1986a). These are outlined in Table 4.3. Are these similar outcomes by different mechanisms? Or do we have an opportunity to decipher the mysteries of improved exercise performance at all ages by understanding the maturational changes that occur in exercise physiology during childhood?

Table 4.3 Comparisons of Physiological Responses to Exercise Occurring With Growth During Childhood and After Physical Training in Adults

Physiological characteristic	Response to growth	Response to training
Submaximal heart rate	Decrease	Decrease
Maximal heart rate	No change	No change
Submaximal stroke index	Increase	Increase
Maximal cardiac index	Increase	Increase
Submaximal $\dot{V}_E/\dot{V}O_2$	Decrease	No change or decrease
Running economy	Increase	No change or increase
Submaximal respiratory rate:tidal volume	Decrease	Decrease
Maximal $\dot{V}_E$/kg	No change	Increase
Maximal $\dot{V}O_2$/kg	No change	Increase
Hemoglobin mass	Increase	Increase
Maximal serum lactate	Increase	Increase
Anaerobic capacity	Increase	Increase

SUMMARY

This chapter investigated the ways age and sex-related and genetic factors affect endurance exercise fitness and how aerobic and anaerobic capacity in children contribute to endurance fitness.

- Performance abilities in endurance sports events steadily improve during childhood, but the physiological factors responsible are not altogether clear. Maximal oxygen uptake per kilogram of body weight does not rise during the growing years, implying that the child's ability to deliver oxygen to exercising muscle is not responsible for changes in endurance performance. However, metabolic scope, or the ratio of maximal to resting oxygen uptake, does increase during childhood. This suggests that there are qualitative improvements in the ability of the growing child to use oxygen during exercise.

  The oxygen-uptake cost of running at a given submaximal work load falls progressively during childhood, indicating improvements in running economy. Enhanced performance in endurance events may be linked to improved economy; at a given running speed the child progressively exercises at a lower relative intensity (percent $\dot{V}O_2$max) as he or she grows.

- Recent studies appear to indicate that children are capable of improving maximal oxygen uptake with physical training, given an adequate training intensity. As with adults, greater responses can be expected in subjects with lower pretraining fitness levels.

- The *average* prepubertal boy has greater levels of endurance fitness than the *average* girl. Lower levels of habitual activity, influences of social expectations, or differences in body composition may be responsible.

- Growing evidence indicates a prominent role of genetic determinants in both endurance exercise capabilities and response to training.

- Anaerobic capacity, which is related to short bursts of activity, improves during childhood, even when related to body weight. Deficient glycolytic enzymes may be involved.

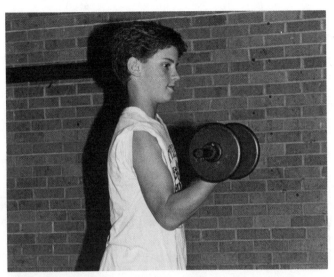

CHAPTER 5

Muscle Strength and Endurance

"Lifting weights" has long held a fascination for many children and adolescents, but until recently resistance exercise has received little support from physiologists, physicians, and physical educators. New information regarding the effectiveness, safety, and health benefits of weight training (also termed "resistance" or "strength" training) in children is now likely to reverse this trend. This chapter examines the current understanding of children's responses to resistance exercise, which can serve as a basis for creating specific weight-training programs for prepubertal subjects (see chapter 13). This chapter reviews the potential advantages gained from weight training in children as well as the risks that may be incurred.

PRINCIPLES OF RESISTANCE EXERCISE

The capacity of muscle to generate high force is associated with several forms of motor performance. *Strength* is a measure of the greatest force that can be produced by a group of muscles. *Muscle endurance* is the ability to contract repeatedly without fatigue, and *muscle power* is the speed at which muscle force can be generated (as in jumping). Activities that are of brief duration and high intensity rely on anaerobic metabolic pathways for energy, either directly from available adenosine triphosphate (ATP) and phosphocreatine in short-burst exercise or from glycolytic metabolism when activities are over 1 to 2 min in duration (Fox, 1984).

Development of Strength in Childhood

Muscle strength is determined principally by the number and cross-sectional area of the muscle fibers involved in a given contraction. Muscle fiber number is largely fixed shortly after birth, but body growth is accompanied by an increase in fiber diameter. As expected, then, strength fitness progresses (at least for boys) throughout childhood (Figure 5.1). Beyond documenting this finding, little attention has been focused on muscle performance in children.

Strength Training

Traditional dogma long held that prepubertal subjects were incapable of increasing muscle strength with resistance training because of the absence of circulating androgens (Vrijens, 1978). Therefore it was believed that there were no health benefits for children from strength training. Recent studies showing significant strength gains in both boys and girls with weight training appear to have dispelled this myth (Servedio et al., 1985; Sewall & Micheli, 1986; Weltman et al., 1986). In addition, these studies indicate that supervised strength programs for children can be conducted safely with little risk and no loss in body flexibility. Based on this information, sound arguments have been made promoting resistance training in youth for enhancing motor performance and preventing injuries (Micheli, 1988b).

Strength Tests

Tests of muscle strength and endurance in large groups of children have usually focused on children's performance with sit-ups, the flexed-arm

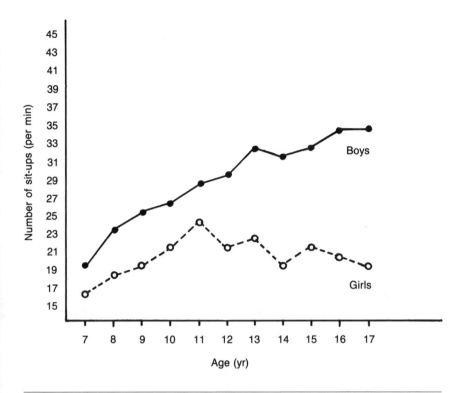

Figure 5.1 Muscular strength and endurance in children as indicated by average number of sit-ups performed in 1 min. *Note.* Data from The CAHPER Fitness Test Manual for Boys and Girls 7 to 17 Years of Age, by F. Hayden and M. Yuhasz, 1965, Toronto: Canadian Association for Physical Health, Education and Recreation.

hang, pull-ups, and jumping ability. More specific techniques for assessing muscle tension include the cable tensiometer (knee extension), handgrip dynamometer, and commercial exercise machines (McArdle et al., 1981). Measurements of isolated muscle groups (such as finger flexors during handgrip testing) may not reflect overall body strength, however, as correlation coefficients may be as low as .4 between different muscle groups. Moreover, these tests rely on subject motivation for valid measurements. Even in well-standardized studies of muscle strength, test–retest standard deviations can be at least 10 percent (Åstrand & Rodahl, 1977).

Sex Differences

As strength improves during growth, males perform better on most test items. A 9-year-old boy, for instance, can complete 20 percent more sit-ups than a girl of the same age (Shephard, 1982). In a pattern reminiscent of aerobic exercise factors, strength performance levels off in females at puberty and does not change appreciably during the adolescent years. Boys continue to accelerate in strength at puberty, associated with increasing muscle mass, and then peak between ages 20 and 30. Average muscle strength for adult men is 50 percent greater than for women of the same age (Åstrand & Rodahl, 1977).

Weight Lifting Versus Weight Training

From the standpoint of the suitability of resistance exercise for children, it is important to distinguish between weight lifting and weight training. *Weight lifting* is a sport in which the contestant seeks to raise the greatest possible weight in a single effort. This activity, defined as a "one-repetition maximum," utilizes free weights and is purely a manifestation of muscle strength. *Weight training*, on the other hand, is performed with a series of submaximal exercises, or "repetitions," against resistances created by free weights, machines, or the body's own weight. The more repetitions, the more likely the training effect will improve muscular endurance; fewer repetitions of higher resistance will have a greater effect on enhancing strength. Weight training is often performed to improve strength and endurance for participation in specific sports. Weight lifting, on the other hand, is itself a competitive sport.

RESISTANCE TRAINING IN ADULTS

Both female and male adults can achieve significant improvements in muscle strength through repetitive exercises of high muscle tension. During resistance training, increased strength of up to 30 to 50 percent can be realized after a 3-month exercise program (Fleck & Kraemer, 1987). This effect is heavily dependent on such factors as the muscle groups exercised, type of resistance, angle and speed of contraction, exercise frequency and intensity, and pattern of motion. In evaluating responses to resistance training it is therefore important to recognize that strength gains may be highly specific to the types of muscle exercises employed in the training regimen.

Resistance exercise can be performed by several means of muscle contraction. In many cases the type of work is defined by the equipment providing the resistance. In *isotonic dynamic exercise*, the muscle shortens against a fixed resistance, typically free weights (barbells) or weight stacks provided by various kinds of exercise equipment. During eccentric exercise the muscle lengthens as it creates tension (as in the work of the thigh muscles while walking downstairs), whereas concentric exercise involves shortening muscles. *Isometric exercise* is typified by highly intense muscle contractions against an unmovable resistance (as in pushing against a wall). *Variable resistance* equipment changes the resistance to match alterations of maximal forces in the range of motion about a joint. *Isokinetic exercise* is provided by equipment that provides a constant velocity throughout the range of motion.

Each of these forms of exercise has its advocates and purported advantages for strength training. Isotonic exercise has been particularly well established as a means of improving performance (in, e.g., the vertical and long jump, shuttle run, short sprint, and shot put) as well as strength. Eccentric training may lead to greater strength improvement because muscle tension is greater than with isometric or isotonic exercises. Eccentric contraction produces more postexercise muscle soreness, however. Proponents of isokinetic exercise note the safety advantages compared to use of free weights, which require balancing skills (Osternig, 1986).

Specificity of Results

It is difficult to compare the different techniques for production of strength and performance gains, because the effects may be highly method-specific. As noted by Fleck and Kraemer (1987), "When training and testing are performed using the same type of resistive equipment, a large increase in strength is demonstrated. If training and testing are performed on two different types of equipment, however, the increase in strength is substantially less, and sometimes nonexistent" (p. 39). As an important principle, then, resistance training for sport participation needs to be designed to mimic the muscle motion patterns employed in the particular athletic activity the individual is training for.

Weight Training and Hypertrophy

Weight training has traditionally been associated with increased muscle bulk, but it is not invariably so. No strong relationship is observed between degree of muscle hypertrophy and strength gains, causing Moritani and deVries (1980) to conclude that mainly nonmuscular factors are responsible for strength increases in the first month of resistance programs. There are no physiological differences between the skeletal muscle of men and women, yet males typically develop muscle enlargement with training while females—with the same strength gains—do not. This difference has traditionally been attributed to the tenfold greater testosterone levels in men. The explanation for improvement in strength without increased muscle size presumably lies in the neural contributions to resistance training, particularly increased neural drive and synchronization of motor unit firing.

Cardiovascular Responses

The acute cardiovascular responses to resistance exercise are very different from those occurring with endurance activities (Petrofsky & Phillips, 1986). Static exercise is typified by significant elevations of both systolic and diastolic blood pressure, creating significant cardiac afterload work. Peak pressures have been reported as high as 480/350 mm Hg during a double leg press by an experienced bodybuilder (MacDougall, Tuxen, Sale, Moroz, & Sutton, 1985). During endurance exercise a modest rise in systolic pressure is observed without much change in diastolic pressure, and mean arterial pressure may remain unaltered (Rost, 1987) (Table 5.1). The cardiac output response to resistance exercise is mild, typically increasing from 5 to about 8 L/min, and this is almost entirely due to a rise in heart rate (which rarely exceeds 120 bpm). If the subject performs a Valsalva maneuver during weight lifting, the hemodynamic picture changes. Intrathoracic pressure can rise dramatically, with a central venous pressure of as high as 178 mm Hg described in weight lifters. Systemic venous return is impeded, and cardiac output may fall by 50 percent (Rost, 1987).

Table 5.1 Maximal Cardiovascular Responses to Resistance and Endurance Exercise

Cardiovascular characteristic	Response to resistance	Response to endurance
Heart rate	↑	↑↑↑
Stroke volume	0/↑	↑↑↑
Cardiac output	↑↑	↑↑↑
Systemic vascular resistance	0/↑	↓
Systolic blood pressure	↑↑↑	↑↑
Diastolic blood pressure	↑↑↑	0/↓
Mean blood pressure	↑↑↑	0/↓

Note. ↑ = increase, 0 = no change, ↓ = decrease.

Chronic adaptive cardiovascular changes to resistance training also vary from those of endurance sports. Echocardiographic studies indicate that weight training is associated with thickening of ventricular walls without chamber enlargement (concentric hypertrophy), whereas the hearts of endurance athletes are notable for ventricular dilatation (Morganroth, Maron, Henry, & Epstein, 1975; Salke, Rowland, & Burke, 1985). Whether the myocardial hypertrophy of weight lifters is simply a reflection of their increased body size cannot be clearly determined from available studies. It has been proposed that ventricular wall thickening in these individuals is a response to repetitive increases in afterload created by the exaggerated rises in systemic blood pressure occurring with resistance exercise (Fleck & Kraemer, 1987).

Although resistance exercises cause a significant acute rise in blood pressure, the resting blood pressure levels of competitive weight lifters are usually normal (Longhurst, Kelly, Gonyea, & Mitchell, 1981). Because increases in heart rate from weight lifting are limited, improvement in maximal aerobic power would not be expected with resistance-training programs (Gettman & Pollock, 1981). Programs employing lower resistance and high-repetition lifting, however, have led to improvements in $\dot{V}O_2$max of 5 to 8 percent over 8 to 20 weeks. Changes in body composition in such programs are not dramatic. Most studies indicate reductions in percent body fat and increased lean body mass of approximately 1 to 2 percent (Fleck & Kraemer, 1987).

Other Effects of Strength Training

Strength training has been thought to decrease flexibility, slow exercise speed, and be less effective when combined with endurance training. There is no scientific validity for the first two concerns. Resistance training generally causes either improvement or no change in flexibility (Massey & Chaudet, 1956), and muscle contraction time is not altered (DeLorme, Ferris, & Gallagher, 1952). There are experimental data, however, to support the third claim. Dudley and Fleck (1987) reviewed published studies regarding the effect of combined strength and endurance training. They concluded that concurrent training reduced the optimization of muscle strength, particularly at fast velocities of contraction. Athletes involved in strength sports should therefore not engage in extensive endurance training. The converse, however, does not appear to be true. Combined strength and endurance training does not affect improvements in aerobic power.

RESISTANCE TRAINING IN CHILDREN

Recommendations for resistance-training programs for children and young adolescents have revolved around three basic issues:

- Is there evidence that these programs effectively improve strength before puberty?
- Even if gains in strength were possible, are there any good reasons children *should* participate in resistance training? Are there real benefits to be gained?

- Are the growing bones, joints, and muscles of children placed at risk by the stresses of weight training? Do the dangers outweigh any possible advantages?

The following sections review these issues.

Effectiveness of Weight Training

Increasing information indicates that both boys and girls demonstrate significant gains in strength after weight training. The traditional concept held that weight training was futile for children because children lack circulating testosterone. This notion was based on the assumptions that testosterone was associated with increased skeletal muscle mass and strength in males at puberty (true), that women had little testosterone and therefore could not increase muscle strength with training (false), and that increase in muscle bulk was a necessary concomitant of improved strength after training, as witnessed in adult males (false).

Weltman et al. (1986) measured responses to a 14-week, three-times-per-week program of hydraulic resistance training in 6- to 11-year-old boys. Each session comprised three circuits of 10 stations each, including exercise of all major muscle groups as well as sit-ups and stationary cycling. At each station the subjects performed up to 30 repetitions over 30 sec. Isokinetic strength increased 18 to 37 percent with training, significantly better than changes recorded in a nontraining control group. Performance in the vertical jump as well as measures of body flexibility also improved. Musculoskeletal scintigraphy disclosed no indication of damage to epiphyses, bones, or muscles. Interestingly, $\dot{V}O_2$max on a treadmill protocol increased by 14 percent, a change felt to be related to the high numbers of repetitions used in the program. Comparable gains in maximal aerobic power during circuit training were described by Docherty, Wenger, & Collis (1987) in 12-year-old boys utilizing a similar training schedule.

Sewall and Micheli (1986) evaluated changes in strength after 9 weeks of resistance training of knee extensors and shoulder flexors and extensors in eight boys and two girls ages 10 to 11 years. The schedule involved three sets of 50 to 100 percent of maximum for 10 repetitions, using different resistance machines. Improvements were greater in each function compared to controls, but differences were statistically significant only for shoulder flexion. In this study, too, there was no evidence of decreased joint flexibility with training. The authors emphasized that specific stretching exercises before and after each session were important to maintain range of motion and flexibility.

Olympic-style, maximum-load weight lifting has not been considered appropriate for children (see later in this chapter), but Servedio et al. (1985) demonstrated that training by this technique did increase strength in prepubertal boys. Sessions three times a week for 8 weeks resulted in significant gains in shoulder flexion strength, compared to controls, with no injuries or loss of flexibility.

These results, plus those of unpublished studies (Duda, 1986) and therapeutic programs for children with muscular diseases (Bar-Or, 1983), indicate that strength gains can be achieved by both boys and girls before puberty and are not reliant upon the presence of high serum testosterone levels. Whether the degree of improvement in strength with training is comparable in children and postpubertal subjects is not clear. Pfeiffer and Francis (1986) placed prepubertal, pubertal, and postpubertal subjects in a 9-week strength-training program to assess maturity-related responses. The exercise protocol was similar to that of Sewall and Micheli (1986). Of the 14 post-tests that showed strength improvements, no differences were observed in the amount of improvement in the three age groups in 11 of the post-tests. On the remaining 3, the prepubertal subjects demonstrated *greater* strength gains. These findings are at variance with those of Vrijens (1978), who showed that postpubertal subjects showed more improvement in strength with training than prepubertal children.

Values of Weight Training

Growing attention has focused on the positive health benefits of resistance exercise for children and adolescents. These benefits extend to both sport performance and health maintenance.

Sports

A properly designed weight-training program will improve performance in sports calling for muscle strength, endurance, or power. Resistance training has also been considered important for protecting against injuries that occur during athletic training and competition, even in those activities not demanding high levels of muscle tension. Athletes involved in such sports as tennis, baseball, and swimming add resistance exercises to their training regimens for this purpose (Micheli, 1983). It should be noted that although intuitively attractive, this assumption has not been subjected to close scientific scrutiny in either children or adults (Fleck & Kraemer, 1987).

Health Benefits

Are there advantages to strength training beyond the values related to sport participation? Is there a role for resistance exercise as part of a general fitness program for nonathletic children? Resistance training has traditionally been viewed as involving short bursts of energy, with little increase in $\dot{V}O_2$ and exaggerated rises in blood pressure; these activities have been considered inappropriate for prevention and treatment of obesity or systemic hypertension and of no value for improving cardiovascular function. Newer information, however, may modify these concepts.

When weight training consists of low resistances at a high number (12 to 15) of repetitions, significant improvements in $\dot{V}O_2$max can be achieved by both children and adults (Docherty et al., 1987; Fleck & Kraemer, 1987; Weltman et al., 1986). This suggests that health-related benefits of exercise training usually related to aerobic exercise might also be gained from this type of resistance program.

Significant decreases in blood pressure have been observed in mildly hypertensive adolescents who underwent weight training after a period of running exercise (Hagberg et al., 1984). Fripp and Hodgson (1987) demonstrated favorable changes in serum lipids in 14 adolescent males after a 9-week program of resistance exercise. Significant increases in high-density lipoprotein cholesterol with a decline in low-density lipoprotein cholesterol were reported compared with nonexercising controls. No changes were observed, in that study, in body composition or $\dot{V}O_2$max with training. Hurley and Kokkinos (1987) reviewed the serum lipid findings in weight-training adults. They concluded that subjects utilizing moderate resistance with a relatively high number of repetitions were more likely to have favorable lipoprotein profiles.

Resistance training may increase bone mineral content and serve as a preventive measure against osteoporosis. Women are more prone to this lifelong disease of decreased bone density, and it is sometimes recommended that weight training be a routine part of girls' physical education (Loucks, 1988). Although this is not well documented, strength training also may help protect against future back disease. In addition, social and psychological benefits may be gained; the mental discipline and enjoyment of weight training are similar to those involved in team sports (Rians et al., 1987).

Many children take up weight training in the hope of improving their physical appearance by increasing muscle bulk. It can be pointed out to these youngsters that, although they can gain strength, it is unlikely that muscle size will increase with resistance training before puberty.

Risks of Weight Training

A properly structured weight-training program is safe for children, but weight lifting poses risks that make maximal lifts inappropriate for pediatric subjects. No long-term studies of injuries from resistance exercise have been performed in prepubertal children, but acute and chronic injuries reported in adolescents give cause for concern (Brown & Kimball, 1983). These have included wrist growth-plate fractures, sprains and strains, and damage to shoulder, low back, and knee (American Academy of Pediatrics, 1983b). Typically such injuries involve unsupervised lifting of maximal weight, often over the head, and usually in the home setting. These reports have spurred the following recommendations (Fleck & Kraemer, 1987; Legwold, 1982):

• Training should be supervised.
• Maximal lifts should not be performed until at least 16 or 17 years of age.
• No child should train with weights that she or he cannot lift through at least 7 to 10 repetitions.

High repetitions at low resistance appear to be safest for prepubertal subjects. Limited information suggests that normal children are not at risk for serious acute rises in blood pressure, syncopal episodes, loss of joint flexibility, or growth retardation with this type of protocol (Rians et al., 1987). Systolic blood pressure rises only 15 to 18 mm in black children performing handgrip exercise at 50 percent of maximal effort for 30 sec (Strong, Miller, Striplin, & Salehbhai, 1978). Similar changes have been reported in adolescents holding handgrip at 25 percent of maximum voluntary contraction for 4 min (Laird, Fixler, & Huffines, 1979). Despite this limited blood-pressure response, resistance exercise may be contra-indicated in children with certain chronic cardiovascular conditions such as Marfan syndrome or aortic valve disease (see chapter 11).

SUMMARY

This chapter focused on the risks and benefits of resistance training for children.

• Contrary to previous dogma, proper weight-training programs in both prepubertal boys and girls can produce significant gains in muscle strength.
• Muscle-strength improvement is important for enhancing sport performance and protecting against injury. There may be benefits from weight training besides athletic participation, including prevention of osteoporosis and lower back disease.
• Risks of strength training generally relate to the unsupervised lifting of heavy weights. To ensure safety, strength training in children should involve high repetitions at low resistance.
• Comprehensive physical fitness programs for children and adolescents should include a properly conducted component on weight training.

PART II

The Influence of Exercise on Health

A man falls into ill health as a result of not caring for exercise.
Aristotle, 300 B.C.

For we all need health, not only for the functions of life which diseases impede, interrupt or destroy, but also that we may avoid disease.
Galen, 200 A.D.

Anyone who lives a sedentary life and does not exercise . . . even if he eats good foods and takes care of himself according to proper medical principles— all his days will be painful ones and his strength shall wane.
Maimonides, 1199

This robust and strong exercise has a tendency to expel excrements and to calm all sorts of humours.
Tuccaro, 1589

*If some of the advantages accru-
ing from exercise were to be pro-
cured by any one medicine,
nothing in the world would be
in more esteem than that medicine would be.*

Fuller, 1704

*[In exercise we have] an agent
with lipid-lowering, antihypertensive, positive inotropic, negative chronotropic, vasodilating,
diuretic, anorexigenic, weight-
reducing, cathartic, hypoglycemic, tranquilizing, hypnotic, and
antidepressive qualities.*

William Roberts, 1985

The belief that keeping physically active is essential to good health is
nothing new. Recorded human history is filled with allusions to the key
role exercise plays in the "total being," both in preservation of wellness
and treatment of disease. In the review from which most of the above
quotations are gathered, Ryan (1984) notes that as far back as the 9th century B.C., Ayur-Veda recommended exercise and massage for the treatment of rheumatism. The idea that the greatest benefit is gained from
starting regular physical activity early in life cannot be claimed to have
originated with present-day advocates either. Exercise has long been promoted in children for the development of "mind, body constitution, and
human spirit," and Alberti (1404-1472) and Andry (1658-1742) both recommended that regular exercise begin during early infancy (Ryan, 1984).

It is interesting, then, that only in the last 2 decades has any reasonable scientific evidence been put forth supporting the salutary effects of
exercise. Indeed, there is still no absolute proof establishing most of the
aspects of the exercise–health connection, nor is it likely there ever will
be. The resulting doubt has produced skeptics eager to dispel the "exercise myth" (Legwold, 1985). The bulk of accumulating evidence com-
pellingly suggests, however, that regular physical exercise can be a vital
factor in both prevention and treatment of disease. This section is devoted
to reviewing that information, particularly as it provides a rationale for
the promotion of physical activity in children. Most data are derived from
reports about adults, and only limited numbers of studies have yet evaluated health-related outcomes from exercise specifically in the pediatric

age group. The broad picture of benefits derived from a lifetime of regular exercise becomes apparent, however, underscoring the importance of beginning a physically active lifestyle during the childhood years.

Perhaps the ultimate question should be addressed first: Can regular exercise be expected to prolong one's life? Most studies examining the effect of physical activity on longevity have viewed this question from the narrow perspective of life spans of athletes compared to nonathletes. Although the data are conflicting, most reports appear to indicate that, in fact, athletic individuals on the average live approximately 2 to 3 years longer than nonathletes (Stephens, Van Huss, Olson, & Montoye, 1984).

In the study of Harvard alumni by Paffenbarger, Hyde, Wing, & Hsieh (1986), regular physical activity after college reduced mortality and extended life span by 1 to 2 years compared to sedentary individuals or athletes who had ceased exercising. Further support for this view comes from animal studies. Five of six studies of rats indicate that exercising animals live longer than sedentary subjects, even when such factors as diet and other environmental influences are controlled (Spirduso, 1986).

Although the issue of exercise and longevity remains problematic, there is clear-cut evidence that regular exercise can delay functional aging. Muscle strength and endurance, cardiovascular function, and psychomotor performance all typically decline with advancing years, but each can be improved through increased physical activity in older individuals (Spirduso, 1986).

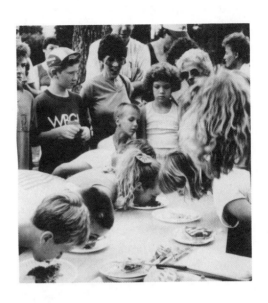

CHAPTER 6

Exercise and Coronary Artery Disease

The sobering statistics have become familiar to an increasingly health-conscious American public: The combined mortality from all forms of atherosclerotic vascular disease accounts for nearly 1 million deaths annually, exceeding that of all other causes combined. One of five American males will develop coronary artery disease (CAD) before age 60; over one fourth of initial coronary artery events in these individuals will be manifest as sudden death. And the survivors of myocardial infarction will have a 5-times greater chance than healthy persons of dying in the ensuing 5 years. The cost of cardiovascular disease is staggering, estimated to be nearly 50 billion dollars annually in the United States (Fraser, 1986; Watkins & Strong, 1984).

But there is good news as well. Mortality rates for adult cardiovascular diseases (including CAD and stroke) began to decline beginning in the late 1960s; by 1982 the death rate was 36 percent lower than it had been in 1963. This same period witnessed significant advances in the diagnosis and treatment of CAD as well as improved health habits in the American population: Male and female cigarette smokers declined 25 and 14 percent, respectively, the percentage of individuals with high serum cholesterol levels fell 12.5 percent in men and 22.5 percent in women (between 1960-1962 and 1971-1974), dietary intakes shifted from saturated fats to more vegetable fats and oils, and the recognition and management of systemic hypertension improved (Kannel & Thom, 1984). Which of these factors has been the most instrumental in the decline of cardiovascular mortality is unclear, but this trend has been viewed with optimism by those advocating a preventive approach to CAD. Here was evidence that atherosclerosis was not simply an inevitable process of aging; instead, the downward mortality curve suggested that preventive medicine was an effective strategy for improving cardiovascular health.

DEVELOPMENT OF ATHEROSCLEROSIS

Physicians caring for children became engaged in these efforts after studies in the 1950s clearly portrayed atherosclerosis as a lifelong process beginning during the pediatric years (Figure 6.1). Autopsy examinations reveal that virtually all children exhibit fatty deposits, termed "fatty streaks," in the intima of the aorta, by the age of 3 years (Holman, McGill, Strong, & Geer, 1958). These streaks are felt to be precursors of fibrous plaques—intimal lesions, consisting of thick caps of fibrous tissue with lipid cores, that begin to appear during the teenage years. Both fatty streaks and fibrous plaques are present in the coronary arteries about 10 years after they appear in the aorta.

Fatty streaks appear to be reversible and innocuous, but fibrous plaques are the initial stages of more advanced lesions that eventually may calcify, ulcerate, and occlude coronary arteries. The end result is myocardial infarction, angina pectoris, and other clinical manifestations of CAD by the fifth decade of life (McGill, 1980). The often-quoted autopsy study of soldiers killed in the Korean war at an average age of 22 years indicated that this process is well established by early adulthood. Over three fourths demonstrated coronary fibrous plaques, and lesions producing

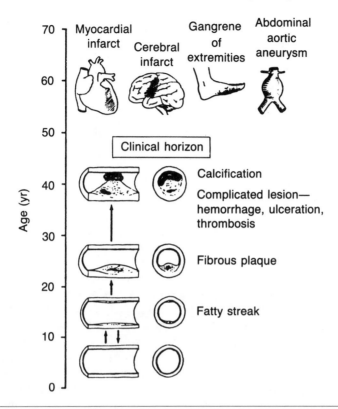

Figure 6.1 The natural history of the atherosclerotic process. *Note.* From "Natural History of Human Atherosclerotic Lesions" by H.L. McGill, J.C. Geer, and J.P. Strong. In *Atherosclerosis and Its Origins* (p. 42) by M. Sandler and G.H. Bourne (Eds.), 1963, New York: Academic Press. Copyright 1963 by Academic Press. Reprinted by permission.

a 70 percent lumen obstruction were evident in 1 of 10 hearts (Enos, Beyer, & Holmes, 1955).

Based on this natural history, efforts to reduce the incidence of CAD might optimally be focused on preventing the development of fibrous plaques. Programs of preventive medicine must then be targeted on individuals well under 20 years of age (Newman & Strong, 1978).

Identifying Risk Factors

The other major impetus behind preventive cardiology, of course, has been the identification of those factors that place an individual at an increased statistical risk for CAD. Large-scale epidemiological studies have established a continuously graded increased incidence of atherosclerosis in individuals with these conditions:

- Hypercholesterolemia
- Hypertension
- Cigarette smoking

Lesser risks are associated with these conditions:

- Obesity
- Diabetes mellitus
- Behavioral traits
- Sedentary lifestyle

Although these factors can be altered through changes in behavior, others are fixed: Mortality from ischemic heart disease is twice as great in males, and the risk is higher in those with a positive family history.

Not much is known about how risk factors influence the formation of atherosclerotic lesions and how age affects this process. A report from the Bogalusa Heart Study, which was designed to evaluate risk-factor variables in a population of 31,000, provides some interesting information. Cardiac autopsies were performed on 35 individuals 3 to 26 years old who died (mostly from accidents, homicides, and suicides) after previously participating in the study. Total serum cholesterol levels correlated with degree of fatty streaks in the aorta in males and in coronary arteries in females. Although failing to reach statistical significance, the amount of fibrous plaques tended to be related to systolic blood pressure and serum lipid levels (Berenson, 1986).

Several excellent books and monographs have addressed the incidence of coronary artery risk factors in children (Berenson, 1986; Lauer & Shekelle, 1980; Strong, 1978; Watkins & Strong, 1984). The facts are not encouraging (Figure 6.2). Serum cholesterol levels are higher in American children than in young residents of countries with a low incidence of adult CAD. One fourth of schoolchildren in the Bogalusa Heart Study had serum cholesterol levels over 175 mg/dl, a value associated with an increased risk for later ischemic heart disease based on epidemiological considerations (Berenson, 1986; Lauer, Conner, Leaverton, Reiter, & Clarke, 1975). Children with high cholesterol levels live in families that have more adults with myocardial infarction. Obesity (defined as over 125 percent of ideal body weight) has been identified in 13 percent of boys 8 to 12 years old (Wilmore & McNamara, 1974). CAD risk factors cluster in children, particularly obesity, abnormal serum lipids, and hypertension (Webber & Freedman, 1986). Mitchell (1973) cautioned that "the applicability of adult risk factors to children at present rests on belief not data," but available information suggests that these factors track (maintain same ranking compared to other subjects) reasonably well during the growing years (Webber, Freedman, & Cresanta, 1986). This would

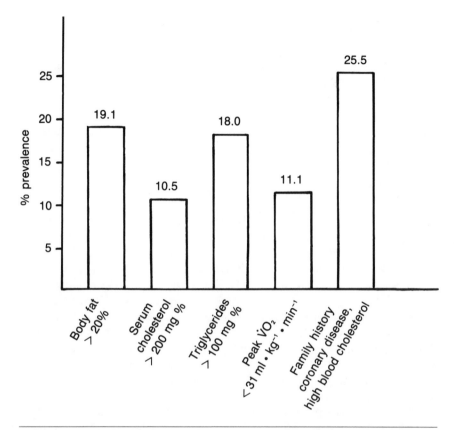

Figure 6.2 Prevalence of coronary artery disease risk factors in children aged 7 through 12 years. *Note.* Data from Gilliam, Katch, Thorlund, and Weltman (1977).

support concerns that the high-risk child will carry this burden into adulthood.

Prevention Strategies

Strategies for preventing CAD draw upon the following conclusions:

• Atherosclerosis is a lifelong process having its origins in childhood.
• Certain identifiable factors appear to increase the risk for atherosclerotic vascular disease.
• Many of these factors are modifiable through changes in lifestyle.

It logically follows that efforts to diminish risk factors during childhood can be expected to pay long-term dividends in preventing or ameliorating adult cardiovascular disease. This conclusion has prompted providers of health care to children to promote diets low in fats and salts, prevent obesity, identify early hypertension, and deter smoking habits in their young patients. In the past, regular exercise has not received great attention in this scheme, because information identifying a sedentary lifestyle as an important risk factor for CAD was considered inconclusive. But recent studies have more convincingly indicated a strong link between physical activity and decreased cardiovascular morbidity and mortality. These have provided a new impetus for the promotion of regular exercise habits in childhood and throughout life.

CORONARY ARTERY DISEASE AND PHYSICAL ACTIVITY IN ADULTS

Early retrospective and cross-sectional studies in adults generally suggested a protective relationship between levels of physical activity and incidence of CAD (Rigotti, Thomas, & Leaf, 1983). These data were flawed, however, by several complicating variables. Most studies used occupation as an indicator of activity, ignoring leisure-time exercise (on this basis, Clarence DeMar, multiple winner of the Boston Marathon, would have been classified as sedentary). Documentation of CAD, which often relied on death certificates, was often inadequate. Moreover, it was difficult to separate cause and effect. Persons free of cardiac disease, for instance, would be expected to engage in physical activity more than those with significant disease. And the influence of other risk factors (such as hypertension, obesity, and smoking), which often cluster with sedentary lifestyle, was often disregarded.

Recent prospective studies designed to avoid these pitfalls have more convincingly demonstrated an inverse relationship between amount of regular physical activity and CAD risk. High-intensity work activity was demonstrated to decrease the incidence of coronary sudden death in San Francisco longshoremen (Paffenbarger et al., 1970). The chance of fatal CAD decreased progressively with energy expenditure on the job, such that risk was decreased by 50 percent with double the work intensity (Figure 6.3).

Effects of Leisure Activity on Coronary Artery Disease

The importance of leisure-time exercise was emphasized by a questionnaire evaluation of daily physical activity in 17,944 middle-aged British civil servants (Morris, Everitt, Pollard, Chave, & Semmence, 1980). During an 8-year follow-up, the incidence of coronary events was 50 percent less in those with a more active lifestyle.

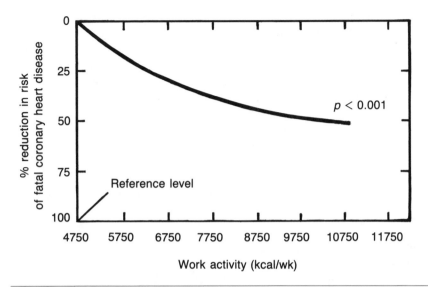

Figure 6.3 Estimated decline in risk of death from coronary artery disease in San Francisco longshoremen related to work energy output. *Note.* From "Exercise in the Prevention of Coronary Heart Disease" by R.S. Paffenbarger and R.T. Hyde, 1984, *Preventive Medicine*, 13, p. 7. Copyright 1984 by Academic Press. Reprinted by permission.

A study of Harvard alumni indicated that regular activity needs to be maintained throughout life to provide a protective effect (Paffenbarger & Hyde, 1984). Daily activities of stair climbing, walking, and sport play were assessed by questionnaire in 16,936 men and related to outcome indicators of CAD. Incidence of angina pectoris, myocardial infarction, and sudden death declined consistently with increased daily energy expenditure, reminiscent of the findings in the longshoremen. Importantly, the decreased risk of CAD was associated only with physical activities continued during adulthood. The risk for sedentary subjects who had previously participated in sport activities during college was no different from the risk for those who had never been physically active. Other studies that support a relationship between levels of physical activity and diminished risk for coronary heart disease have been extensively reviewed (Leon, 1985; Paffenbarger & Hyde, 1984; Rigotti et al., 1983).

Influence of Physical Fitness

How the incidence of cardiovascular disease might be influenced by physical fitness, on the other hand, has received less attention. Peters, Cady, Bischoff, Bernstein, and Pike (1983) compared performance on cycle ergometry in Los Angeles firefighters and policemen with the frequency of first symptomatic myocardial infarction during an average 5-year follow-up. Infarction occurred twice as often in those with poor fitness, and in those with low fitness, high serum cholesterol, smoking, and high blood pressure, the rate of heart attack was 6 times that of the fit men.

Cooper, Pollock, Martin, White, Linnerud & Jackson (1976) evaluated the relationship of coronary risk factors to physical fitness (treadmill endurance time) in 3,000 adult men. In this cross-sectional study, fitness was inversely correlated with resting heart rate, body weight, percent body fat, serum cholesterol and triglyceride levels, glucose, and systolic blood pressure. Ekelund et al. (1988) reported that a lower level of physical fitness (endurance time and submaximal heart rate on treadmill testing) correlated with a higher risk of coronary heart disease in adult men.

Results From Animal Studies

The effect of exercise on experimentally induced atherosclerosis in a variety of animal species has produced conflicting results. Studies performed on primates fed an atherogenic diet, however, strongly suggest that exercise can retard CAD. Monkeys trained on a treadmill for 1 hour three times a week demonstrated significantly less coronary atherosclerosis and wider coronary arteries than nonconditioned animals (Kramsch, Aspen, Abramowitz, Kreimendahl, & Hood, 1981).

Paffenbarger and Hyde (1984) summarized the evidence for a beneficial influence of regular exercise on atherosclerosis risk:

• Lower risk for developing CAD has been described for both occupational and leisure-time activities.
• The relationship between exercise and coronary risk is dose-dependent over a wide range of energy expenditure.
• The findings are consistent by several markers of CAD (angina pectoris, myocardial infarction, sudden unexpected death, and total CAD death).
• The influence of exercise is independent of other variables associated with coronary risk, although these risk factors (cigarette smoking, hypertension, and obesity) tend to clump in individuals.
• Experimental evidence in primates indicates that moderate exercise inhibits the development of coronary atherosclerosis.

What is missing, of course, is a prospective, well-controlled clinical trial in which subjects reduce their rate of CAD after the initiation of a long-term program of physical exercise. The logistical dilemmas of such a study dictate, in fact, that it probably will never be performed. Going one step farther, attempts to link preventive interventions during childhood (exercise as well as dietary, body-composition, and behavioral changes) with adult cardiac disease outcomes will also be extremely difficult to conduct. *Proof* that these measures retard atherosclerotic disease may never be at hand. Nonetheless, persuasive arguments for a positive effect of exercise in reducing risks of coronary disease can be made from the data just reviewed. In addition, the data suggest that a lifetime of regular exercise, begun during the growing years, is the most promising means of gaining this benefit.

By what mechanisms might exercise provide this protective effect? Regular exercise stimulates changes of heart rate and stroke volume that presumably reflect improved myocardial efficiency, but there are no data directly linking cardiac function and extent of coronary atherosclerosis. The study in monkeys noted above suggests a primary effect of exercise on delaying the development of atherosclerotic plaques. Other reports on exercising animals have described decreased arterial collagen deposition and rise in arterial enzymes that catabolize cholesterol (Wolinsky, Goldfischer, & Katz, 1979; Wong, David, & Orimilikwe, 1974). The information in the box that follows summarizes the possible effects of exercise on CAD risk factors.

How Exercise May Affect Coronary Artery Disease Risk

- Reduces blood pressure
- Lowers serum cholesterol, LDL-cholesterol
- Increases HDL-cholesterol
- Lowers circulating catecholamines
- Potentiates fibrinolysis
- Decreases adiposity
- Improves psychosocial profile
- Improves health attitudes and practices (e.g., smoking cessation)

Mechanisms in Humans

In humans, several other means have been suggested by which exercise might directly slow the atherosclerotic process. If regular exercise can reduce anxiety, hostility, and time urgency (the so-called type A personality), physical activity might decrease exaggerated responses to stress of blood pressure and plasma catecholamines typically observed with this behavior (Glass, Krakoff, & Contrada, 1980). Norepinephrine released during emotional upset causes an increase in plasma free fatty acids, which could accelerate atherosclerosis (Carruthers, Taggart, & Somerville, 1970). Physical training may result in increased fibrinolysis, which could serve to reduce growth of atherosclerotic lesions (Williams et al., 1980). Also, runners have lower blood viscosity, which has been postulated to play a positive role by improving myocardial blood flow (Letcher, Pickering, Chien, & Laragh, 1978).

It appears likely, however, that exercise protects against coronary disease indirectly through its influence on other risk factors. The observation that these factors are abundantly evident during childhood provides further reason for promoting early habits of regular exercise.

The following sections review information about the effect of exercise on three of the principal coronary risk factors in both children and adults. Regular physical activity may play an important role in ameliorating risks from elevated serum lipids, systemic hypertension, and cigarette smoking. The relationship between exercise and obesity will be discussed in the next chapter.

SERUM LIPIDS

Early concern about total serum cholesterol as a coronary risk factor has evolved to a fuller understanding of how subtypes of cholesterol influence the atherosclerotic process. Subsequent attention has focused on factors that alter serum concentrations of these substances and presumably affect one's chances for developing CAD. A principal means by which exercise decreases this risk may, in fact, be through favorable changes in the blood lipid profile.

In large population studies, high levels of total serum cholesterol are clearly associated with an increased incidence of coronary disease (Scrimshaw & Guzman, 1968). The risk is a continuous one—the more the cholesterol level rises above 180 mg/dl, the higher the danger. Cholesterol does not dissolve in blood and thus must be linked with protein in one of several forms to allow for hematogenous transport. The result is a family of lipoproteins, each member playing a different role in cholesterol transport as well as in the pathogenesis of atherosclerotic lesions (Dufaux, Assmann, & Hollman, 1982).

Lipoproteins

Low-density-lipoprotein cholesterol (LDL-C) and very-low-density-lipoprotein cholesterol (VLDL-C) are formed by the liver and serve to transport cholesterol and triglycerides to peripheral cells. Because they act to promote the deposition of intracellular lipid, these fractions (particularly LDL-C) have been incriminated as important factors in the atherosclerotic process. Epidemiological data support this concept, as a close relationship exists between LDL-C values and the incidence of CAD. On the other hand, high-density-lipoprotein cholesterol (HDL-C) appears to provide a protective effect, perhaps related to its role as cholesterol "scavenger," removing cholesterol from the cells and transporting it to the liver. In large population studies, individuals with coronary disease demonstrate lower levels of HDL-C. HDL-C level predicts the development of atherosclerotic disease 8 times better than does total cholesterol (Gordon, Castelli, Hjortland, Kannel, & Dawber, 1977). An imbalance of cholesterol deposition and removal from vascular walls is key to the growth of atherosclerotic lesions—thus the designation of "good" (HDL) and "bad" (LDL) cholesterol. Whether triglycerides play a role in increasing coronary risk is controversial.

After the first year of life, serum lipid levels remain relatively constant throughout childhood and adolescence (Figure 6.4). The mean cholesterol value is approximately 160 mg/dl in both boys and girls, with the 95th percentile at 210 mg/dl. In young people aged 16 to 17, levels begin a progressive rise through the middle adult years. HDL-C values average 50 to 60 mg/dl from ages 2 to 14 and then fall about 10 mg/dl to adult levels (Cresanta, Srinivasan, Webber, & Berenson, 1984; Fraser, 1986).

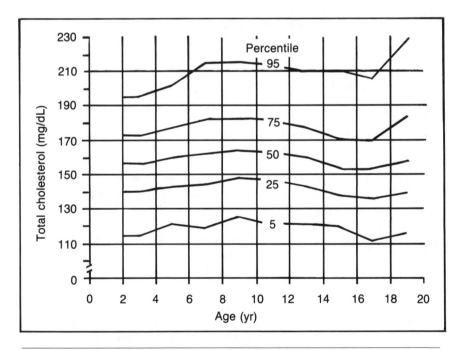

Figure 6.4 Norms for serum total cholesterol level in children aged 2-19 years in the Bogalusa Heart Study. *Note.* From "Serum Lipid and Lipoprotein Cholesterol Grids for Cardiovascular Risk Screening of Children" by J.L. Cresanta, S.R. Srinivasan, L.S. Webber, and G.S. Berenson, 1984, *American Journal of Diseases of Children*, **138**, p. 380. Copyright 1984 by the American Medical Association. Reprinted by permission.

Abundant evidence in adults indicates that regular exercise is associated with increased HDL-C levels. Although cross-sectional studies have been confounded by factors that alter HDL-C (e.g., alcohol consumption, diet, and smoking) virtually all have demonstrated significantly higher HDL-C levels in endurance athletes compared to sedentary individuals (Leon, 1984). This has been evident in both males and females, with mean values approximately 40 to 50 percent greater than for nonathletes.

The picture of the relationship of total serum cholesterol and LDL cholesterol to physical activity or fitness is less clear. Goldberg and Elliot (1985) reviewed both epidemiological and prospective studies and concluded that no direct relationship had been conclusively established between exercise and total cholesterol concentrations.

Studies evaluating longitudinal changes in serum lipids with physical training of adults have produced conflicting results (Dufaux et al., 1982). Findings in the meta-analysis of Tran, Weltman, Glass, and Mood (1983) help explain some of these inconsistencies. The authors examined the results of 66 training studies and found that the average exercising subject demonstrated a fall in total cholesterol of 10 mg/dl, LDL-C of 5.1 mg/dl, and triglycerides of 15.8 mg/dl. Mean HDL-C increased 1.2 mg/dl (statistically insignificant), and the ratio of total cholesterol:HDL-C fell .48. Several factors were shown to influence these results. Most favorable changes in lipids with training were observed in the following persons:

- Older subjects
- Those who had greater abnormalities in lipids before training
- Those who had longer training programs
- Persons who exhibited the largest improvement in $\dot{V}O_2$max during training (typically those with the lowest initial $\dot{V}O_2$max levels)

That is, studies of fit individuals with normal cholesterol and its subfractions showed fewer changes with training than sedentary subjects with more deranged lipid levels.

These factors may also help explain studies indicating that women do not increase HDL-C with training, because some of the studies evaluated females with high initial HDL-C levels (Brownell, Bachorik, & Ayerle, 1982). Others have reported rises in HDL-C in women with a physical conditioning program and increased running mileage (Farrel & Barbariak, 1980; Rotkis, Boyden, Pamenter, Stanforth, & Wilmore, 1981).

Resistance training typically has not been considered an effective means of improving blood lipid profiles (Farrel et al., 1982). However, Goldberg, Elliot, Schutz, and Kloster (1984) demonstrated reduced total cholesterol: HDL-C ratios by 14.3 and 21.6 percent, respectively, in women and men after a 16-week weight-training program. Other studies have also indicated that resistance exercise can improve blood lipid levels (Hurley et al.,

1984; Johnson et al., 1982). Fleck and Kraemer (1987) suggested that favorable changes in blood lipids from weight training were more likely in resistance exercise with short rest periods and high repetition volume.

Exercise and Lipids in Children

Will exercise (or at least the avoidance of a sedentary lifestyle) effect favorable changes in serum lipids in children? A positive answer would certainly serve as an impetus for promoting physical activity during childhood to help forestall CAD in the adult years. The available data are encouraging but not conclusive (Linder & DuRant, 1982; Montoye, 1986).

Cross-Sectional Studies

Table 6.1 summarizes the results of cross-sectional studies assessing habitual activity levels and serum lipids in children ranging from elite distance runners to physically active nonathletes. The consistency of elevated HDL-C values in the more active subjects is similar to that reported in adults, and in two of the pediatric studies that did not support this association the ratio of HDL-C to total cholesterol was significantly higher in the active children (DuRant, Linder, & Mahoney, 1983; Thorland & Gilliam, 1981). These reports indicate no significant differences in total cholesterol and LDL-C between active and inactive subjects. In some of the studies but not all, triglyceride levels were higher in the more sedentary children.

When markers of physical fitness and blood lipids are compared in children, no strong relationship emerges. Total work per kilogram of body weight performed on a maximal cycle test by boys aged 14 to 16 correlated weakly with HDL-C levels ($r = .39$, $p < .01$), but no significant relationship was observed in female subjects (Wanne, Viikari, & Valimaki, 1984). Similar coefficients were described by Atomi, Kuroda, Asami, and Kawahara (1986), in 10- to 12-year-old boys using $\dot{V}O_2max$ by treadmill testing to measure fitness ($r = .38$, $p < .05$), and by Valimaki, Hursti, Pihlakoski, and Viikari (1980), utilizing total cycle work output per kilogram of body weight in boys aged 11 to 13 years ($r = .53$, $p < .05$). Sady et al. (1984) studied the relationship of maximal aerobic power and HDL-C in 108 5- to 12-year-old children. $\dot{V}O_2max$ correlated directly with HDL-C ($r = .18$, $p < .05$), but this relationship became insignificant after considering age, sex, body fat, and triglyceride level. DuRant, Linder, Harkess, and Gray (1983) used peak work level on a cycle ergometer as the fitness variable and found no correlation with HDL-C values in boys 11 to 17 years old. A review of 10 studies of children revealed no relationship between physical fitness and total serum cholesterol level (Montoye, 1986).

Table 6.1 Cross-Sectional Lipid Studies in Active Children

Reference	Subjects	N	Sex	Age	Total cholesterol	HDL-C	LDL-C	Triglycerides
Smith, Metheny, Van Huss, Seefeldt, & Sparrow (1983)	Track athletes	28	M/F	10-15	0	↑	0	↓
Nizankowski-Blaz & Abramowicz (1983)	Sports school	38	M/F	14	0	↑	0	↓
Valimaki et al. (1980)	Track athletes	9	M	11-13	0	↑	0	0
		7	F	11-13	0	↑	0	↓
Viikari et al. (1984)	Active normals	61	M/F	12	0	↑	0	0
Wanne et al. (1984)	Trained	14	M	14-16	0	↑	0	↓
		16	F	14-16	0	0	0	0
DuRant, Linder, Harkess, & Gray (1983)	Active normals	62	M/F	7-11	0	0	0	0
DuRant, Linder, & Mahoney (1983)	Active normals	50	M	11-17	0	0	0	0
Atomi, Kuroda, Asami, & Kawahara (1986)	Soccer	21	M	12	↑	↑	-	0
Thorland & Gilliam (1981)	Active normals	28	M	8-12	0	0	-	↓

Note. ↑ = greater than controls, ↓ = less than controls, 0 = no difference, - = not reported.

Training Studies

The argument for a positive effect of exercise on lipids would be more convincing if improvements in blood lipid profiles could be demonstrated following a period of physical training. In this regard the available literature is disappointing. Of six controlled studies in children, only one demonstrated increased HDL-C levels with physical training. Fisher and Brown (1982) evaluated 38 seventh graders divided into exercise, exercise/diet, and control groups. After 12 weeks of physical conditioning, the exercise group showed significantly increased treadmill endurance times, higher HDL-C levels, and lower total cholesterol values compared to the controls. Differences in body composition may have influenced the HDL-C changes, however; skinfold measurements decreased in the exercisers, but the control subjects became fatter.

Linder, DuRant, and Mahoney (1983) measured serum lipoprotein levels in 21 boys 11 to 17 years old during an 8-week aerobic training program. The exercise-trained subjects did not show any differences in blood lipid concentrations compared with nontrained controls despite improvement in their levels of fitness. In an earlier study Linder, DuRant, Gray, and Harkess (1979) could demonstrate no changes in lipids in children who exercised for 4 weeks compared to untrained controls. Gilliam and Freedson (1980) found no effects of a 12-week school fitness program on either $\dot{V}O_2$ or serum cholesterol and triglyceride levels in children 7 to 9 years old. These findings may be partly explained by the selective, fit nature of the group: 39 of the initial 62 children in the study (63 percent) were excluded because they either did not attend enough classes or did not satisfy criteria for maximal effort on treadmill testing.

Savage et al. (1986) described a significant *decrease* in HDL-C levels following a 10-week training program in 12 pubertal boys. This ''particularly interesting'' finding was attributed possibly to the high baseline HDL-C values (over the 75th percentile for age). That study also included a group of adult men, who demonstrated a similar decline in HDL-C with training compared with controls.

In an uncontrolled study, Gilliam and Burke (1978) measured the response of serum lipids in girls 8 to 10 years old to a 6-week physical activity program. Posttraining HDL-C values were significantly higher compared to baseline levels (36.4 mg percent vs. 30.0 mg percent, p < .05). Total cholesterol did not change during the study.

Strength Training Studies

Weltman, Janney, Rians, Strand, and Katch (1987) demonstrated that high-repetition strength training can be associated with lipid profile changes in children. In a 14-week circuit resistance exercise program, 32 boys aged 6 to 11 years decreased both total cholesterol and total cholesterol:HDL-C ratios. No significant changes were observed in either HDL-C or triglyceride levels.

Conclusions From Studies

Favorable blood lipid profiles are more often observed in active children, but increasing exercise by the intensity and duration involved in the studies described appears to have little effect in changing lipid levels of normal subjects. The latter observation is consistent with the meta-analysis in adults by Tran et al. (1983), which indicated that younger subjects with higher $\dot{V}O_2$max and less-abnormal lipid levels can expect to experience limited changes in HDL and other lipoproteins with exercise training. It should be noted that the studies assessing lipid changes with training have principally involved fit, healthy, motivated children. In other categories of youngsters, such as obese or sedentary individuals, increases in physical activity may prove to have a greater beneficial effect on blood lipid profiles (Ylitalo, 1984) (see chapter 7).

SYSTEMIC HYPERTENSION

In the United States, as in most populations of the world, systolic and diastolic blood pressure levels are observed to rise inexorably throughout the course of an individual's lifetime. The rate of increase is pronounced enough that by age 70 the systolic pressure has doubled over values measured in the first weeks of life (Fraser, 1986). Persons are identified as having "hypertension" when, in the course of this progression, certain threshold limits of blood pressure are exceeded, placing the individuals at increased risk for complications of stroke, myocardial infarction, congestive heart failure, and renal vascular disease. Estimates are that 20 percent of the adult American population fits this definition, amounting to 30 million persons when pressures exceeding 160/95 are used as the criterion (Kaplan, 1986). The risk to these individuals is not insignificant, as the incidence of CAD in men 45 to 62 years old with this level of blood pressure is 5 times that of men with average readings for age (Fraser, 1986).

The goal of physicians caring for children is to prevent, or at least moderate, the rise of blood pressure with age. There is a critical need, then, to identify those youngsters who are at higher risk of developing adult hypertension and create preventive strategies to modify the factors that place these children at risk.

In fact, no particular level of blood pressure separates normal from abnormal. The morbidity and mortality rates from atherosclerotic vascular disease rise progressively across the entire range of systolic and diastolic blood pressures, with an increased risk of 30 percent for each rise of 10 mm Hg in systolic pressure. In terms of prevention of cardiovascular disease, then, the lower the pressure, the less the risk. This observation also suggests that the "normal" rise in blood pressure with age does not represent a natural course of events.

Epidemiological Studies

Further support for this conclusion is drawn from studies of some 20 populations in the world whose blood pressure values remain low throughout life, usually not exceeding systolic pressure of 125 mm Hg. These groups, which are all unindustrialized and live apart from Western society, provide an opportunity to pinpoint factors that might be responsible for the climb in blood pressure and vascular complications in more civilized nations (Page, 1980b). Although they are essentially free of cardiovascular disease, these peoples do not all exhibit good health (many suffer from undernutrition and chronic infections) or altogether beneficial lifestyles (the Masai of Tanzania consume a diet rich in animal proteins and dairy fat).

But certain characteristics they do have in common:

- All are highly physically active, and the levels of fitness in some of these cultures is extraordinary.
- Dietary sodium intake is limited in all low-blood-pressure populations, rarely exceeding 70 mEq per day (approximately one fifth that of the typical adult American diet).
- Individuals in these groups are typically short and lean, with little increase in weight with advancing years (Page, 1980b).

The Tarahumara Indians of northern Mexico and the Masai illustrate at least the first point. Living a virtually prehistoric lifestyle at an 8,000-ft elevation, the Tarahumara rely on their physical powers for survival in the mountain wilderness but still engage in distance running as their favorite recreation. The principal sport is a 75- to 150-mile race over mountain trails, during which the participants continuously kick a small ball. Observing these feats of endurance, Groom (1971) noted that the runners typically do not become dyspneic but instead their performance is limited by leg pain. High levels of physiological fitness were also reported during treadmill testing of Masai men (Mann, Shaffer, & Rich, 1965). Estimated $\dot{V}O_2$max in this highly active population *averaged* nearly 60 ml • $kg^{-1}min^{-1}$ in individuals as old as 40 years.

The importance of environmental factors in maintaining low blood pressures is indicated by the observation that their blood pressures rise when these groups enter advanced cultures. Which changes in lifestyle are most influential in causing elevated blood pressures when primitive peoples are "acculturated" remains unclear, but diet, particularly salt intake, is among the most significant (Page, Friedlander, & Moellering, 1977). It should be noted, however, that not all epidemiological studies have reported such convincing data linking salt intake and hypertension, and efforts to demonstrate such a connection within population groups have generally failed (Fixler, 1978).

Analysis of low-hypertension populations does imply that the relentless rise in blood pressure with age in advanced cultures is a reflection of environmental rather than genetic influences. Moreover, these data suggest that alteration of dietary and physical activity behaviors might alter the risk of systemic hypertension in adulthood. One cannot expect to turn American children into Tarahumarian Indians, but this information suggests that regular exercise, low-salt diet, and avoidance of obesity might be important means of avoiding adult hypertension.

Intervention Targets

Systemic hypertension in adults can be defined by the blood pressure levels associated with vascular complications, but during childhood, long before these pressures can do their damage, a hypertension label can be assigned only by a person's percentile ranking in the population. Thus a child or adolescent is usually considered to be hypertensive if his or her blood pressure values are above the 95th percentile for age on successive readings. The relationship between blood pressure levels in the child and the subsequent risks of hypertension complications during the adult years is not known, however, and the wisdom of targeting youngsters with hypertension for preventive intervention hinges on the degree to which a child with such blood pressure levels can be expected to become a hypertensive adult. Tracking, or the tendency of blood pressure levels to maintain the same percentile ranking with age, has subsequently received a good deal of attention in large-scale epidemiological studies in children (Fixler et al., 1984; Webber et al., 1986).

Values of systolic blood pressure in children compared at 4- to 6-year intervals correlate with coefficients of .24 to .50; the relationship of serial diastolic values is lower. In the Muscatine study, a child with pressures in the upper 20th percentile had a 60 percent chance of remaining in the upper 40th percentile during this period of time (Lauer, Conner, Leaverton, Reiter, & Clarke, 1975). But the chance of remaining in the top 20th percentile group over serial examinations was 17 and 9 percent for systolic and diastolic pressures, respectively. In adults, 6-year followup correlation coefficients are typically .60 for systolic and .50 for diastolic pressures (Lauer & Clarke, 1980; Lieberman, 1986).

In the Evans County study 11 percent of adolescents were found to have blood pressures over 140/90; on follow-up examination 7 years later only one third were still hypertensive. There is thus great variability in individual pressures during childhood, and "labile" hypertension is not uncommon in adolescence. These transient elevations of blood pressure are not necessarily benign, though, because up to half of these individuals may go on to sustained hypertension in adulthood (Fraser, 1986).

Based on these data, one can conclude that blood pressure does track in children to a limited degree but not to the extent observed in adults. Blood pressure levels in youngsters are not strongly predictive of adult values, and limiting preventive interventions to children above certain percentile levels may not be appropriate. As Fixler et al. (1984) commented,

> longitudinal data indicate that movement into and out of the upper quintile rank is common. Also, many youths who will develop hypertension may not have had pressures in the upper ranks in childhood. Therefore, identification of the proper target population for intervention may be difficult in childhood. If we are to adopt a pediatric primary prevention policy for essential hypertension, it would probably be more effective to direct prevention efforts at all youths, rather than limit efforts to an ill-defined population at risk. (p. 49)

Risk Factors

The family history also contributes to assessment of risk, because the incidence of hypertension is increased in first-degree relatives (Feinleib, Garrison, & Havlik, 1980). The chance of a child developing elevated blood pressure levels doubles if one of his or her parents is hypertensive. Significant correlations are observed in measurements between infants and their mothers as early as the newborn period, and this familial aggregation persists as children grow, with typical regression coefficients of .33 between siblings (Zinner & Kass, 1984). Studies of twins suggest that the genetic contribution to this family clustering is approximately 25 percent (correlations for identical twins are approximately .55 compared to .25 for fraternal twins) (Kaplan, 1986).

Strategies to diminish the risks of hypertension—whether for selected groups or for the pediatric population at large—have focused largely on body weight (and adiposity) and salt intake. These factors have the following characteristics (Kaplan, 1986; Page, 1980a; Stamler, 1980):

- They increase tracking correlations.
- They are related most closely with familial blood pressure patterns.
- They differentiate populations with high and low blood pressure.
- They can be manipulated to effect changes in blood pressure levels.

Body Weight

Body weight stands out in all epidemiological studies as the most significant environmental factor contributing to systemic hypertension. The relationship between obesity and hypertension is so strong that it has been estimated that the incidence of whites with hypertension in the United States could be reduced by half simply by controlling excess weight (Tyroler, Heyden, & Hames, 1975). In the Muscatine Study, one fourth of overweight children had blood pressures above the 90th percentile (Lauer et al., 1975), and body weight was the only predictive factor of persistent high blood pressure levels in a 7-year follow-up study of adolescents and young adults (Hames et al., 1978). Weight loss has been associated with a reduction of blood pressure in hypertensive individuals (Reisen et al., 1978).

Salt Intake

The importance of salt restriction as a means of preventing or reducing high blood pressure is based on the previously described population studies of low-blood-pressure cultures. Attempts to correlate salt intake with the incidence of hypertension in individuals in advanced societies has been disappointing. Still, moderate salt restriction will frequently lower blood pressure levels in hypertensive individuals, usually by about 10 mm Hg for both systolic and diastolic values (Fraser, 1986). Considering the body's basic sodium requirement as well as salt consumption in populations with low blood pressure, an appropriate daily intake of sodium for children is approximately 26 mEq (600 mg) per 1,000 kcal. Most American children consume about 63 mEq per 1,000 kcal daily, so a 62 percent reduction would be required—a limitation that can be reached by adding no salt at the table or during cooking, plus avoidance of heavily salted foods (Prineas, Gillum, & Blackburn, 1980). The problems of excessive salt intake and body weight and their relationship to hypertension have been extensively reviewed elsewhere (Dustan, 1980; Fraser, 1986; Page, 1980a).

Physical Activity

The influence of physical activity or fitness on the natural course of blood pressure with age has not been systematically studied in the same manner. But, as noted previously, regular exercise could be expected to help lower blood pressure levels, based on the high levels of physical activity in populations devoid of hypertension. No study has yet been performed to determine whether regular exercise during the growing years will suppress the rise in blood pressures with increasing age. But conclusions affirming the salutary effects of physical activity on blood pressure can be drawn from reports that indicate the following:

- Many physically fit individuals have lower blood pressure values.
- A fall in resting blood pressure levels is observed in some non-hypertensives after a period of physical training.

• Regular exercise can effect modest reduction in blood pressure in subjects with hypertension.

Exercise and Blood Pressure in Adults

Evidence in adults is suggestive but not conclusive that physically active or fit individuals have lower resting blood pressure levels (Cooper, Pollock, Martin, White, Linnerud, & Jackson, 1976; Montoye, Metzner, Keller, Johnson, & Epstein, 1972; Tipton, 1984). Most cross-sectional studies demonstrate this association, particularly in fit populations of individuals who are active in endurance sports, with pressure differences in the range of 4 to 15 mm Hg (Tipton, 1984). Others, such as the Framingham study, have failed to support a relationship of blood pressure and physical activity. In the Framingham study, subjects were interviewed regarding hours per day spent in sedentary, moderate, and strenuous activities. No significant correlation was found between habitual physical activity and blood pressure levels (Dawber, Kannel, & Kagan, 1967).

Paffenbarger, Wing, Hyde, and Jung (1983) demonstrated a significantly lower risk of hypertension in male college alumni who engaged in regular vigorous exercise (such as running, swimming, or handball). Previous participation in collegiate athletics and habitual lighter activities (such as yard work, golf, and climbing stairs) did not influence the incidence of high blood pressure levels. Physical fitness levels in a study of 4,820 men and 1,219 women aged 20 to 65 years were found to predict risk of hypertension after an average 4-year follow-up (Blair, Goodyear, Gibbons, & Cooper, 1984). After adjustments for body habitus, age, sex, and baseline blood pressure, the excess risk in the low-fitness subjects (measured by treadmill testing) was calculated to be 52 percent. This compares to a value of 35 percent in the alumni reported by Paffenbarger et al. (1983) who did not participate in vigorous sports.

Longitudinal studies of blood pressure responses to physical training in normotensive adults have produced conflicting results, but most have demonstrated only insignificant changes in resting values (Bonanno & Lies, 1974; McMahon & Palmer, 1985; Seals & Hagberg, 1984). These individuals may, however, have decreased blood pressure responses to a given exercise workload (Åstrand & Rodahl, 1977).

Blood pressure responses to training in adult hypertensive subjects are more promising. Seals and Hagberg (1984) reviewed 11 studies published between 1967 and 1983 and found, in two thirds, significant reductions in resting systolic and/or diastolic blood pressure after training. The average decline was 9 and 7 mm Hg for systolic and diastolic pressure, respectively, after programs consisting typically of running, cycling, or walking for 4 to 6 months. Blood pressure was also significantly reduced during submaximal exercise in 6 of 9 of the studies. These studies were beset with numerous methodological problems, however, most prominently the absence in many cases of control subjects. Intensity of exercise was rarely documented, nor was information provided regarding program adherence.

Exercise and Blood Pressure in Children

Few comprehensive studies have been conducted comparing habitual physical activity and blood pressure in children. Seliger, Cermak, & Handzo (1971) could find no significant differences between the systolic pressures of Czechoslovakian athletes and their nonactive peers, either at 12 or 15 years of age. Similarly, highly active Dutch boys and girls had blood pressure levels comparable to a sedentary group of the 13- to 14-year-old subjects studied by Verschuur, Kemper, and Besseling (1984). On the other hand, a study of elite distance runners aged 9 to 15 years showed lower resting and submaximal treadmill systolic pressures than nontrained controls (Van Huss et al., 1988). Reports in older teenage athletes, however, indicate that at comparable submaximal heart rates (instead of work loads), trained subjects have higher blood pressure responses to exercise than untrained (Dlin, 1986).

Several authors have reported a relationship between measures of physical fitness and resting blood pressure during childhood. Fraser, Phillips, and Harris (1983) described lower systolic and diastolic pressures in prepubertal and adolescent subjects with greater levels of fitness as indicated by heart rate response to submaximal treadmill exercise (Figure 6.5). When these results were adjusted for body fat, height, and age, the relationship persisted for systolic pressure in preadolescent boys and in teenagers of both sexes. Negative correlations between blood pressure and physical fitness have also been reported in children with fitness determined by step test (Hofman, Walter, Connelly, & Vaughan, 1987; Panico et al., 1987) and treadmill $\dot{V}O_2max$ (Wilmore & McNamara, 1974).

The response of resting blood pressure in training studies involving healthy, normotensive children is not impressive. Only one of five reports has indicated any significant change, that being a 6.4-mm drop in diastolic pressure after 12 weeks of exercise training in seventh graders (Fisher & Brown, 1982). As reviewed by Montoye (1986), other investigators have shown no alteration in resting pressures after training programs ranging from 8 to 16 weeks (Bryant, Garett, & Dean, 1984; Dwyer, Coonan, Leitch, Hetzel, & Baghurst, 1983; Eriksson & Koch, 1973; Linder et al., 1983).

Exercise may, however, play a useful role in the management of children and adolescents with mild to moderate hypertension. Hagberg et al. (1983) studied the effects of a 6-month aerobic exercise training program on 25 adolescents with persistently borderline blood pressures (mean

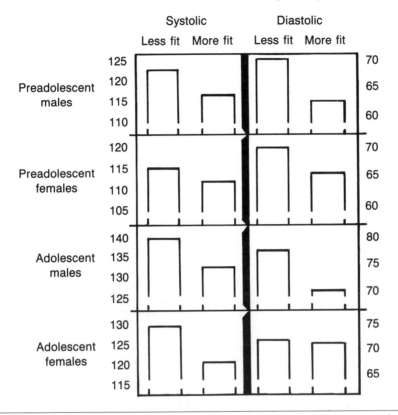

Figure 6.5 Relationship between physical fitness and blood pressure in the Loma Linda Children's Blood Pressure Study. *Note.* From "Physical Fitness and Blood Pressure in Children" by G.E. Fraser, R.L. Phillips, and R. Harris, 1983, *Circulation,* **67**, p. 405. Copyright 1983 by the American Heart Association. Reprinted by permission of the American Heart Association, Inc.

137/80). Systolic and diastolic pressures both fell, with an average post-training value of 129/75. Pressures were recorded again 9 months after cessation of the program, when levels approximated pretraining values. No changes in blood pressures were observed in nontraining controls over the same period of time (Figure 6.6).

Most programs showing an effect of physical training on blood pressures have utilized endurance (aerobic) sports. Resistance training has not typically been associated with these changes. It is intriguing, then, that 5 of the subjects who began weight training after completing the aerobic exercise program of Hagberg et al. (1983) maintained or further decreased their blood pressure after 5 months. The average final systolic pressure in these subjects was 17 mm Hg lower than at the start of the first program (Hagberg et al., 1984).

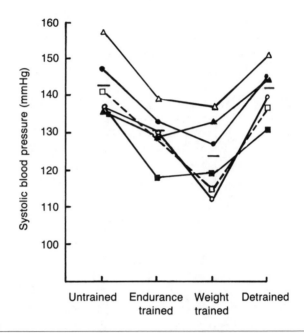

Figure 6.6 Changes in blood pressure with endurance and weight training in adolescent subjects. *Note.* From "Effects of Weight Training on Blood Pressure and Hemodynamics in Hypertensive Adolescents" by J.M. Hagberg, A.A. Ehsani, O. Goldring, A. Hernandez, D.R. Sinacore, and J.O. Holloszy, 1984, *Journal of Pediatrics*, **104**, p. 149. Copyright 1984 by the C.V. Mosby Co. Reprinted by permission.

Based on previous successes in adults (Bhasin, Khullar, & Weissler, 1980), efforts have been made to use blood pressure responses during exercise testing in children to predict future hypertension. Fixler, Laird, and Dana (1985) performed both dynamic and isometric exercise tests on teenagers who 1 year before had been identified as hypertensive (i.e., having pressures over the 95th percentile on three measurements). Blood pressure responses to testing and earlier resting blood pressure levels were compared with pressures recorded 1 year later. Stepwise regression analysis revealed that the first resting blood pressure determination was the best predictor of the systolic pressure 2 years in the future. Blood pressures obtained during exercise testing did not contribute significantly to that prediction.

Reduction of Hypertension Through Exercise

The mechanism by which regular exercise might depress blood pressure levels has particular relevance to children and adolescents. According to

Poiseuille's law, increases in blood pressure must be accounted for by either a rise in cardiac output or peripheral vascular resistance (or both). Some evidence indicates that a hyperkinetic phase of augmented heart rate and cardiac output can be identified early in the natural course of hypertension. Later on in life, these findings are replaced by those of high peripheral resistance and normal cardiac output, characteristic of older individuals with established hypertension (Kaplan, 1986). The early hyperkinetic phase is associated with increased levels of circulating epinephrine and augmented sympathetic tone (McCrory, Klein, & Fallo, 1984), a response directly opposite to that achieved by aerobic exercise training. It might be expected, then, that regular endurance exercise would be particularly effective in reducing blood pressure levels in those younger hypertensive individuals by decreasing epinephrine levels at resting and submaximal exercise.

Experimental data support this assumption. Duncan, Hagan, Upton, Farr, and Oglesby (1983) demonstrated a fall in blood pressure with exercise training in adult subjects with mild hypertension. Those with elevated catecholamine levels experienced a greater reduction in blood pressures than subjects with normal plasma catecholamine concentrations, and the change in catecholamine values related directly with fall in blood pressure. Other studies in adults have suggested that milder degrees of hypertension are more responsive to the influence of exercise training (Seals & Hagberg, 1984). These findings suggest that exercise might optimally suppress the rise of blood pressure in the earlier years of life and that physical training is most effective as a therapeutic measure for hypertension in adolescents and young adults.

The potential of exercise as one alternative to drug therapy for hypertensive children and adolescents with mild or labile hypertension is a particularly attractive one. The prospect of a lifetime of antihypertensive medication with its toxic side effects, expense, and psychological impact for a condition with an uncertain progression is an unsettling one. Some data in adults, on the other hand, indicate that it is important to reduce blood pressure levels even in those individuals with diastolic pressures as low as 90 mm Hg (Freis, 1982). This dilemma of "when to treat" is comfortably avoided if control of obesity, decreased salt intake, and institution of regular endurance exercise can effect small but persistent depression of blood pressure in young subjects.

The preceding discussion addresses subjects with essential hypertension, or elevated blood pressure levels of unknown cause, which constitutes 90 percent of adult hypertension. In children and adolescents the incidence of secondary hypertension from renal, adrenal, or cardiovascular disease is greater; in general, the younger the child and the higher the blood pressure, the more likely an identifiable disease process is responsible. Evaluation of the role of exercise in the management of these cases (e.g., chronic renal disease) has been limited. A decline in resting blood pressure has been reported after physical training in adult patients on hemodialysis, but other studies have reported no change (Painter, 1988).

SMOKING

Despite the cheering news that teenage smoking is on the decline, one of five high school seniors still consumes a pack of cigarettes a month. Most adult smokers took up the habit during adolescence (half of teenage girls started before the age of 13), and over one fourth of the adult population in the United States continues the habit. Why? Cigarette smoking *each year* is responsible for 350,000 deaths in the United States from CAD, cancer, and chronic lung disease, a number almost equal to the total number of American lives lost in all of World War II (Fielding, 1985). Adolescents know that smoking has risks. In one survey 94 percent of the subjects stated that they were aware that smoking is harmful to health (Green, 1980). Yet family role models and social pressures apparently bear more immediate influence than unforeseeable health consequences decades in the future. Teenagers smoke because their parents, siblings, or friends do. They smoke out of boredom, to calm their nerves, for peer acceptance and conformity, and for a feeling of importance and of acting grown up (James, 1978; McAlister, Perry, & Maccoby, 1979).

Could increasing participation in physical activities help prevent this trend? Most studies have indicated that smoking has an adverse effect on exercise performance, which could serve as a motive to quit smoking for those committed to athletic excellence (Shaver, 1972). In a study of Navy volunteers enlisted for underwater demolition training, Biersner, Gunderson, & Rahe (1972) reported that smoking habits correlated negatively with physical fitness and sports interest. Cross-sectional studies in adults generally indicate a lower incidence of smokers among those who are highly physically active (Rigotti et al., 1983), but completing a physical training program has not necessarily resulted in a decrease in smoking (Bonanno & Lies, 1974).

A questionnaire study of 2,831 Finnish children indicated that more active children smoked significantly less than those who were inactive (Laakso, Rimpela, & Telema, 1979). Shaver (1972) reported that physical fitness scores were lower for high school female smokers than for non-smoking controls. It is not clear, of course, whether this means that smokers are not interested in athletics or whether physical activity reduces the need or desire to smoke.

Athletic participation may play an important role in antismoking strategies aimed at youth. Regular exercise may stimulate improved motivation for health-oriented behaviors and block the motivation to smoke by serving as an alternative means of gaining peer support and improved self-confidence. Many of the personality characteristics that lead to teenage smoking (a need to feel grown up, desire for peer acceptance, release from boredom) might equally well be satisfied by sports participation.

SUMMARY

Based on epidemiological and experimental data, it is possible to confidently make some rather sweeping generalizations about the effect of human behavior on atherosclerotic vascular disease.

- *If* dietary lipids were limited sufficiently to decrease serum cholesterol by 8 percent, the risk of ischemic heart disease would fall by 20 percent (Lipid Research Clinics Program, 1984).
- *If* obesity could be controlled, the incidence of systemic hypertension would be halved (Tyroler et al., 1975).
- *If* everyone consumed only the amount of salt required by the body, hypertension might be eliminated altogether (Page, 1980a).
- *If* no one smoked, the mortality from coronary artery disease would be reduced by one third, saving 170,000 lives per year (Fielding, 1985).

The evidence cited in this chapter suggests that regular physical activity contributes to these efforts and perhaps even has a primary effect of its own. The signal to health caretakers of children is a strong one: Getting youngsters started early in habits of regular exercise can provide a lifelong means of helping to prevent chronic cardiovascular disease in adulthood.

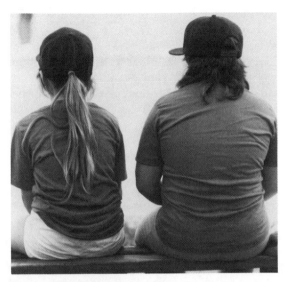

CHAPTER 7

Obesity and Physical Activity

Trying to understand childhood obesity is a "trying" experience. This condition has been termed "the most serious nutritional disease in the United States" (Dietz, 1983, p. 676) as well as "the leading chronic pediatric disorder" (Ward & Bar-Or, 1986, p. 44). Yet there is no agreement on its definition, the affliction having been described as "undefinable" by several authors (Williams, 1986), nor on how it can best be identified. The laws of thermodynamics notwithstanding, the cause of obesity is not at all obvious. Fat children may consume more food than lean individuals, which conforms to popular opinion (Waxman & Stunkard, 1980), but then again, they may eat less (Thompson, Jarvie, Lahey, & Cureton, 1982). Likewise, obese subjects have been reported to exhibit degrees of physical activity less than or similar to those of the non-obese (Bullen, Reed, & Mayer, 1964; Stunkard & Pestka, 1962). The treatment of the obese child is equally controversial: "There is no reason to believe that there is any theoretical upper limit to the amount of weight which can be lost by sufficiently prolonged dietary restriction" (Garrow, 1986, p. 68). But "dietary counseling, as practiced, is rather ineffective in the long run" (Ylitalo, 1981, p. 24). All agree, however, that reported long-term results of treatment by any method are "dismal."

The relative contributions of heredity and environmental factors to the obese state are no more clear. "The fact that there are 'obese families' gives a misleading impression that genetic factors are of decisive importance" (Simic, 1980, p. 8), but "the importance of the genetic component should not be underestimated" (Mayer, 1980, p. 207). Can an obese child be expected to become an obese adult? The Committee on Nutrition of the Mother and Preschool Child of the Food and Nutrition Board (1978) concluded that there was no convincing evidence that the obese child was at risk for becoming an obese adult; however, Abraham and Nordsieck (1960) reported that over two thirds of overweight teenagers carry their obesity into adulthood.

Studies of fat-cell development suggest that there are critical periods during the pediatric years that determine the risk for future obesity. These points in time would serve as logical targets for preventive efforts to reduce the chances of adult obesity. But when are they? Suggestions from multiple authors have included the last trimester of pregnancy, the first 6 months of life, before ages 2 to 4 years, age 6, the preadolescent years (ages 7 to 11), and adolescence (Knittle, 1972; Williams, 1986). From these data, it appears that only the 5-year-old child rests (transiently) in an oasis of low-risk fat security!

The primary care physician is thus faced with managing a frequently occurring, medically significant condition with vague definition and diagnostic criteria, obscure etiology, and uncertain natural history. But out of this confusion must come a rational approach to a problem that appears to be growing in the pediatric population and that, if left unchecked, diminishes quality of life and increases morbidity and mortality during the adult years. Despite the frustrations of dealing with these patients, it remains essential that continued efforts be made to find effective means of both preventing and treating childhood obesity. Considering the nearly intractable nature of obesity once it is fully established, the key to success may lie in impeding, before they get started, the energy imbalances that lead to fat accumulation. The role of regular exercise and prudent diet during the growing years may be more importantly one of preventing rather than treating childhood obesity.

THE MEANING OF OBESITY

The tendency for human beings to accumulate fat is not, of course, altogether sinister, at least in terms of evolutionary process. The ability of both plants and animals to store reserve energy substrates for the lean times when food supplies are short has a clear-cut survival value. Plants accumulate carbohydrate (thankfully, for we would otherwise be deprived of such items as apples, raisin bran, and French fries), while animals' mobility requires the more compact, calorie-dense stores provided by fats. The fact that this fat-storing capacity is hardly appropriate for most humans living in affluent societies has unfortunately had little impact on the physiological mechanisms of fat deposition.

Development of Fat Stores

The human fetus contains virtually no fat until the middle of gestation, but adipose tissue then grows rapidly to account for 16 percent of body weight at delivery. The curve of absolute body fat content is slowly progressive throughout childhood and adolescence but after age 6 is always higher on the average in females. Relative body fat remains essentially stable at approximately 15 percent in boys from age 6 to puberty; thereafter it decreases by 2 or 3 percent with growth of muscle tissue. Percent body fat progressively rises in girls from 15 to 20 percent before the age of 10 years to 20 or 25 percent during adolescence (Burmeister, 1966; Parizkova, 1977).

The problem of obesity begins when the control mechanisms for this process of fat deposition go awry. The mechanism causing this miscalculation appears to persist; that is, obese children tend to become increasingly obese with time. Just how much extra adipose tissue qualifies an individual as obese depends on the means of assessing body fat content. Body densitometry by underwater weighing has been regarded as the "gold standard" for determinating relative fat content, but variability in tissue densities with growth weaken the validity of this technique in children. In addition, many children cannot cooperate with the motionless underwater breathholding necessary for underwater weighing. Adolescents with body fat over 20 percent in boys and 25 percent in girls have been classified as obese by this method (Huenemann, Hampton, Behnke, Shapiro, & Mitchell, 1974).

Body-Fat Indices

Four indices of body fatness have been commonly used in the clinical setting:

• Body weight
• Body mass index (BMI)
• Skinfold thickness
• Direct observation

Body weight is an easy, precise measure, and values greater than 120 percent of the average expected for height and sex have been considered indicative of obesity in many studies (Williams, 1986). The difficulty here is that extra weight for height can be fat or muscle, and it may therefore be "impossible to gauge the presence or extent of obesity by comparing a set of numbers to a table of weights and heights" (Mayer, 1980, p. xi). Judging responses to dietary–exercise treatment programs by this method is also fraught with potential error, because significant fat can be lost and muscle mass gained with little change in overall body weight.

The use of the **body mass index (BMI)**, or weight/height^2, is based on the finding in adults that height is independent of obesity and that this index correlates reasonably well with other measures of body fat. When weight is expressed as kilograms and height as meters, a BMI of over 30 has been associated with significant obesity in both adult men and women (Thomas, McKay, & Cutlip, 1976). The BMI has also been reported to correlate with subscapular skinfold thickness in children (Rollard-Cachera et al., 1982), but Roche (1984) argued against its use in this age group because there is a tendency toward tall stature in obese youngsters (Hampton, Huenemann, Shapiro, Mitchell, & Behnke, 1966).

Determination of **skinfold thickness** by calipers provides a localized estimate of subcutaneous fat, which has been used as an index of total body adiposity. Standardized techniques and norms for scapular and triceps measurements in children have been presented in several reports. Generally values above the 75th to 95th percentile are considered indicative of obesity (American Alliance for Health, Physical Education, Recreation and Dance, 1980; Parizkova, 1977; Ross, Dotson, Gilbert, & Katz, 1985; Tanner & Whitehouse, 1975). The precision of this technique for determining body fat is uncertain, however, particularly in children (Committee on Nutrition, 1968). Variability in fat distribution, skin thickness and compressibility, and limb length may significantly affect skinfold measurements independent of body fat. In a lean individual, for instance, the dermal thickness may account for over half of the skinfold measurement; the proportion will be less in the obese. In addition, the ability to accurately and reproducibly measure skinfold thickness is difficult in subjects with marked obesity. If skinfolds are used to judge obesity, the thickness value itself should be used as the criterion, because insufficient data are available to reliably convert these measurements into relative body fat.

That leaves **direct observation**, which in the end may be the simplest way to effectively identify the obese individual (Dietz, 1983; Heald, 1972; Mayer, 1980). The ability of the physician to diagnose obesity because the patient "looks fat" correlates well with skinfold measurements (Rauh, Schumsky, & Witt, 1967). This method will be of little help, however, in assessment of the amount of body fat with time or response to therapy.

By these several techniques it has generally been estimated that significant obesity affects from 10 to 25 percent of children in the United States (Dietz, 1983; Ward & Bar-Or, 1986). As Heald (1972) has emphasized, "Although the statistical data are crude, there is substantial evidence that a significant amount of obesity is found at every age in both sexes, no matter how it is defined" (p. 103).

Some information suggests, as well, that childhood obesity is on the rise (Figure 7.1). Skinfold measurements in the National Children and Youth Fitness Study in 1985 indicated an increase in subcutaneous fat since the early 1970s (Safrit, 1986). Other studies have indicated gains in body weight and fatness in European children over recent 7- to 20-year time spans (Durnin, Lonergan, Good, & Ewan, 1974; Sunnegardh, Bratteby, Hagman, Samuelson, & Sjolin, 1986). Interestingly, these and other reports indicate that average caloric intake in these populations has *decreased* over the same time period, a trend attributed to (undocumented) lower levels of habitual physical activity (Rasanen, Ahola, Kara, & Uhari, 1985; Whitehead, Paul, & Cole, 1982).

THE HEALTH IMPLICATIONS OF OBESITY

It has often been claimed that unless body fat is truly extreme there are no significant medical complications of obesity during the childhood years. Morbid obesity in children and adolescents can be associated with musculoskeletal problems (e.g., slipped capital femoral epiphysis) as well as cardiopulmonary complications (e.g., respiratory failure, pulmonary hypertension), but these are unusual. Bar-Or (1983) pointed out, however, the morbidity that hypoactivity might create for these patients, noting that a diminished level of physical activity is not uncommonly the *result* of obesity as much as it may be a cause. The hypoactive, overweight child becomes indifferent to physical exercise, resulting in even greater degrees of obesity and, in turn, an increasingly sedentary lifestyle.

Low Physical Fitness Levels

Depressed levels of physical fitness are consequently typical of obese children, which could be the result of sedentary habits (deconditioning) or

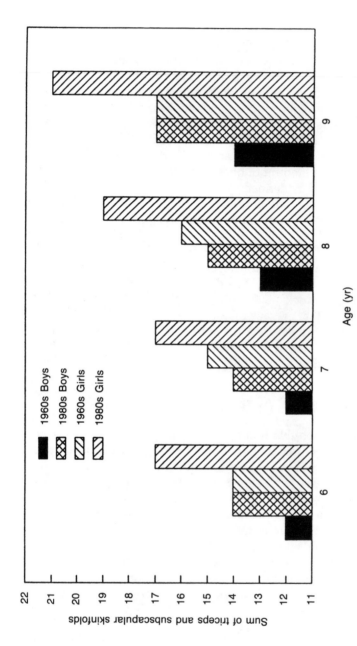

Figure 7.1 Comparison of sum of median triceps and subscapular skinfold measurements between the 1960's and 1980's. *Note.* From "The National Children and Youth Fitness Study II. Changes in the Body Composition of Children" by J.G. Ross, R.R. Pate, T.G. Lohman, and G.M. Christenson, 1987. This article is reprinted with permission from the *Journal of Physical Education, Recreation & Dance,* November/December, 1987, p. 77. The *Journal* is a publication of the American Alliance for Health, Physical Education, Recreation and Dance, 1900 Association Drive, Reston, VA 22091.

the extra work load imposed by excessive body fat (Epstein, Koeske, Zidansek, & Wing, 1983). Fitness indicators with exercise testing can be improved following weight loss in obese subjects (Epstein et al., 1983; Sprynarova & Parizkova, 1965; Ylitalo, 1981).

Medical Risks

The medical dangers of obesity increase with age. Simonson (1982) listed 26 conditions associated with excessive body fat during the adult years, including coronary artery disease, hypertension, diabetes mellitus, arthritis, and kidney disease. Weinhaus (1969) calculated that life expectancy is decreased 1 year for each 5 lb above ideal body weight. Even during childhood, obesity clusters in individuals with other risk factors for coronary artery disease, particularly systemic hypertension and detrimental serum lipid profiles (Aristimuno, Foster, Voors, Srinivasan, & Berenson, 1984; Williams, 1986; Ylitalo, 1981).

The medical risks to obese children can therefore be defined by the extent to which the children can be expected to carry their obesity into adulthood. Consequently a good deal of research has examined this question, and the results reveal a fairly consistent picture: In general, the older the patient, and probably the greater the obesity, the more likely that obesity will persist. Only equivocal data relate birthweight with later obesity, and most studies have failed to reveal any connection between the two (Heald, 1972). At the later end of the growing years, adolescent obesity is a stronger predictor of adiposity in adulthood. Abraham and Nordsieck (1960) and Lloyd, Wolff, and Whelen (1961) reported that up to 80 percent of adolescents in their early teens will sustain their obesity in the young and middle-aged adult years.

There appears to be a graded risk between these age extremes. Most fat infants do not go on to become fat young adults, but there is a two- to threefold-increased chance that this will happen to an obese baby compared to a lean infant (Charney, Goodman, McBride, Lyon, & Pratt, 1976). Forty percent of overweight British 11-year-olds were still obese at age 26 in the report by Stark, Atkins, Wolff, and Douglas (1981). Most adult obesity (about two thirds) does not have its origins in the pediatric years, however (Mullins, 1958).

Psychosocial Effects

Psychosocial consequences of obesity may powerfully affect the self-image and social standing of the overweight child during critical phases of emotional development. Studies evaluating the influence of obesity on mental health portray a disturbing picture of depression, low self-esteem, poor body image, and social isolation (Allon, 1980; Williams, 1986). The failure to achieve success with dieting and other therapeutic interven-

tions may potentiate these negative feelings, and the inability to participate in physical activity and discrimination by peers and adults are further
additive influences. The morbidity of obesity during the childhood years
from these psychological issues should not be underestimated.

ENERGY BALANCE
AND THE ETIOLOGY OF OBESITY

The laws of thermodynamics dictate that the energy entering a system
minus the energy leaving equals the energy stored in the system. Which,
applied to humans, means that food energy consumed must be equally
expended, or the excess will be stored as body fat (Figure 7.2). Obesity
must then ultimately be considered a mismatch of energy-in versus
energy-out, a statement that Mayer (1980) has termed "purely tautologi-
cal." A hasty trip to the dictionary reveals that Mayer finds this account
to be logically true but empty of any useful content because it sheds no
light on the etiology of this imbalance. But the concept *is* a useful one,
for it signifies that somewhere between caloric intake and the several factors responsible for energy expenditure lies an answer (or answers) to
why people become fat—and presumably a means of both preventing and
treating obesity.

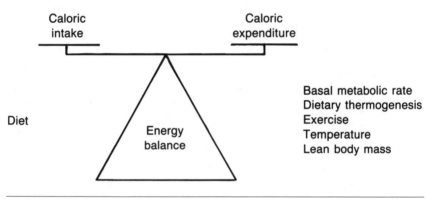

Figure 7.2 Contributions to energy balance.

In the search for the "lesion" in the energy equation that leads to
obesity, researchers have been hampered by two major obstacles. First,
studies of groups of obese and non-obese individuals are made long after
the event that initially triggered the energy in–out imbalance. These
studies may, in fact, be assessing features that either maintain or are the
result of obesity rather than its cause. Second, measurement techniques
for investigating energy intake and expenditure are too crude to reveal
those small mismatches that over time lead to fat accumulation. Wilmore

(1983) pointed out that it would be impossible, using current methods, to detect a net daily change of 100 cal, yet such an imbalance, when consistent, would yield a 10-lb weight gain or loss over a year's time.

Energy Intake

In the popular image, the obese individual is a gormandizer whose excess poundage reflects a certain lack of willpower to control his or her appetite. But do obese individuals really eat more than lean subjects? Certainly there appears to be the well-recognized phenomenon of the thin person who "can eat anything" without gaining weight while with others "everything turns to fat." Studies of caloric consumption in non-obese compared to obese subjects have produced conflicting results. Early studies in overweight children did not reveal an excess of food intake in obese youngsters (Huenemann et al., 1974; Johnson, Burke, & Mayer, 1956; Stefanik, Heald, & Mayer, 1959); these relied on self-reporting questionnaires, however, a method that may result in underestimation in fat subjects.

Waxman and Stunkard (1980) reported direct observation of eating patterns in four families, each with an obese child and a non-obese brother within 2 years of each other. In each case, the obese children were served more food, consumed more calories, and ate more quickly. Pi-Sunyer and Woo (1985) cautioned against drawing conclusions from studies in which food intake is carefully weighed and portioned, however, because the very act of measuring food intake may alter caloric consumption by the study's subjects.

Thompson et al. (1982) reviewed studies of caloric intake in obese subjects of all ages and could find only 2 of 13 who reported that the obese ate more than non-obese individuals. Based on these investigations of *established* obesity there is little to support the idea that specific eating habits are of primary importance in causing or maintaining excessive body fat (Dahlkoetter, Callahan, & Lindton, 1979).

Energy Expenditure

On the energy-out side of the equation, basal metabolic rate (BMR), thermogenic effect of food (specific dynamic action), and physical activity all contribute to caloric expenditure. An average 70-kg man who lies in bed all day will use up approximately 1,650 cal (the basal metabolic rate). With eating, the metabolic rate rises, presumably due to chemical reactions involved in the digestion and absorption of food. Typically this thermogenic effect of eating contributes another 200 cal to the daily total. If another 200 to 400 cal is added as the energy cost of sitting in a chair all day, the expected expenditure for doing nothing is about 2,000 cal for the adult male (Guyton, 1966).

Energy expenditure above this level is determined by the level of physical activity (Table 7.1). Exercise can dramatically increase metabolic rate, from 50 times normal for a few seconds of vigorous activity to 20 times baseline for exercise that can be sustained for several minutes. A person involved in heavy labor over the course of a day usually expends 6,000 to 7,000 calories, or 3.5 times the BMR. Through choice of daily exercise, then, an individual has the ability to substantially affect total energy outgo.

Table 7.1 The Influence of Physical Activity on Caloric Expenditure for a 70-kg Man

Activity	Caloric expenditure (kcal/hr)
Lying in bed	70
Playing violin	180
Playing basketball	500
Soldier marching	600
Running marathon	1,020
Lumberjacking	1,320

Do obese individuals exercise less, or expend fewer calories in physical activity, than the non-obese? Again inadequate methodology prevents a full answer to the question. The best way to measure energy output—by measuring heat production or oxygen consumption in laboratory chambers—is obviously unsatisfactory. Field methods (such as heart rate monitoring or mechanical motion devices) may be too imprecise to measure differences in caloric expenditure that would differentiate the obese from the non-obese. Questionnaires, interviews, and activity diaries are even more likely to be inaccurate.

With these pitfalls in mind, the evidence can be examined. Most observational studies have indicated that obese subjects are less active than their lean peers (Thompson et al., 1982). Bullen et al. (1964) filmed obese and control girls during volleyball and other sports participation and reported significantly lower levels of activity in the overweight subjects. Corbin & Pletcher (1968) used similar techniques to show a correlation between skinfold thickness and activity in fifth-grade students. Other studies using pedometer readings or subject recall have indicated no differences in the activity levels of obese and non-obese subjects (Stefanik et al., 1959; Stunkard & Pestka, 1962; Wilkinson, Parkin, Pearlson, Strong, & Sykes, 1977). When Waxman and Stunkard (1980) observed obese children and their non-obese siblings, the overweight subjects were less active at home but not at school. However, when caloric cost of their activities was estimated, the obese children demonstrated a greater energy expenditure (because the caloric cost of a given activity is greater for obese subjects). From these data it is difficult to conclude whether obese children expend fewer, the same, or more calories during daily physical activity.

The accumulation of adipose tissue in obese children would be neatly explained if their BMR were lower. There are little convincing data to that effect, however. Overweight individuals tend to have *higher* BMRs (because of greater amounts of fat and lean body mass), but values are generally equal to those for non-obese subjects when corrected for body surface area (Bray, 1983; Dietz, 1983). Ravussin et al. (1988) demonstrated, however, that metabolic rate at rest could be used to predict body weight gain over a 4-year follow-up in a group of adult Native Americans. Katch, Marks, & Rocchini (1983) reported lower absolute and surface-area-related BMR in adolescent males and females who had twice the percent body fat as control subjects.

If overweight children do not obviously eat more or exercise less, could their energy imbalance result from a greater energy efficiency? This phenomenon is observed in animals, which can be selectively bred to maintain weight on less dietary intake (Ravussin et al., 1988). Furthermore, when obese animals are fed the same diet as lean animals, the obese gain more weight (Bray, 1983). Attractive as this explanation is, similar proof that obese humans have superior energy efficiency has been elusive. Bray (1983) reviewed several potential means by which biochemical processes may be more or less energy efficient, but there is no clear documentation that these are important in causing human obesity. A number of studies have indicated that thermic response to food is greater in lean than in obese persons (Pittet, Chappius, Acheson, DeTechtermann, & Jequier, 1976; Shetty, Jung, James, Barrand, & Callingham, 1981). These findings bear significance, because thermogenic effect may add up to 40 percent of BMR during the hours after food consumption. They imply that given the same caloric intake and physical activity, the obese subject will have extra energy for storage compared to the lean subject who burns off these calories in response to the digestion of food. But— the reader should be prepared for this by now—others have failed to document differences in the thermogenic responses to a meal between obese and non-obese individuals (Bradfield & Jourdan, 1973).

Pre-Obesity Studies

The reports cited all suffer from having examined potential etiological factors after the fact of established obesity, leading others to attempt to analyze energy imbalance early in life before the onset of fat accumulation. Rose and Mayer (1968) measured dietary intake, triceps skinfold thickness, and physical activity in babies from the newborn period to age

6 months. They found that extremely thin infants exhibited significantly greater activity levels while consuming less food than their obese counterparts. This pattern, similar to that reported in adolescents (Johnson et al., 1956), thus appeared to be fixed at or shortly after birth, suggesting a genetic predisposition to obesity as well as a primary role of physical inactivity.

Roberts, Savage, Coward, Chew, and Lucas (1988) recorded energy expenditure, postprandial metabolic rate, and caloric intake in infants shortly after birth and related findings to weight gain in the first year of life. Fifty percent of babies with overweight mothers become obese (weight for length greater than 90th percentile), compared to none of the infants whose mothers were non-obese. Among those babies who were obese at age 1 year, the weight, skinfold thickness, thermogenic response to food, and caloric intake were not different at age 3 months from that for babies who were eventually non-obese. However, the daily energy expenditure at 3 months of age was 20.7 percent lower in those who became overweight. The authors concluded that reduced physical activity may be a significant factor in determining weight gain in the first year of life.

Realizing that a child with obese parents is at high risk for obesity, Griffiths and Payne (1976) examined energy intake and expenditure in two groups of 4- to 5-year-old children, one with obese parents and one without. No significant differences in height, weight, or percent body fat was observed between the two sets of children, but those with an obese parent were less active and had a lower daily caloric intake.

These studies of subjects early in life suggest the possibility that physical inactivity is of primary importance in excessive fat accumulation. They do not, of course, provide any explanation of the ultimate development of childhood and adult obesity.

The Fat-Cell Number/Size Hypothesis

The possibility that overfeeding during infancy and other critical points of childhood might cause obesity arose during the 1970s from evolving concepts of fat-cell development (Knittle, 1972). Based principally on animal studies, this idea has not received a full examination in humans, and its methodology has been questioned (Hammar, 1980; Ylitalo, 1981). But it does provide a model that might be useful in the prevention of long-term obesity.

According to this concept, body fat accumulates by an increase in fat-cell size or number. Thus overweight individuals can have *hypertrophic* (engorgement of fat cells) or *hyperplastic* (proliferation of cells) obesity. Which process causes a person to become obese is important in terms of potential reversibility and response to therapy, because once fat cells are created they cannot be eliminated. Hyperplastic obesity is therefore typically much more resistant to treatment, as obesity is more or less fixed by the increased number of cells.

Obesity during childhood is characteristically hyperplastic in nature, and these fat cells are created particularly at times of rapid growth (during the last trimester of gestation, the first 2 or 3 years of life, and at adolescence). Cellular proliferation might be decreased or eliminated by nutritional intervention at these points, specifically by the avoidance of overfeeding (Knittle & Ginsberg-Fellner, 1980). These ideas have stimulated dietary recommendations for infants that hopefully will suppress fat-cell hyperplasia: an emphasis on breast feeding (during which a baby is presumably more likely to self-limit intake), avoidance of forced bottle feeding, and delayed introduction of solid foods. There is currently no evidence, however, that any of these measures relate to the incidence of future obesity (Wolman, 1984).

Genetics Versus Environment

Obesity clearly runs in families. Mayer (1980) reported that a child's chance of becoming obese is only 7 percent if neither parent is obese, 40 percent if one parent is obese, and 80 percent if both are. The extent to which this clustering is genetically or environmentally determined has been vigorously debated (Mayer, 1980; Simic, 1980).

Stunkard, Foch, and Hrubec (1986) studied a large population of monozygotic adult twins and reported an estimate of BMI heritability of .84. This compares favorably with values of .64 to .88 in other studies and led the authors to "suggest that human fatness is under substantial genetic control" (p. 51). Mayer (1980) noted that studies indicating close correlations of obesity within families do not hold when adopted children and their adoptive parents are examined. Other supportive evidence for the importance of heredity comes from studies indicating a strong genetic influence on BMR and familial aggregation of energy expenditure (Fontaine et al., 1985; Ravussin et al., 1988). Others have been less convinced of the extent of genetic determination of obesity, citing the influence of social factors on fatness as one example of the strength of environmental influences (Ylitalo, 1981). Then, too, there is the fascinating observation that fat pet-owners tend to have fat pets (Mason, 1970).

THE EFFECTS OF EXERCISE ON ENERGY BALANCE

The control and prevention of obesity must by necessity involve changes in diet and exercise, these being the most easily modifiable factors in the energy-balance equation. Attempts to force low-calorie diets on children and adolescents have been highly unsuccessful in achieving long-term weight loss, and there is serious concern that such diets may interfere with normal growth processes (Williams, 1986). Exercise may be helpful in both regards. Increasing physical activity serves as a valuable complement to dietary restriction, not only in expending additional calories but also by acting to counteract loss of lean body mass, decline in BMR, and other disadvantageous responses to caloric deprivation (see the boxed information). In fact, as the following information shows, regular exercise may favorably affect all components of the energy in–out equation.

Potential Effects of Exercise on Obese Children

- Decreased percent body fat
- Increased lean body mass
- Potentiated dietary thermogenesis
- Reduced blood pressure
- Improved cardiovascular fitness
- Benefits to psychosocial health
- Prevention of obesity (unconfirmed)

Direct Energy Expenditure

Regular daily physical activities account for approximately half of all calories expended, so increasing exercise can significantly influence the energy-out side of the ledger. How much extra activity does it take to effect meaningful weight loss? A pound of fat is equivalent to 3,500 cal, and that turns out to be the number burned by chopping wood for 10 hr, walking for a day and a half, or playing volleyball for 32 hr (Katch & McArdle, 1983). The caloric "debt" of a large hamburger, french fries, and a milk shake can be erased by running about 9 mi. Which all seems like a great deal of work for little profit and would certainly be very discouraging to a child 30 lb overweight setting out to lose body fat. Fortunately, the effect of exercise on caloric expenditure is accumulative, and with time smaller amounts of activity can add up to significant weight loss. For instance, walking 1 mi a day or running 2 mi three times a week—both achievable goals—can account for 10 lb of fat over a year's time. Add to this the effect of limited caloric restriction, and the prospects for successful weight loss become realistic, particularly if the physician and patient have the patience to view the treatment of obesity as a long-term project. Fat accumulates by small disturbances in energy balance over many years. The undoing of this condition may be best accomplished by the reverse—creating small negative energy imbalances over time with exercise and dietary manipulations of modest proportions that create no physical discomfort or major changes in eating habits.

The exercise for shrinking adipose tissue must rely on aerobic metabolism for its energy source, because fats are not utilized as a fuel in glycolytic anaerobic pathways. Walking, swimming, running, cycling, and cross-country skiing at intensities that can be endured for at least 20 to 30 minutes are most appropriate for weight loss. It should be appreciated, however, that it is not necessary to satisfy exercise criteria for improving cardiovascular fitness in order to reduce body fat. In fact, the intensity and duration of activities required to improve $\dot{V}O_2$max might prove overly fatiguing to the obese subjects, perhaps disillusioning such individuals and leading them to drop out from exercise programs altogether.

Exercise appears to reduce body weight by removing fat from cells rather than decreasing the number of adipocytes (Björntorp, 1978). The ability of physical activity to achieve weight loss may therefore be dependent on the number of fat cells; that is, the patient with hyperplastic obesity is less likely to respond to treatment than the individual with hypertrophic obesity.

Besides the energy expended during exercise, a bout of physical activity may increase the BMR for several hours after exercise has stopped, adding to the total energy cost. A rise in BMR as high as 25 percent for 15 hr after strenuous exercise has been reported (Ylitalo, 1981). The cause of this extended elevation of metabolic rate is unknown. Garrow (1986) argued that this benefit is not accrued by overweight patients because "that exercise level which obese subjects might be able to tolerate has no detectable effect on metabolic rate a few minutes after the exercise has ceased, although there may be a prolonged effect on metabolic rate after more severe exercise continued to exhaustion in well-trained subjects" (p. 71). Thompson et al. (1982) notes, however, that no study testing the differential effects of exercise intensity and duration on postexercise metabolic rate had been performed; based on a report by deVries and Gray (1963), they concluded that light exercise in an adult would produce a rise in metabolic rate after exercise of approximately 40 to 50 cal.

Exercise and Appetite

Does physical activity stimulate appetite? The benefits of running 2 mi would be eliminated if afterward the hungry child balanced the effort with a milk shake and fries. Skeptics have frequently cited this compensatory effect of increased appetite as an argument against the utility of exercise for preventing or treating obesity. A review of the experimental data on this question reveals, however, that such a conclusion is unwarranted: Regular exercise may or may not suppress appetite in obese subjects, but in general any increases in caloric intake that do occur will not match those expended by exercise activities (Epstein & Wing, 1980).

In lean subjects, energy expenditure is closely matched by caloric intake, although that balance may take several days to become apparent (Edholm, Fletcher, Widdowson, & McCane, 1955; Epstein & Wing, 1980). That is, there appear to be prominent control mechanisms in these individuals whereby the body "defends" its usual composition (Pi-Sunyer & Woo, 1985). On the other hand, obese patients do not typically raise their food consumption sufficiently to balance energy losses from exercise. Because of the imprecision of measuring physical activity and food intake, this conclusion has been drawn recognizing that body weight declines in exercise programs for obese subjects when calories are not restricted. In their meta-analysis of 16 such studies, Epstein and Wing (1980) discovered that although exercise without planned diets resulted in weight loss, the extent of that loss was less than expected by the exercise performed. This phenomenon, which was greater in the more obese subjects, could be explained by either a noncompensatory increase in food intake or a decrease in physical activities outside of the exercise program.

Woo, Garrow, and Pi-Sunyer (1984) confirmed the dissociation of physical activity and caloric intake in the obese by careful measurements of overweight adult women in a metabolic ward setting. The subjects were sedentary for one period and for two other periods walked on a treadmill to raise daily energy expenditure by 10 and 25 percent. No significant increase in caloric intake was observed with the added levels of physical activity.

Increased Lean Body Mass

The relationship of exercise and lean body mass (LBM) has particular importance for the management of childhood obesity. The significance of LBM to energy expenditure lies in the fact that the metabolic rate of nonfat tissue (particularly muscle) is triple that of adipose tissue. At the same time, maintenance of LBM is essential for the normal growth and development of children, including those with excess adiposity. Strategies for weight reduction that diminish LBM in addition to fat are therefore inappropriate during the growing years. Instead, methods to reduce body fat while *increasing* LBM in obese children will pay extra energy dividends by raising the basal metabolic rate.

During growth, dietary protein requirements are increased, and dietary restriction may thereby result in a catabolic effect on LBM. The obese adolescents studied by Brown, Klish, Hollander, Campbell, and Forbes (1983) demonstrated a decline in lean body mass that accounted for

36 percent of weight loss after institution of a very low-calorie diet. Decreases in LBM can be observed in obese teenagers even when diets are rich in protein (Heald & Hunt, 1965). Although the effects of these changes on growth have not been evaluated, sufficient concern exists to caution against severe caloric restriction in children, particularly any that would create a weight loss of greater than 1 lb per week (Williams, 1986).

Physical activity, on the other hand, tends to increase muscle mass while fat is burned for energy. In studies where diet and exercise are combined, the loss of LBM is approximately 5 percent; if physical activity is used alone to treat obesity, LBM usually increases (Eisenmann, 1986). From the standpoint of preventing the catabolic effects of dieting, then, exercise should play a key role in the management of the overweight child (Table 7.2).

Table 7.2 Exercise Versus Dietary Effects in Control of Obesity

Effect	Exercise	Diet
Weight loss	Yes	Yes
Decrease in fat	Yes	Yes
Lean body mass	Gain	Loss
Growth retardation	No	Possible
Improved exercise fitness	Yes	No
Weight-loss rate	Slow	Fast
Basal metabolic rate	Possible increase	Possible decrease

Limiting Dietary-Reduced Basal Metabolic Rate

Caloric restriction characteristically depresses the BMR, a response that may originally have been a survival mechanism for enduring times when less food was available. Whatever its evolutionary roots, this phenomenon is an anathema to the obese patient and is probably partly responsible for the high long-term failure rate of dietary approaches to obesity. The fall in BMR with dieting appears to be independent of changes in body fat or LBM. It could be the result of the decreased concentrations of thyroid hormones or the reduced activity of the sympathetic nervous system that occur with fasting (Bray, 1983).

Although not supported by experimental data, it has been suggested that regular exercise tempers the reduction of BMR with dieting in the obese patient (Thompson et al., 1982). This makes physiological sense, considering that exercise increases or maintains lean body mass.

Increasing Dietary Thermogenesis

The increased caloric expenditure following consumption of food may be augmented by exercise. Studies examining this question have produced conflicting results. In one of the few reports in which both lean and obese subjects were evaluated, Segal and Gutin (1983) showed that body composition may influence this effect. Thermic effect of food at rest was not different in obese and lean adult women, but eating followed by exercise potentiated the thermic effect of food only for the lean subjects. Conversely, there is suggestive evidence that low-calorie diets may suppress the thermic effect of eating as well as the BMR (Thompson et al., 1982).

Improved Serum Lipid Profile

Becque, Katch, Rocchini, Marks, & Moorehead (1988) studied serum lipids, blood pressure, and physical fitness before and after treatment of 36 obese adolescents. Subjects were randomly assigned to either a 20-week program of diet therapy and behavior change, these two interventions plus exercise, or a nontreatment control group. Caloric intake was planned to reduce weight by 1 to 2 lb per week. The exercise program consisted of aerobic activities at 60 to 80 percent of maximal heart rate for 15 to 40 min three times a week. Reduction of body fat by approximately 3 percent was observed in both treatment groups. A significant rise in mean HDL-cholesterol (HDL-C) (35.4 to 43.4 mg/dl) and reduction in both systolic and diastolic blood pressure levels were observed only in the subjects who exercised.

Similar results were reported by Sasaki, Shindo, Tanaka, Ando, and Arakawa (1987) in 41 obese 11-year-old children. These youngsters were involved in a 2-year, school-based exercise program consisting of 20 min of running 7 days a week without dietary intervention. After 1 year HDL-C increased 16 percent in the boys and 19 percent in the girls. No changes in serum cholesterol values occurred.

The 14 obese children studied by Widhalm, Maxa, and Zyman (1978) showed a significant decrease in LDL-cholesterol after a 3-week program of caloric restriction and intense physical activity at an obesity camp. HDL-C values, however, did not change. Findings were less impressive in obese Finnish schoolchildren provided a diet–exercise program in an outpatient setting. After 2 years, the total cholesterol had decreased but there were no mean changes in HDL-C for the group (Ylitalo, 1981).

Improved Physical Fitness

Exercise programs may improve physical fitness in obese youths by reducing the fat load, increasing cardiovascular efficiency, allowing more economical locomotion, or decreasing the oxygen cost of ventilation. Golebiowska and Bujnowski (1986) found decreased submaximal heart rates and more rapid recovery rates in 9 to 16-year-old overweight children after 32 weeks of combined exercise and dietary treatment. The 18 obese children reported by Hayashi, Fujino, Shindo, Hiroki, and Arakawa (1987) demonstrated decreased resting heart rates and increased left-ventricular end-diastolic dimension by echocardiography after 1 year of exercise training.

Epstein et al. (1983) found a positive relationship between weight loss and physical fitness (heart rate recovery) in obese children after a 6-month program of diet and unstructured home exercise. Sprynarova and Parizkova (1965) demonstrated that obese boys could increase treadmill endurance time following a 7-week exercise–diet program that resulted in significant weight loss. Changes in $\dot{V}O_2max$ per kilogram of body weight or LBM were not significant, however. The training program of Becque et al. (1988) noted earlier also resulted in no changes in $\dot{V}O_2max$ per kilogram of body weight.

EXERCISE IN THE MANAGEMENT OF CHILDHOOD OBESITY

Extensive experience has demonstrated that exercise can be an effective means of reducing fat in obese children, with or without specific dietary restriction. Most of these reports have involved programs of increased physical activity in the school setting. Ward and Bar-Or (1986) reviewed 13 school-based interventions of regular aerobic exercise lasting from 9 weeks to 18 months. Percent overweight fell in all these published studies, typically 5 to 10 percent, whereas little change was observed in nonexercising control subjects. In some reports, improvement in weight loss was more prominent in the more obese subjects. Only one program introduced structured dietary restriction, although most involved nutrition education as well as behavior counseling. Structured exercise programs for obese children have also been successful in other settings, including summer camps (Sprynarova & Parizkova, 1965; Widhalm et al., 1978), hospitals (Becque et al., 1988; Cecere, 1983; Pena, Barta, Regoly-Merei, & Tichy, 1980), and at home (Epstein et al., 1983; Ylitalo, 1981).

The durability of weight loss following the completion of these programs is considered poor, but it has been examined in only one follow-up study. Seltzer and Mayer (1970) demonstrated slower rates of growth in weight and skinfold measurements in 350 obese students during a 10-month program of exercise, nutrition education, and psychological counseling compared to controls. When these subjects were reevaluated 3 years later, these effects were no longer evident (Mayer, 1980).

Weight loss during exercise programs for obese children is similar to that observed in adults. Numerous short-term studies demonstrate that participants in regular physical activity (without dietary control) can expect to lose body fat, although there is a large variability in this response (Epstein & Wing, 1980). In adult studies, males and subjects who are more obese, for instance, tend to be more successful (Eisenman, 1986). The fat loss in these reports is small (usually about 2 percent of body weight) but is greater if there is concomitant caloric restriction (Björntorp, 1978; Dahlkoetter et al., 1979; Hagan, 1988; Wilmore, 1983).

The relative contributions of dietary restriction and exercise to weight loss in programs for obese children have been examined in three studies. Marks et al. (1986) reported changes in body composition in 51 obese adolescents randomly assigned to exercise and diet, diet alone, and control groups. After 6 months the exercise-and-diet group lost 2.4 percent more body fat than the diet-only subjects, and the controls experienced small gains. Comparable findings were reported by Pena et al. (1980) after an intense 15-day program that involved dietary restriction with and without 2 hr of walking daily plus stair stepping. Percent body fat fell, but the decline was significantly greater in those who were treated with combined diet and exercise compared to diet alone.

These findings indicate an independent effect of weight reduction by exercise that is additive to results obtained by caloric restriction. However, Epstein et al. (1982) found that combined diet and exercise programs produced no greater weight loss than exercise alone over a 17-month period in obese 8- to 12-year-old children.

It should be noted that these studies reporting successful weight loss in children with exercise and/or diet are highly structured, heavily staffed programs that generally do not involve subjects with extreme obesity. In this regard, Garrow (1986) expressed a more pessimistic viewpoint regarding the role of exercise in treating obesity: "Although exercise is most important in the normal range of body weight, it becomes less important with increasingly severe obesity. Above a BMI of 40, obese patients are incapable of exercising enough to affect energy balance or body composition significantly" (p. 72). Nevertheless, Foss, Lampman, and Schteingart (1980) were able to successfully employ a progressive walking-jogging regimen into a treatment program for markedly obese adults (average entry weight 416 pounds). These subjects, who were hospitalized and restricted to a 600-cal intake per day, lost an average of 73 lb over 9 months.

CAN OBESITY BE PREVENTED?

Efforts to sustain long-term weight reduction after treatment for obesity, by *any* method, have not met with a great measure of success (Hammar,

1980). In adults, no more than 20 percent can be expected to maintain initial fat loss on follow-up several years after dietary therapy (Coates & Thoresen, 1978). The outlook for fat children after successful exercise programs is not any brighter (Mayer, 1980). Failure to succeed with these interventions may only add to the obese patient's feelings of inadequate self-worth and poor social confidence.

Prevention sounds like a better idea. But can the processes leading to fat accumulation really be reversed before obesity becomes entrenched? The answer, given the unknown nature and timing of these mechanisms, is "definitely maybe."

The Pessimist's Perspective

The pessimistic perspective is something like this: The tendency toward obesity is controlled principally by immutable hereditary factors that influence fat accumulation through greater degrees of energy efficiency in fat individuals. There is no evidence that overeating is the cause of obesity; instead, physical hypoactivity may serve as a primary mechanism, as observed by Roberts et al. (1988), as early as the first 6 months of life. This physical activity is unlikely to be related to environmental influences. Instead, it is a manifestation of central control mechanisms that regulate energy balance and are not easily influenced by behavior.

A model for this process is observed in studies in which lesions in the ventromedial hypothalamus cause rats to markedly increase food intake and gain excessive body fat. Several months afterward, the food intake normalizes and weight stabilizes at the higher point. In effect, the homeostatic set point for body fat is reset at a greater level (Keesey, 1980).

In humans the body also staunchly defends its fat composition. It is extremely difficult to maintain a weight significantly above or below a person's usual weight. Caloric restriction is interpreted by the body as starvation, with compensatory responses to conserve energy (i.e., a fall in BMR). All this supports the presence of a genetically determined weight-regulatory center in the brain that controls appetite and exercise level to defend against changes in body composition. Therefore, neither preventive nor therapeutic effects are likely to have any long-term effect on reducing body fat.

The Optimist's Outlook

The optimistic view, on the other hand, goes somewhat as follows: Evidence supports efforts early in life to prevent progressive obesity by limiting caloric intake and increasing the level of physical activity. The difficulty in achieving weight loss in the obese individual is determined by the number rather than the size of adipose cells. Interventions early in life to prevent proliferation of adipocytes should effectively forestall progressive fat deposition. Knittle and Ginsberg-Fellner (1980) demonstrated that a combined exercise–diet program in young obese children can stabilize fat-cell number as well as long-term weight gain. Early dietary restriction has also been shown to diminish the number of fat cells in young rats (Knittle & Hirsch, 1968).

Exercise early in life may also prevent future obesity by the same mechanism. Young rats in a regular swimming program during the first month of life have been demonstrated to have lower fat-cell counts than either dieting or control animals (Oscai, Babirak, & Dubach, 1974).

The existence of a set point, or "adipostat," that controls body composition through altering appetite and physical activity is not questioned, but the "immutability" of this point is. In fact, sustained exercise programs could conceivably lower the set point (Katch & McArdle, 1983). As Roberts et al. (1988) pointed out, there is no evidence that increasing the physical activity of their obesity-prone infants would not have prevented eventual gains in body fat.

From this viewpoint, the high failure rate of treatment programs doesn't mean that obesity *can't* be controlled. Rather, this is only indicative that effective therapeutic techniques have yet to be developed. Genetic factors may predispose to obesity, but overeating and hypoactivity are still directly responsible, and these can be modified through changes in lifestyle.

WHY DOES OBESITY THERAPY FAIL?

Many obese individuals will experience early success in treatment programs, but few will sustain their weight loss for any extended period of time. Why? What factors are responsible for this high failure rate? Effective strategies for managing obesity will need to be designed specifically in response to these problems. It makes no sense to persist in methods that have proven fruitless in the past (Coates & Thoresen, 1978). Growing experience in the treatment of obese children and adolescents has identified the following points to consider.

• **Obese young people lose interest in therapy.** Dropout from obesity therapy has been linked with insufficient self-discipline, inadequate time, boredom, discomfort and injuries, and slowness of weight loss (Sheldahl, 1986). Certainly, the ability to maintain interest and conform to a prolonged, disciplined regimen of any type is not characteristic of the pediatric age group. Focusing efforts on obesity treatment in the school setting may alleviate some of these problems.

• **Implementing caloric restriction by itself is ineffective.** Diets don't work; they waste physician time and may create a "failure experience" for the already-tenuous ego structure of the obese child (Coates & Thoresen, 1978). Greater success is achieved through a combined approach of exercise, diet, behavior modification, and education. Physicians play a vital role in the detection, evaluation, and counseling of the obese child, but such a comprehensive approach can seldom be conducted in the office setting.

• **Weight reduction is a family problem.** Neglecting the total family structure to focus only on the child dooms therapeutic interventions. The family provides the food, emotional support, and behavioral role models that intimately determine a child's response to obesity treatment. It is particularly important to appreciate that parenting abilities (such as the strength to set limits) can be limiting factors to successful therapy (Dietz, 1983).

• **Obesity is not a character deficiency.** Viewing obesity as a lack of personal courage or willpower, or as the fault of the parent, will not win the physician any admiration from the obese child and his family, who are already concerned, frustrated, and feeling guilty. As Dietz (1983) has noted, "Although a more compassionate and empathetic approach is no guarantee of success, it is unlikely that therapy will be successful in its absence" (p. 681).

• **Treating obesity is a two-phased process.** Techniques useful for achieving *induction* (initial weight loss) may be different from those for *maintenance* (sustaining fat reduction). Programs aimed only at short-term weight loss have little hope of producing prolonged results. Optimally, weight reduction should be viewed as a long-term project. The youngster who is 40 lb overweight would best plan on reducing weight over years, not weeks or months. In this way the severity of dietary restriction and added physical activity can be kept at acceptable levels that do not interfere significantly with normal lifestyles. Unfortunately, it is not common for children and their parents to comply with such a long-range approach in the absence of observable weight-loss success.

• **Recommendations to "eat less" or "exercise more" will have little impact.** Children and their families require very specific guidelines, presented as simply as possible, if any compliance is to be expected.

ORGANIZING A WEIGHT-REDUCTION PROGRAM

The objective of an obesity therapy program is to introduce balanced interventions of dietary manipulation, aerobic exercise, and behavioral modification, all modest enough to be acceptable to children and adolescents, yet still sufficient to successfully limit or reduce body fat. The creation of realistic weight-loss goals is an important initial step. In adults and older adolescents weight loss up to 2 lb per week is appropriate, but the potential negative effects of caloric restriction on growth has prompted more conservative recommendations for children. A well-balanced nutritional program plus aerobic exercise should not cause weight loss to exceed 1 lb per week in the obese adolescent (Williams, 1986). Before puberty, weight stabilization or even small *gains* in weight are appropriate goals for treating the rapidly growing obese child (Hoerr, 1984; Ylitalo, 1981). This concept needs to be made clear to the parent and child at the onset to prevent unrealistic expectations. Nonetheless, it may be difficult to achieve compliance with dietary or exercise interventions unless some weight loss is achieved.

What is the best way to assess the response to obesity treatment? As noted above, body weight is the parameter most commonly used because it is both convenient and accurate to measure. But body mass is composed of water and muscle as well as adipose tissue. It is not uncommon for weight to decline significantly during the initial phases of an exercise program simply due to loss of body water, and small gains in muscle mass from exercise may partially offset weight reduction in fat. Body weight might not, therefore, be altogether indicative of decrease in fatness in response to exercise activities, particularly in short-term programs, and should be interpreted cautiously. Skinfold and limb-circumference determinations do not offer sufficient precision in most obese subjects to compare body fat on repeated measurements. Underwater weighing for recording body density and percent fat offers greater serial accuracy and reproducibility but is not usually available in the clinical setting.

Obese children typically possess very negative attitudes toward physical activity. By gradually being introduced to enjoyable forms of exercise, these children can lose these opinions, hopefully developing more physically active lifestyles. In this process, obese children begin to feel more confident about their capabilities, and their self-images and sense of self-mastery can improve (Eisenman, 1986). Physical fitness can improve as well, allowing obese children to participate more fully in activities with peers and to gain more social acceptance. Exercise interventions for obesity, therefore, have broader goals and implications than simply helping arrest accelerated gains in body fat.

Although obesity treatment programs have been conducted in various kinds of sites, the advantages offered by the school setting have received increasing attention (Collipp, 1980a; Ward & Bar-Or, 1986). Considering all the problems inherent in sustaining motivation in therapeutic interventions, the school seems to offer the best hope for achieving long-term success. Children are captive subjects 5 days a week, eliminating the problem of dropouts. Transportation by parents to the program is not an issue. School is in session 9 months of the year, providing the opportunity to conduct both induction and maintenance phases with sustained guidance and support for years, not months. Moreover, the personnel and facilities of the school are ideal resources for organizing physical activities and nutritional guidance for obese children. Concern that fat children might suffer from the stigma associated with special classes for the obese does not appear warranted (Brownell & Kaye, 1982). In fact, the organization of these programs in a familiar setting may provide a more comfortable environment than hospital clinics or physicians' offices.

Usually—but perhaps not always—treatment directed by the physician from the office setting appears to be inadequate for the comprehensive approach necessary for optimal obesity management. Time and personnel constraints preclude the necessary degree of nutritional and psychological counseling, exercise prescription, and follow-up assessment. An unstructured exercise program, also, is less likely to be successful than those that are supervised (Rowland, 1986). Beyond recognizing obesity and ruling out its organic causes (such as hypothyroidism and Cushing's syndrome), the physician's role in obesity management might most importantly be to ensure that community resources are made available for treatment of these children. Physicians need to be particularly aware of the existence and potential of obesity treatment programs in the schools (Ward & Bar-Or, 1986).

Types of Exercise

The ideal form of exercise for the obese child would be aerobic, involving high caloric output, no special skills or equipment, little risk for injury or discomfort, and opportunity for socialization (Epstein & Wing, 1980). Endurance activities such as walking, cycling, running, and swimming come closest to meeting this description and have been employed most frequently in weight-loss programs (Sheldahl, 1986).

Walking is perhaps the most frequently recommended exercise for obese subjects. It is convenient, can be performed anywhere, and involves a tolerable degree of intensity and stress. Its major drawback is the time required to expend an acceptable amount of calories compared to more vigorous activities. If done alone, walking can also be very boring. Running is like concentrated walking: The time is shorter and the boredom less, but the trade-off is in greater amounts of stress and fatigue, which may be unacceptable to the overweight individual. Cycling is more non-weight-bearing, with little stress on bones and joints. A stationary cycle ergometer has the advantage of allowing exercise in private as well as during inclement weather. Boredom can be alleviated by placing the ergometer in front of the television set, but local muscle fatigue, heat stress (there is no cooling from convection because of the stationary position), and the discomfort of prolonged sitting may limit acceptance.

Conceptually, swimming is the most ideal form of exercise for the obese patient. It is totally non-weight-bearing, caloric expenditure can be high, and the water offers an excellent mechanism for cooling. The disadvantages are that the individual must possess swimming skills, finding and traveling to a pool may be inconvenient, and obese patients are often embarrassed to be publicly exposed in a swimming suit. Boredom can be prevented by interspersing water games (e.g., polo and basket-ball) and dance with lap swimming (Sheldahl, 1986).

Other forms of exercise generally are ineffective in expending calories for weight loss. Calisthenics are too brief (although they are useful as a warm-up exercise to improve flexibility). Weight lifting and other high-resistance exercises are short-burst, anaerobic activities that cannot be expected to reduce fat, but by increasing muscle bulk (at least beyond puberty) they may be useful in raising body metabolism. Resistance exercises performed with a high number of repetitions may be more useful in burning calories (Katch & McArdle, 1983).

It is important to use great care when selecting an exercise regimen for the obese child. These patients generally do not tolerate physical activity well, they tire easily, both physically and mentally, and if uncomfortable will rapidly become discouraged and drop out of the program. When a start-up exercise regimen is prescribed, it should be remembered that for many patients *any* physical activity may be new.

With this in mind, Epstein et al. (1982) offered an alternative approach to structured exercise for obese children. Instead of prescribing programmed aerobic activities, the authors described changes in daily activity behaviors that increase caloric expenditures. In this study of obese 8- to 12-year-old children, subjects were given instruction on ways to increase body motion in their daily lives, such as walking instead of riding, decreasing reliance on energy-saving devices, and performing errands by walking. Weight changes from this lifestyle program were compared with those achieved by children involved in programmed aerobic exercise. No differences were observed over an 8-week period, but lifestyle subjects maintained weight loss better during a maintenance phase and follow-up.

The Program Plan

With these concepts as background, a realistic program for helping the obese child can be constructed through exercise in combination with diet and psychological support. It must be acknowledged that chances for long-term success are not high, but an optimistic, supportive approach by the physician will provide the best chance of achieving effective weight loss. The following guidelines, based on the contributions of several authors, may be helpful in beginning that process, whether in the office, clinic, camp, or school setting (Bar-Or, 1983; Katch & McArdle, 1983; Lindner, 1980; Walberg & Ward, 1983; Williams, 1986).

Obesity treatment programs begin with an educational session in which the director reviews concepts regarding the origin and treatment of obesity as well as the structure and goals of the program. Ideas presented in this chapter might serve as an appropriate checklist for this discussion, as outlined in the "Patient Education Checklist."

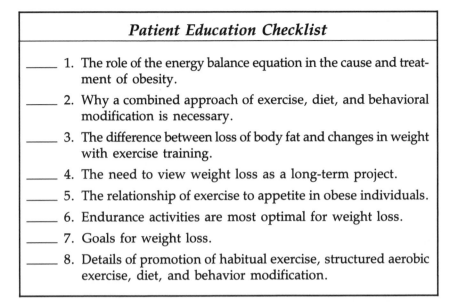

	Patient Education Checklist
_____	1. The role of the energy balance equation in the cause and treatment of obesity.
_____	2. Why a combined approach of exercise, diet, and behavioral modification is necessary.
_____	3. The difference between loss of body fat and changes in weight with exercise training.
_____	4. The need to view weight loss as a long-term project.
_____	5. The relationship of exercise to appetite in obese individuals.
_____	6. Endurance activities are most optimal for weight loss.
_____	7. Goals for weight loss.
_____	8. Details of promotion of habitual exercise, structured aerobic exercise, diet, and behavior modification.

The exercise program is designed to assist weight loss and strengthen confidence. Although high caloric expenditure is desirable, an excessively intense regimen will defeat both purposes. The goal is to introduce gradual but regular changes based on the child's existing habits and preferences. The intensity of exercise prescribed will therefore vary depending on the patient's age, degree of obesity, previous level of physical activity, and motivation. The program planned for a reluctant, very obese 9-year-old will be very different from that for the older adolescent who wishes to lose weight to improve his or her physical appearance.

Before the start of the program, a 3-day diary of regular physical activities recorded by the child can be helpful in the same way that a food-intake diary is useful for nutritional counseling. Opportunities for increasing exercise (such as walking to school) can be identified, and poor habits (such as excessive television watching) corrected.

For the child with low fitness levels and/or significant obesity, the approach outlined by Epstein et al. (1982) of increasing lifestyle activities is a logical initial step, preceding a more structured plan of aerobic activities. These can be listed in a handout similar to the one that follows, that is to be completed and signed by the patient at each weekly visit. This gentle approach will allay the child's fears about the rigors of "working out" and create a more positive attitude toward subsequent programmed exercise.

In the organized phase of an exercise program, a goal of expending 100 cal per day above that of usual activities is reasonable. Exercise sessions five times weekly in conjunction with minimal caloric restriction

Exercise Lifestyle Changes			
	No	Occasionally	Yes
1. For activities during which I used to sit, I stood up.	0	1	2
2. I stood when talking on the telephone.	0	1	2
3. I used stairs instead of an elevator or escalator.	0	1	2
4. I did not ride when I could walk.	0	1	2
5. I did more chores at home.	0	1	2
6. I used a rocking chair while reading, watching TV.	0	1	2
7. I helped someone move heavy objects.	0	1	2
8. I paced while waiting for the bus, etc.	0	1	2
9. I got up and down from my chair more often.	0	1	2
10. I danced or played sports more vigorously.	0	1	2
11. I remembered to "think activity" at every chance.	0	1	2
12. New ideas for activity:			

_____

_____

From "Techniques of Management for the Inactive Obese Child" by P. Lindner, 1980, in P.J. Collipp (Ed.), *Childhood Obesity* (2nd ed.), Littleton, MA: PSG Publishing. Copyright 1980 by PSG Publishing. Adapted by permission.

(100 to 300 cal per day) will result in a weight loss of approximately 1/2 lb per week or 13 lb over a 6-month period. This calculation assumes that the exercise regimen does not lead to a compensatory decline in routine daily physical activities, another reason why excessively fatiguing exercise should be avoided in treatment programs. Such goals do not need to be attained immediately. Starting with 5 to 10 min per day of gentle walking, for instance, might be very appropriate for some patients. Direct observation and feedback by the patient are important in setting guidelines for amount and progression of exercise intensity. Guidelines for prescribing an exercise program for obese children are given in the following box.

Whenever possible it is best to have the patient select the mode of exercise; compliance is much more likely if he or she finds it enjoyable.

Exercise Prescription Guidelines for Obese Children

- Exercise should be part of a multifaceted program that includes nutritional counseling and psychological support.
- Set realistic weight-loss goals. Stabilization of weight (i.e., preventing excessive gains) may be more appropriate than weight loss in children. A decrease of not more than 1 lb per week is advised for most obese adolescents.
- Body weight is the easiest parameter to follow in assessing response to therapy. The influence of loss of body water and gain in muscle mass from exercise training needs to be considered in serial weight measurements.
- Exercise intervention for obesity is best conducted in an organized program setting (school, YMCA, etc.).
- Exercise intervention should be initiated with easily tolerated activities such as walking, swimming, and games. Improvement in daily physical activity can add substantially to caloric expenditure. Endurance exercise is optimal for energy loss, but intensity needs to be tolerable for the obese child to assure compliance.

Dancing in one's room to rock music behind closed doors, or skipping rope with a friend are just as acceptable as the more traditional exercises reviewed earlier. In institution-based programs, interspersing aerobic games and floor sports can add variety to running laps or cycle exercise. In all these activities children should become accustomed to an initial 5- to 10-minute warm-up of stretches and calisthenics, then the regular exercise period followed by a similar short cool-down at the end.

Some programs have emphasized the importance of teaching subjects to take their pulse as a means of assessing proper exercise intensity. This is based on recommendations that target rates at a certain percent of maximal rate are necessary for improving physical fitness (American College of Sports Medicine, 1978). However, there is no good evidence that fitness guidelines are equally applicable for weight loss. Likewise, target heart rates are based on maximal values in non-obese subjects, and those in obese patients are frequently much lower. Unless an obese subject has undergone a maximal test, the proper target rate is unknown; basing this on an estimated maximum of 220 minus age will almost certainly overestimate the target rate for the obese child and lead to exercise recommendations that are overly intense.

The key to success for obesity programs is compliance, and a number of factors reportedly are influential in sustaining motivation and adherence. A greater chance for success is provided if the child can observe some effective weight loss. Prescribing enjoyable exercise that avoids embarrassment is essential, and having the child keep weekly exercise records is particularly useful. Enthusiastic leadership, parent support, well-defined goals, lack of expense, and easy accessibility have all been identified as important in successful programs.

Tangible rewards such as T-shirts, headbands, jump ropes—even money—have all been employed (without apologies) by program directors who have found by experience that these are strong motivating factors for children and adolescents. By enticing the child to persist in the program, these rewards may lead to more intrinsic motivating factors, such as feelings of pride and desires for achievement, with more lasting value.

The scope of this book does not allow a full discussion of dietary and behavioral approaches to childhood obesity, and the reader is referred to extensive reviews of these subjects (Collipp, 1980b; Katch & McArdle, 1983). In general, the emphasis during childhood has been on better nutrition, not fewer calories. Instruction on a well-balanced diet, use of low-calorie alternatives (such as for milk, soda pop, and salad dressings), and proper selection of snack foods will frequently lower caloric intake by the 100 to 300 cal daily goal without amounting to drastic changes in usual eating habits. In patients with advanced degrees of obesity, more aggressive dietary therapy may be indicated.

Finally, a word about ego support. Obese children consulting the physician for help have lived in an endless sea of negativism. Teased by their peers, hounded by their parents, unable to participate in sports activities, failing in efforts to diet, knowing that obesity creates a risk for strokes, heart attacks, and early death—it comes as no surprise that these children possess poor self-concepts. There is an important message here that physicians can help impart: Being overweight (or thin or bald or tall or short) has no bearing on the worth of the individual. "You are a good person, even if you have more weight" is an idea that the obese patient may never have heard before. Helping the child and his or her family find ways to support a positive self-image are important. Perhaps the child is good at art—find ways to promote it. Maybe she or he can grow a fine garden—support it. Providing alternative means of ego support other than body weight may help the child cope better with his or her obesity and perhaps aid the child in complying with dietary and exercise strategies.

SUMMARY

Despite the frustration of treatment failures, the growing significance of obesity as a health risk demands that physicians continue their efforts to control body fat in their patients. Much adult obesity originates in childhood and adolescence, which underscores the importance of early attention to this problem during the pediatric years.

- Greatest success in obesity treatment can be expected with a combination of diet, exercise, and behavior modification. During childhood, concern about the effects of caloric restriction on normal growth makes physical activity a particularly attractive therapeutic modality.
- Treatment of obesity must be viewed as a family problem, requiring cooperation and support by all members.
- Exercise programs for obese children are best conducted in group sessions, involving activities sufficiently intense to increase caloric output but avoiding excessive bodily stress.
- Management of obesity in children must balance intervention efforts with ego-supportive measures that avoid the negative implications of treatment failure.

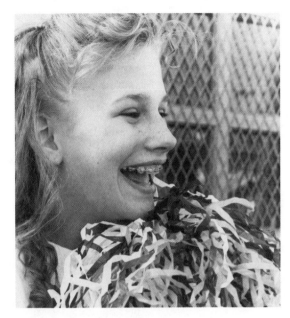

CHAPTER 8

Physical Activity and Psychological Health

This chapter explores the influence of exercise on mental health and its implications for children and adolescents, examining information about the relationship between physical activity and both emotional well-being and psychopathological states. Available data suggest that exercise has a positive effect on a wide variety of these conditions, which supports the use of regular activity as a both therapeutic and preventive measure.

THE PROBLEM OF MENTAL ILLNESS

Health care providers for children seek to ensure that their patients thrive in the journey through the growing years to become happy, healthy adults. It is often forgotten what a remarkably safe trip, from a historical standpoint, this has become. In advanced cultures, most children will almost certainly escape death from infectious disease or dehydration; congenital anomalies are surgically remedied, and metabolic diseases such as diabetes mellitus are effectively controlled. Rickets, scurvy, and other nutritional deficiencies are virtually unheard of. The medical profession can feel justly proud of the therapeutic, technological, and public health advances that have made this progress possible.

In the midst of this success, there are still some discomforting statistics (Dishman, 1986):

- An estimated 29 to 38 percent of Americans experience psychiatrically significant mental problems during their lifetimes.
- Mental illness ranks first in cause of hospitalization days (30 percent of the total in 1975) and is the third-leading cause of social security disability.
- Interview studies indicate that over a 6-month period 29 million American adults experience mental disturbance, most commonly anxiety disorder, substance abuse, and depression.
- The financial cost of mental disease is estimated at 40 billion dollars annually, accounting for 8 to 15 percent of the nation's health budget.

In American school-age children, the prevalence of psychiatric disorder is felt to be approximately 10 to 20 percent. Nearly 2,000 children and adolescents in the United States commit suicide each year, 3 times the number reported 35 years ago. There are an estimated 50 to 220 suicide attempts for each of these deaths (Earls, 1982; Shaw, Sheehan, & Fernandez, 1987).

In the final analysis, then, the major obstacles to a healthful, fulfilled adult life may be created by breakdowns in emotional as much as physical well-being. The identification, prevention, and treatment of mental disorders therefore deserves a high priority from those responsible for the health care of children and adolescents. In the same way that the origins of adult atherosclerosis, hypertension, and obesity lie in the pediatric years, emotional disorders during childhood and adolescence can also serve as preliminaries to significant mental illness in adult life.

The idea that physical activity and mental health are intimately linked is deeply rooted in human history. The ancient Greeks advanced the concept of body wholeness (*Mens sana in corpore sano,* a healthy mind in a healthy body), the breakdown of which is nowhere more obvious than in the contemporary physician's office: Mental illness becomes manifest as physical disease just as powerfully as organic illness precipitates secondary emotional disorders.

Classic psychological theory places heavy emphasis on the roles of play and motor activity in the cognitive development of children. Far from being simply a way to release physical energy, play is a central means by which social, moral, and intellectual growth is achieved. Piaget, Mead, Erikson, Bruner, and Freud all viewed the contributions of physical activity to these functions from different perspectives, but considered exercise to be an essential element in the development of personality and cognitive capacity (Sage, 1986a).

Considering this heritage, it is not surprising that physical activity has been considered an important tool for both maintaining mental health and managing emotional disorders (Taylor, Sallis, & Needle, 1985). There is little question that exercise has a positive effect on mental function. Most people, in fact, participate in physical activity simply because it is enjoyable; there is a sense of well-being associated with athletic participation that is probably the single most influential factor sustaining interest in regular exercise. But beyond this there is evidence that exercise can effect changes in self-perception, mitigate responses to external stimuli, affect cognitive function, and produce changes in human behavior. The mechanisms responsible for these effects are unknown; either physiochemical or psychological processes or both may be involved.

The experimental data reviewed in this chapter provide a rationale for the use of exercise to sustain mental well-being and as a treatment modality for a wide variety of psychological disorders. This role for exercise in children and adolescents is just beginning to be explored, and much of the information available on this subject is limited to adults. Still, the inferences for pediatric subjects appear clear.

Before examining this information, several caveats are in order. The conclusions in many of these studies indicate an *association* between exercise and improvements in mental health. The questions of *causality*, however, is not resolved in these reports; it may be just as likely that mentally stable individuals are more likely to exercise as that physical activity induces emotional well-being. Then there is the problem of the Hawthorne effect, a phenomenon initially described in a study of the effects of illumination levels on the work output of factory workers (Cook, 1962). The surprising results: Productivity increased *equally* when illumination was increased or decreased. The Hawthorne effect explains this apparent paradox by pointing out that simply knowing that they are part of an experimental process causes subjects to focus attention and increase concentration on the trait in question. *Any* experimental intervention might therefore change subject behavior because of the subjects' awareness of special treatment created by the conditions of the experiment (Corder, 1966).

STRESS IN CHILDHOOD

A certain level of psychological stress is important to meaningful living, and high degrees of it are even sometimes sought for their pleasurable effects (as in riding a roller coaster or viewing a horror film). But excessive stress is detrimental to mental well-being and interferes with enjoyment of life; responses to stress influence physical health as well and may contribute to risk for coronary artery disease (Dishman, 1986).

But do children experience stress? After all, youngsters are not burdened by anxieties concerning professional failure, marital discord, and financial insecurity. They don't feel the pain of adult disillusionment, fear of growing old, or despair about crabgrass growing in the lawn. Children don't worry about those things—they just eat, play, and watch television, right? Wrong, unfortunately. It comes as no revelation to physicians caring for children that, although difficult to quantitate, childhood stress is probably no less common than adult. The daily contributions to the office schedule of children's behavioral problems, psychogenic symptoms, and stress-related organic illness attests to the impact of anxiety and depression in the pediatric age group.

Children experience stress when environmental influences create a loss of security and threaten their sense of being a worthwhile person. The mentally healthy adult possesses sufficient self-esteem through accumulated life experiences to feel intrinsically comfortable with his or her value. Children, on the other hand, rely on external support mechanisms for these perceptions of security and self-worth, and when love and emotional support are perceived to be withdrawn, anxiety and depression result. These in turn can be manifest to the physician as behavior problems (e.g., hyperactivity, rebellion, destructiveness) or organic symptoms (e.g., headache, chest or abdominal pain, fatigue).

In many ways it may be more difficult for children to tolerate stress than for adults. Older individuals can often tolerate transient stressors by appreciating their insignificance in the long term. Children do not see this "big picture" and are less likely to handle stress well in the immediate situation. Many stresses in adulthood are managed easily simply through avoidance. Unpleasant jobs can be changed, moves can be made from disagreeable neighborhoods, and obnoxious or threatening individuals can be evaded. Children do not possess the freedom or financial means to avoid stress by these methods. Family, teacher, school, and peers are all fixed for youngsters, and there is no easy way to escape stress in these settings (Chandler, 1985).

THE ROLE OF EXERCISE
IN STRESS MANAGEMENT

Participation in physical activities has long been recognized to induce subjective improvements in emotional well-being. Only recently, however, have scientific investigations more objectively evaluated these responses and the effect that exercise might have in reducing the emotional effects of environmental stress.

Anxiety

Acute bouts of physical exercise serve as an effective tranquilizer. EMG studies indicate that half an hour of aerobic exercise in adults reduces anxiety-related muscle tension as much as does a 400-mg dose of meprobamate. This relaxation effect of physical activity is manifest by subject self-reports, electroencephalographic changes, and reduction in peripheral deep-tendon reflexes. The reduction in tension is most marked in individuals with high levels of resting anxiety, but it occurs in asymptomatic individuals as well. The relaxing effect of acute exercise is not related to muscle fatigue; EMG activity becomes increased rather than depressed in fatigued muscle. The influence of exercise on reducing muscle tension is therefore felt to be a central (corticospinal) effect (Dishman, 1986).

Morgan, Roberts, and Feinerman (1971) could demonstrate no changes in self-report measures of anxiety after walking 1 mi at intensities that resulted in a mean heart rate of 125 bpm in adult male and 144 bpm in adult female subjects. This and other studies have suggested that exercise must be fairly strenuous before it can effectively reduce anxiety. The tension reduction following acute exercise lasts for up to 4 to 6 hours. Because of this, Morgan (1981) suggested that regular physical activity might be best employed to lower anxiety levels on a daily basis and thereby help prevent the development of chronic anxiety.

The tranquility effect of acute exercise does not appear to be greater than that of other methods, however. Wilson, Berger, and Bird (1981) demonstrated similar reductions in pre- and postanxiety levels by questionnaire in young adults who were in a running group, an organized exercise class, and a group eating lunch. Similarly, the tranquilizing effects of rest breaks, meditation, and beer drinking may be equally as effective as acute exercise in reducing anxiety (Morgan, 1981).

Whether chronic exercise training will lower resting-anxiety levels is not so clear, because experimental data have provided conflicting results. Case reports have indicated that regular physical activity may be helpful in the treatment of panic attacks and phobias (Morgan, 1981).

Data examining the effect of exercise on anxiety in children are limited. Hanson concluded that daily half-hour movement training for 10 weeks reduced anxiety in healthy 4-year-olds, based on teachers' reports and psychological testing (cited by Brown, 1982).

Response to Stress

Physiological responsiveness to stress has typically been analyzed by examining reactions of subjects to stressors such as cognitive puzzles (e.g., mazes or arithmetic problems), viewing films of accidents or medical operations, or physical discomfort (e.g., holding a limb in ice water). To test whether physical activity would dampen physiological responses to these insults, Crews and Landers (1987) performed a meta-analysis of 34 studies addressing this issue in the adult literature. This procedure, which statistically combines the results of the reports, showed that regardless of modifying variables, subjects who were aerobically fit demonstrated decreased psychosocial stress responses compared to control groups. Some of these studies indicated that blood pressure, pulse, or other physiological markers were lower in the exercising group; others indicated that fit subjects experienced a more rapid recovery from stress.

This protective effect of exercise appears to carry over to the real world outside the laboratory (DeBenedette, 1988). Negative life events (such as a death in the family, family discord, or failure in school or on the job) have been correlated with a higher incidence of physical illness. Roth and Holmes (1985) confirmed this effect and found in addition that physically fit college students experienced fewer health problems in response to psychological stressors than unfit subjects. Brown and Lawton (1986) demonstrated similar findings in 220 girls age 11 to 17 years attending a private school. Life stress events such as failing a course, breaking up with a boyfriend, or family instability were assessed by questionnaire and related to physical health over the previous year as well as to extent of habitual physical activity. The students' somatic health was seen to correlate directly with increased stress from negative life events, but this effect was less in those with higher levels of regular physical exercise. The authors cautioned against concluding that exercise acted as a protective buffer against stress, however, because the study design did not establish a causal relationship.

But exercise itself is a stressful event, so couldn't physical activity, particularly participation in competitive sport, *add* to psychic tension rather than relieve it? Volumes have been written regarding the pros and cons of competitive athletics during childhood in light of the stresses of competition, creating an emotional cross fire the present author wishes to duck (Feltz & Ewing, 1987; Magill, Ash, & Smoll, 1982; Martens, 1978).

The accumulated information on this subject might be summarized as follows: Emotional responses to competitive sport may vary significantly from one child to the next (as they do in adults). Most youngsters do experience stress during athletic competition, but for most, it is mild and transient (and enjoyable?). Participants who are at risk for more adverse emotional reactions to sport participation include those with diminished levels of self-esteem or low performance expectations (Scanlan & Passer, 1978). Individual sports such as wrestling and gymnastics generate more stress than team sports, but overall the emotional reactions to competitive sport are no greater than other children's activities (e.g., band competitions, academic tests) (Simon & Martens, 1979). Only in situations where individual performance and outcome of the contest become linked (consciously or unconsciously) by parents and coaches to the self-worth, personal integrity, and virtue of the players does competition in athletics become a truly destructive force.

Depression

In adults, chronic aerobic exercise has been valued for its ability to reduce mild-to-moderate degrees of depression. Again, if one ignores the anecdotal nature or inadequate experimental design of much of the research data, abundant evidence supports this effect of physical activity (Dishman, 1986; Monahan, 1986; Rape, 1987). Exercise has been demonstrated to be comparable to psychotherapy and meditation–relaxation techniques for treating moderate depression, so the effect does not appear to be specifically related to improvements in physical fitness. Physical activity does not appear to be useful in the management of depression in psychotic individuals, however (Dishman, 1986).

Studies in older teenagers tend to support the use of exercise for management of adolescent depression. Rape (1987) compared scores on the Beck Depression Inventory between 21 runners and an equal number of nonexercisers 18 to 25 years old. Runners demonstrated both significantly greater fitness (by step test) and lower depression ratings. Improvement in depression scores has also been described following an aerobic exercise program in college students (Sharp & Reilley, 1975). However, Folkins et al. (1972) could find such a result only in females, and a comparison of 42 runners and 43 nonrunners ages 12 to 15 revealed no differences in depression levels between the two groups (Buchanan, cited by Brown, 1982). Sage (1986b) has pointed out that exercise appears to be less effective in improving measures of depression in adults and college students who are already in the normal range on depression test scales when they start exercise programs.

Possible Mechanisms

The means by which repetitive muscular activity alters psychological states remains a mystery, but certainly not one begging for theorists. If one were convinced of the ancient Greeks' view that mind and body are bound together in a holistic sense, there would be no difficulty expecting the body's responses to physical stress to influence mental state. More intriguing are contemporary concepts that provide insights—albeit limited—into the basic physiological and psychological means by which humans react to their environment.

"Time Out" Theory

Reduced anxiety, euphoria, and relief of depression all may result from exercise simply because the subject's attention is diverted away from environmental stressors. This "time out" theory is supported by findings in several studies that anxiety reduction is no greater with acute exercise than with passive interventions (e.g., relaxing in an easy chair in a sound-filtered room). Others have suggested that the social interaction provided by many sport events may provide positive feedback from exercise activities. According to Ransford (1982), however, experimental evidence indicates that psychological improvements are more commonly noted in individual than in team sports.

Self-Significance

Society has characterized physical activity as "good" and provides messages that athleticism might just be equated with moral integrity and self-significance (cf. the Boy Scout Oath, with which one pledges to be "physically strong, mentally awake, and morally straight"). Identifying oneself as an "athlete" can be a strong statement to both oneself and others that counters insecurity and feelings of helplessness from environmental stressors. In a similar vein, regular exercise provides a sense of self-mastery, competence, and control that may provide very beneficial gains from physical activity. This theory, although not well-tested, suggests that sports in which improvement can be most easily measured (and achieved) might be expected to stimulate the most positive psychological effects.

Control

Many of the psychosocial stresses in society are diffuse, difficult to confront because of their ambiguity, and devoid of distinct positive feedback (e.g., confronting troublesome relatives, public speaking, working with a critical employer). The stresses created by exercise, on the other hand, are concrete and the results easily charted. The ability to know that "working" hard will improve running time or swimming distance and that overcoming these obstacles can be clearly measured provides a strong attraction to these types of sport.

Biochemical Changes

The ancient Greeks would probably be more interested in explaining the exercise–psyche connection by shifts in body "humors." Contemporary research does, in fact, provide abundant support for the idea that biochemical and physiological changes occurring with exercise may be responsible for variation in one's psychological state. Alterations in central neurotransmitters, cortisol levels, body temperature, cerebral blood flow, and endogenous opiates have all been suggested to link exercise and affect (Morgan, 1985; Ransford, 1982). These factors are established determinants of psychological state and, at the same time, vary in response to physical exercise. To establish a causal connection between the two is difficult, but animal studies have provided some evidence that such a relationship exists. Direct experimental evidence in humans, who resist serial brain biopsies, is not unexpectedly scant.

Psychological function is strongly influenced by levels of norepinephrine, dopamine, serotonin, and other amines within the brain. These substances serve as neurotransmitters, carrying electrical signals between neurons, and their depletion in the central nervous system (CNS) has been associated with depression and other mood disorders. Because amines are increased in the peripheral circulation with exercise, the ameliorating effects of physical activity in these conditions could occur through a restoration of normal CNS neurotransmitter levels.

Support for this concept has come mainly from animal research. Chronic running or swimming regimens in rats decrease emotionality, and evidence indicates that both acute and chronic exercise increase brain norepinephrine and serotonin levels. In humans, circulating sympathetic amines increase 2 to 6 times over resting levels after one half hour of vigorous exercise. But how this relates to brain amine content is uncertain.

The role of endorphins, or endogenous brain opiates, as possible mood elevators with exercise has gained popular attention because these substances can produce "morphine-like" effects of pain reduction and euphoria (Morgan, 1985). Does the concentration of these substances increase in the brain in response to exercise, and are they responsible for "runner's high" and other positive postexercise emotional states? Research information conflicts on this point. Exercise results in an increase in brain opiate receptor occupancy in rats, from which Pert and Bowie (1979) conclude anthropopathismistically (a phrase offered with apologies) that "cessation of running must therefore be correlated in rats with a euphoric feeling induced by increased opiate receptor occupancy" (p. 100). Mood elevations after exercise in human subjects have been reduced by naloxone, a narcotic antagonist, in some studies but not others, a difference that might result from variation in naloxone dose (Morgan, 1985). Plasma endorphin levels have been shown to increase with physical activity in humans, but brain and circulating concentrations may not be well correlated.

SELF-CONCEPT

Positive self-concept, the feeling that one has value in the world, is a hallmark of good mental health. With the depersonalizing effects of modern civilization, the individual's ability to sustain a sense of worth is a requisite for happiness in all phases of life. For the child, self-esteem appears to be a central component of success in academic achievement, classroom participation, social skills, and leadership potential (Sonstroem, 1984). As noted previously, children depend for this positive self-identity largely on external factors, particularly a supportive family environment. The failure to develop self-esteem, on the other hand, results in a vulnerability to anxiety, depression, and more serious psychiatric illness.

For this reason, participation in regular exercise might be expected *a priori* to improve self-esteem: Elevated mood and feelings of well-being as well as relief of depression and anxiety—effects all related to physical activity—are also associated with a positive self-concept. In adults, chronic exercise has not been shown to promote measures of overall self-esteem in all studies. But because body image is linked to self-concept, self-esteem has been demonstrated to increase in subjects who value physical competency and increase their fitness or athletic ability through an exercise program. The failure of some adult subjects to improve self-concept with regular physical activity has been explained by the multiplicity of factors contributing to self-esteem in this age group (Dishman, 1986). Society permits individuals to achieve success and develop a positive self-concept by many different means (e.g., social identity, occupation, avocation); being physically fit is not particularly valued by all people (Sonstroem, 1984). But if the role played by an individual is that of an athlete, and if that identity is a positive one, the individual has adopted a strong means of improving self-esteem.

Development of Self-Concept

The perception one has of oneself is developed during childhood. Nonexistent at birth, self-concept is formed as the child grows, and mature self-esteem is typically reached by the time of adolescence. Much research indicates that self-concept grows largely by social experiences and therefore is derived from one's cognitive, social, and physical success in relation to peers. In this process experiences in physical activity, particularly sport participation, are expected to influence the development of healthy self-esteem, particularly considering the value placed by society on athleticism and sports skills (Sage, 1986b).

Abundant experimental evidence supports the concept that physical fitness and self-concept are related in elementary age children. Gruber (1986) reviewed 84 studies between 1966 and 1986 exploring the relationship of physical activity and self-esteem in this age group. Meta-analysis revealed that, overall, physical fitness activities were significantly related to improvements on test scores of self-concept. This held true for healthy children as well as for those who were emotionally disturbed, mentally retarded, or perceptually handicapped, but the effect was greater in the latter three groups. The relationship of self-esteem and exercise was also more prominent when aerobic activities were utilized. Significantly less effect was observed for sports instruction, perceptual motor activities, and dance. Although most experimental evidence thus supports the value of exercise in the development of childhood self-esteem, it should be noted that not all studies have found a relationship between fitness and self-concept (Kay, Felker, & Varoz, 1972; Sonstroem, 1978).

Methodology Pitfalls

Sonstroem (1984) has brought attention to the many methodological shortcomings associated with these studies. The following limitations weaken the conclusion that exercise or physical fitness truly influences self-esteem:

- Absence of proper control subjects
- Deficient experimental design
- Lack of random treatment assignment
- Initial group differences
- Improper statistical analysis

After reviewing this literature, Sonstroem (1984) concluded that exercise *programs* are related to improvements of self-esteem *scores* of the participants. But based on these studies, summarized in the box that follows, it is not possible to identify the agent(s) responsible for the association in each of these categories. Specifically, it is difficult to establish that increases in physical fitness are linked with self-esteem per se.

Cross-sectional studies have not provided a clear picture of the influence of participation in organized team sports on self-esteem in children. Information exists to indicate that competing youngsters have more, less, or the same levels of self-esteem as nonparticipants. The few reports of changes in self-esteem during participation do suggest a positive effect (Sage, 1986a). Unfortunately, Iso-Ahola (1976) demonstrated that winning or losing a Little League baseball game influenced self-reports of personal esteem immediately after the contest. And Zeigler (cited by Sage, 1986b) reported that female high school basketball players' feelings of self-esteem were affected by the win–loss records of the team.

Factors Potentially Influencing Self-Esteem in Exercise Programs

Program agents	Esteem score agents
• Improved physical fitness	• Self-preservation strategies
• Achievement of goals	• Defensiveness
• Feelings of well-being	• Social desirability
• Competence, mastery	• Expectancy, suggestion
• Social reinforcement	• Perceived leader or group pressures
• Experimental attention	

From Sonstroem, 1984.

LEARNING AND ATTENTION-DEFICIT DISORDERS

Little research has addressed the effect of physical activity on specific abnormalities in cognitive or behavioral dysfunction in children. Two studies have indicated that a regular jogging program for 10 to 22 weeks may decrease the need for stimulant medications for hyperkinetic children (Shipman, cited by Brown, 1982; Elsom, 1981). Shephard (1983) proposed that these patients suffered from an abnormally high setting of a hypothalamic control center for physical activity. According to this idea, stimulant medications provide effective therapy in these cases by substituting for motor activity as an arousal mechanism. A structured exercise program might therefore be equally useful for the same reason, resulting in a decreased level of spontaneous activity during the rest of the day.

MacMahon and Gross (1987) investigated the effect of a 20-week aerobic exercise program on the self-concept, academic achievement, and cardiovascular fitness of boys 7 to 12 years old with learning disorders. Measures of physical fitness and self-esteem improved following this program, but there were no changes in academic performance compared to subjects participating in a lower intensity, nonaerobic exercise regimen.

PSYCHOTIC STATES

Studies in adult patients indicate that exercise has little direct effect upon psychotic disorders. Small changes have been observed in psychiatric states following physical training in these subjects, but such responses are no greater than those expected simply from social interaction with other patients (Dishman, 1986). However, the National Institute of Mental Health workshops on exercise in 1984 suggested exercise as an adjunct to medication, electroconvulsive therapy, and psychotherapy for psychotic depression (Dishman, 1986).

Katz (1982) investigated the effects of exercise on three 5- to 6-year-old autistic children. These patients regularly jogged hand-in-hand with the experimenter for 5 to 8 minutes, while a "nonaerobic group" played sedentary games, and a third group played quietly. The running children demonstrated a reduction in self-stimulating behavior but no improvements in social function. Watters and Watters (1980) also showed a decrease in self-stimulating behavior following a running program in autistic children. Brown (1982) commented that in studies such as these the child's contact with the experimenter during exercise may have influenced the results.

INTELLIGENCE

Developmental psychologists have asserted that physical activity is essential in promoting normal growth of mental function. If this is true, physical capabilities and/or level of regular exercise might be expected to bear a relationship to intelligence. This association has been extensively evaluated and recently reviewed in depth by Kirkendall (1986).

There is no clear indication that athletes score higher on IQ tests than nonathletes. In fact, when Slusher (1964) compared IQ levels between high school nonathletes and a group of baseball, basketball, swimming, wrestling, and football participants, the athletes demonstrated *lower* scores than the nonathletes. Several studies have indicated, however, that athletes have higher grade-point averages (Eidsmoe, 1951). Kirkendall (1986) pointed out several possible explanations for this finding. Athletes may enroll in easier classes than nonathletes and receive preferential treatment from teachers (the "halo" effect). In addition, individuals with low grade-point averages will not be represented among the athletic subjects because they will have failed to qualify academically for team participation.

In a longitudinal study, Leuptow and Kayser (1973) could find no greater improvement in grades in athletes than in nonathletes during their high school careers. In a second study, Hauser and Lueptow (1978) showed that the nonathletes actually demonstrated greater gains in grade-point averages over the high school years.

Another approach to this question has been to compare the physical abilities of normal children to those with significant degrees of mental retardation. Virtually all studies in this area have indicated that retarded children perform less well than nonretarded subjects in a wide variety of motor tasks. This includes coordination, strength, sports skills, speed, and balance (Francis & Rarick, 1959; Sloan, 1951). At the other end of the intelligence scale, Disney (cited by Kirkendahl, 1986) examined several fitness parameters in high school boys with IQs over 130 and in those with average intelligence. The mentally gifted performed better on 7 of 11 fitness tasks (broad jump, sit-ups, sprint, softball throw, basketball shooting, and tennis and volleyball tests), and there were no group differences in the remainder.

Many studies have attempted to correlate performance or tests of fitness and intelligence, with conflicting results. When statistically significant positive relationships have been reported, the correlation coefficients have generally been low (.16 to .31), precluding the use of physical tests to predict academic success. However, Ismail and Gruber (1967) were able to develop regression equations from an association between IQ-test results and measures of coordination and balance (but not speed, power, or strength) in 10- to 12-year-old boys and girls.

Few studies have examined the influence on intellectual function of instituting a physical exercise program. In the Trois Rivieres study, effects on academic performance of 5 additional hours of physical activity per week in elementary school children were compared to a control group. Despite their classroom time being curtailed by 13 percent, the exercising group showed greater improvement in marks in French, mathematics, English, and science (Shephard, 1983). Ismail (1967) showed that an organized physical education program had no effect on IQ scores in fifth- and sixth-grade children but that academic achievement scores improved. These findings tend to support the studies involving cross-sectional studies in athletes; that is, increased physical activity does not increase basic intelligence but may improve academic performance. The caveats have already been discussed earlier. Despite being unable to draw firm conclusions on this subject, Kirkendall (1986) observed that no study has demonstrated an *impairment* of intellectual performance or development from increases in physical activity.

MENTAL RETARDATION

Most studies have shown little or no gain in intelligence scores when physical activity is increased in mentally retarded subjects. Solomon and Pangle (1966) observed this result after an 8-week structured physical education program in adolescent retarded boys, and Chasey and Wyrick (1970) could find no improvements in academic performance in a similar intervention with 12-year-old institutionalized mentally retarded children.

The increased intellectual function with exercise training observed by Corder (1966) was confounded by the Hawthorne effect. But Brown (1977) demonstrated a rise in mean IQ from 35 to 43 in trainable mentally retarded 12-year-old subjects after a 6-week daily program of mild isometric exercise. Other gains were also observed, including in strength and social skills, that may have contributed to improved scores on intellectual testing. Oliver (1958) evaluated the effects of a 10-week program of progressive exercise on educable mentally retarded boys (IQs 54 to 86) in a residential institution. Significant improvements in intelligence test scores as well as motor abilities were observed compared to a control group. Taylor, Sallis, and Needle (1985) commented that although such results might be explained by factors other than physical activity per se, little follow-up research attention has been paid to these findings.

Although it is unlikely that major gains in intellectual function can be achieved through exercise in mentally retarded subjects, other benefits may follow from a program of physical activity. Physical capacity is typically diminished in these children, as manifested by clumsiness, muscle weakness, and slow speech. Maximal aerobic power, however, may be relatively normal. Exercise performance is additionally impaired by poor attention span, obesity, delayed biological maturation and inability to follow instructions.

Shephard (1982) emphasized, however, that "if a physical education program is presented patiently and in small steps, mentally-retarded students will show surprising progress both in the development of strength and aerobic power and in the improvement of motor skills" (p. 228). Such gains may be particularly important to this group because they might enable them to perform functional work and to secure employment. Skrobak-Kaczynski and Vavik (1980) reduced body fat and improved strength and aerobic power in subjects with Down syndrome using circuit training, 1 hour three times a week. Similar findings were observed by Oliver (1958) and Brown (1977). Improved body image following physical activities has also been described in retarded children (Chasey, Swartz, & Chasey, 1974; Maloney & Payne, 1980).

JUVENILE DELINQUENCY

The belief that participation in sports is a deterrent to juvenile delinquency was initially adopted by public schools in Great Britain during the middle of the 19th century. Athletic activities were instituted in an effort to curb stealing, drinking, and other antisocial behavior, and sports became part of the curriculum in correctional institutions for juvenile delinquents (McIntosh, 1971). The concept that athletics can act as a means of social control has received strong support from sport organizations (such as the American Alliance of Health, Physical Education, Recreation and Dance, and the British Sports Council) and has been a major impetus behind the push for interscholastic athletic programs (Segrave, 1981).

Scientific scrutiny of this relationship has generally indicated that the occurrence of juvenile delinquency among athletic groups is less than in nonathletic youth. The question of causality, however, remains unsettled.

Segrave (1983) has exhaustively assessed this literature, and the following summary is derived from that review.

The first obstacle in examining the relationship between athleticism and antisocial behavior is the definition and identification of delinquency. Some studies have used an official measure (such as an encounter with law enforcement agencies), but most have relied on self-report as a more reliable indication of delinquent behavior. It might be suspected that this technique would be limited by forgetfulness, exaggeration, and falsification, but the validity of self-report as a credible measure of delinquency has been substantiated.

In 1907, a survey in Chicago indicated that the provision of play facilities had reduced the incidence of juvenile delinquency almost by half, and similar results were soon reported in Knoxville, Binghamton, and St. Louis. Outward Bound, a program to improve self-concept and social confidence through vigorous outdoor activities, has been the focus of several studies examining the influence of physical activity on delinquent behavior. These have indicated improved social attitudes and self-concept following activities such as mountain hiking and climbing, camping, and canoeing; in addition, recidivism rates were approximately half the rates for those who did not participate in these programs (Kelly & Baer, 1969; Willman & Chun, 1973). Segrave (1983) concluded that "the adventure and personal challenge offered by Outward Bound are perceived as a particularly effective mechanism for the re-socialization of delinquents. The development of competence and confidence, the opportunity to test one's physical and psychological limits, and the sense of accomplishment are some of the many factors offered in support of Outward Bound experiences" (p. 190).

Most studies have indicated a negative relationship between participation in interscholastic athletics and delinquent behavior, whether measured by official or by self-report methods. From this research, several conclusions appear valid:

- Athletes, on the whole, are less delinquent than nonathletes, for both males and females.
- The negative relationship between athleticism and delinquency is largely restricted to lower socioeconomic groups. Several studies indicate that when social status is controlled for, the inverse correlation between sport participation and delinquency is greatly weakened.
- The relationship between athletics and delinquency is a function of the seriousness of the offense. Antisocial behavior among athletes diminishes even more significantly when acts of vandalism, theft, and physical assault are considered.
- The psychosocial profiles of athletes contrast vividly with those of deviant youth, particularly in the areas of social background, educational achievement, self-image, and peer status.

The difficulty arising from this analysis, particularly considering the last point, is obvious. Could it not be concluded that the well-motivated, socially upright individual is more likely to participate in sport rather than that athletic participation inhibits delinquent behavior? Numerous studies have indicated—as expected—that delinquent subjects are much less disposed than nondelinquents to organized sport programs and extracurricular activities. Interscholastic sports teams may be viewed by the delinquent as representing "small-scale replicas of the larger social order" from which they are rebelling (Segrave, 1983, p. 200). Still, there are some sound psychosocial constructs, including the following, that make tenable a causal relationship between sport participation and decreased delinquent behavior.

• **Recapitulation theory.** According to this theory, children possess innate, animalistic tendencies toward disruptive behavior, which are thwarted by play activities. When physical activity through sport and recreational exercise is not available, delinquency and other antisocial behavior results. The recapitulation theory was a driving force behind the early creation of urban playground and athletic programs.

• **Surplus energy theory.** This theory proposes that children's excess energy needs to be vented, and sport participation provides a healthy way to "blow off steam." Delinquency occurs as an alternative means of releasing physical tension in individuals not engaged in sport play.

• **Personality theory.** According to this theory, athletic participation promotes the development of self-discipline, social adequacy, emotional security, and optimism. By promoting these wholesome traits, athletics helps to inhibit antisocial attitudes. The growth of self-esteem through sport participation may be particularly important, because delinquency often serves as a response to inadequate self-concept. The feelings of achievement and recognition gained in athletics may eliminate the need to seek these rewards in delinquent behavior.

• **Stimulus-seeking behavior.** According to this concept, delinquency occurs because of a heightened need for stimulation. Sport allows individuals to gain their thrills through the excitement of athletic participation rather than antisocial activities.

• **Boredom theory.** Similarly to the previous idea, this theory advocates that delinquency results largely from boredom. In the face of "nothing better to do," antisocial behavior fills the time void. Sport provides an alternative use of spare time; when youth are busy after school and on weekends in athletic activities, they have neither time nor energy to commit crimes.

• **Subculture theory.** According to this theory, delinquent behavior feeds on peer-group norms and expectations. The more frequently youths associate with antisocial individuals, the more likely delinquency is to occur.

The rules, achievement-directed behavior, and sense of cooperation toward common goals that surround athletics, on the other hand, are strong counterbalancing forces against antisocial behavior.

CHARACTER DEVELOPMENT

"There is a deep-seated and pervasive belief that the effects of involvement in physical activities extend beyond the immediate fun and excitement of the moment" (Sage, 1986a, p. 22). The British public school systems of the mid-19th century believed this. They saw team sports as engendering personal virtue and social qualities, serving as a training ground for the discipline and leadership necessary for success in adult life. The idea that "sport builds character"—character that is transferrable to other aspects of life—began there; the idea was that physical activity is a social experience that can powerfully influence attitudes and values. Sportsmanship, cooperation, honesty, selflessness, commitment, and other personality traits were felt to flourish in the context of team sports.

No one ever scientifically validated this deep-rooted premise of the British system. But something was lost in the translation to modern-day organized youth sports in America, where research fails to support the view that these activities contribute to growth of character; indeed, they suggest in many cases that just the opposite effect may occur. The difference, according to Sage (1986a), is a change from student-organized activities typical of the English system to those dominated by adult control in the United States. In the process the emphasis has shifted from social growth to winning, and the role of sport in character development has been nullified. The nihilists and the champions of youth sport have engaged in lengthy debate surrounding this conclusion, which is summarized elsewhere (Magill et al., 1982; Martens, 1978).

Scientific evidence provides little support for those who argue that participation on youth sports teams builds personal virtue (Sage, 1986b). Studies indicate that preadolescent athletes value winning and skill more than do nonparticipants, who view fair play and fun as higher goals (Kidd & Woodman, 1975; Maloney & Petrie, 1972; Mantel & Vander Velden, 1974). Sage (1986b) commented, "Although it is difficult to credit (or discredit) sports participation entirely for greater professionalized attitudes toward play, it seems that sport for fun, enjoyment, fairness, and equity are sacrificed at the altar of skill and victory as children move toward adulthood" (p. 357).

Athletic competition does not appear to promote sportsmanship. In fact, several studies show that individuals with long-time sport experience demonstrate poorer attitudes toward fair play than do nonathletes (Allison, 1982; Kistler, 1957). The explanation: The desire for victory and sportsmanlike behavior are often in direct conflict with each other. Success in competitive athletics rests with aggressiveness, dominance, and nonsociability (Arnold, 1986). As soon as child's play becomes organized by adults with team victory as a primary goal, the rewards for sportsmanship become weakened.

Other character traits suffer the same fate. Prosocial behaviors such as cooperation, friendliness, and generosity are inconsistent with a sport philosophy that places major emphasis on winning. Kleiber and Roberts (1981) demonstrated that traits of cooperation and altruism in males were actually inhibited by sport competition. The authors concluded that "to the extent that competition is allowed to dominate the interpersonal relationships in children's sports, their potential for actually facilitating the development of prosocial behavior is entirely lost" (p. 121). As Ogilvie & Tutko (1971) titled their article regarding sport, "If you want to build character, try something else."

That is not to say that the *potential* for personal growth in qualities like persistence, resourcefulness, self-reliance, and other prosocial traits cannot be provided by sport participation. Arnold (1986) noted that not many activities in everyday life provide such an opportunity for gains in moral virtues as athletics. He challenged teachers of sport to understand and accept this opportunity to assist in the development of moral character of children and youth.

SUMMARY

Information surrounding the impact of exercise on mental function suggests many things, including the following, which were discussed in this chapter.

- Physical activity is a largely untapped resource for the management of emotional illness and maintenance of mental well-being. Experimental methodology is weak in all aspects of this relationship, but the overwhelming bulk of data supporting the salutary effects of exercise is impressive.
- It must be appreciated that exercise is not an emotionally satisfying experience for all individuals. But considering the evidence that physical activity favorably influences mental well-being, it is surprising that the adherence rates to exercise programs are so low, or that so few children enjoy physical education classes. The need for additional research investigating the exercise–mental health link—as well as answering these questions—is obvious.
- It is not at all clear from the available research what type, duration, or intensity of exercise is necessary to achieve positive emotional

benefits. Presumably the exercise prescription might be different depending on the mechanism of action of physical activity as well as its purpose. For instance, if exercise reduces anxiety or depression by acting as a diversion, physical activity of any enjoyable type would be appropriate. On the other hand, exercise to achieve progress or attain certain goals might be more appropriate for improving self-esteem.

• Certain positive psychological responses to exercise may be dependent on changes that occur only in aerobic exercise regimens designed to improve cardiovascular fitness, such as suppression of resting adrenergic tone (DeBenedette, 1988). But subjects training with aerobic or anaerobic activities have been shown to have equal reduction in responses to psychosocial stress (Crews, Landers, O'Connor, & Clark, 1988).

At present, too little is known to identify specific exercise prescriptions, except that these need to be tailored to help ensure compliance and achieve end-points in individual patients. Several options are outlined in Part III of this book.

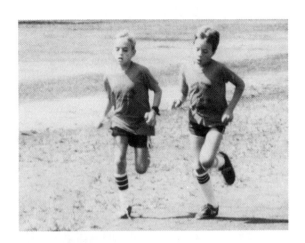

CHAPTER 9

Exercise
in the Management
of Cardiopulmonary
Disease

Exercise programs can play a vital
role in improving the lives of children and adolescents with chronic
cardiac and pulmonary illness.
Some diseases (e.g., cardiac anomalies and cystic fibrosis) interfere
with normal exercise capacity by
impairing oxygen delivery to exercising muscle (Bar-Or, 1986), whereas others, such as postoperative
cardiac arrythmias, may place the
child at risk during physical activity
if not adequately managed. In
either case, the patient may shun
exercise activities from either fear or

disinterest, leading to depressed levels of fitness, more hypoactivity, and an even lower exercise capacity. This cycle of events creates an impaired child whose ability to participate in and enjoy life's everyday activities are reduced much more than by the disease itself (Bar-Or, 1983).

The primary goal of exercise rehabilitation is to reverse this process—to maximize physical potential, reduce the fear of complications of exercise through proper therapy, and minimize the debilitating effects of depressed cardiovascular fitness. The benefits have long been subjectively obvious. These children improve their ability to participate in daily activities while enjoying the company of friends. Their morale and self-confidence are uplifted, and their level of cardiovascular fitness improves. In short, regular exercise improves the *quality* of life for children with all forms of chronic disease.

This chapter addresses the role of exercise in pediatric patients with heart disease, asthma, and cystic fibrosis. The recurrent theme in each of the following sections is that scientific evidence is now available to document many of the salutary effects of physical activity. It is unlikely that exercise will often be shown to modify basic disease processes per se, but abundant information indicates that regular exercise is a valuable adjunct to medical therapy in each of these illnesses.

CARDIAC ANOMALIES

The idea that exercise training might prove beneficial to children with heart disease is a spin-off from the larger experience of rehabilitation programs for adults recovering from myocardial infarction or coronary bypass surgery. These programs have sought to restore physiological and psychological well-being and—as a secondary effect—to prevent subsequent coronary events. Their success rate in this endeavor has been variously interpreted. Proponents identify improvements in work capacity that follow exercise training in these patients, often accompanied by reductions in submaximal heart rate and blood pressure (the rate–pressure product, a marker of myocardial work). Quality of life is further enhanced by improvements in mood, self-concept, and social confidence that follow exercise training—directly countering the devastating emotional impact of the previous coronary event. In short, patients with coronary artery disease (CAD) typically feel better about themselves, can enjoy more physical activities, and make a more rapid return to regular employment after an exercise rehabilitation program (Shephard, 1985).

On the other hand, Froelicher's (1983) review of the literature indicated that it is impossible to conclude with confidence that a program of physical activity has any direct beneficial effects on cardiac function, coronary blood flow, or the arteriosclerotic process itself. Because maximal stroke volume and heart rate do not usually change with exercise training in coronary patients, improvements in work capacity have been related to alterations in peripheral circulation and increased aerobic capacity of exercising muscle.

Exercise cannot be administered in a double-blind fashion; thus the most precise measurable outcome for rehabilitation programs has been subsequent death or recurrence of a coronary event. Shephard (1988) reviewed nine major controlled trials of exercise in postcoronary rehabilitation and reported an overall 20 to 50 percent reduction in mortality rates in exercising subjects. However, a positive therapeutic effect was not observed to be statistically significant in any one study.

Much of the conflict over interpreting the value of these programs arises from a virtual quagmire of methodological difficulties, including the following:

• A tendency for those with a more favorable outlook to enter exercise programs
• The influence of confounding variables, particularly the use of medications
• The variability of the cardiac insult suffered by the participants
• Differences in subject compliance
• The influence of social reinforcement created by these programs
• Variability in program duration, structure, and sample size

Exercise Programs for Children

The ability of exercise training to improve the physical and emotional quality of life in adult coronary patients has stimulated interest in using similar programs to help children with heart disease. Early reports are optimistic (Table 9.1), although many of these studies suffer from the same drawbacks as their adult counterparts (particularly, small subject numbers and absence of matched controls). In general, these few programs have demonstrated the capability of increasing aerobic capacity, improving the ability to tolerate exercise, and strengthening emotional health in a wide variety of congenital and acquired cardiac diseases in children and adolescents.

The following are goals of a carefully regulated and monitored exercise program for pediatric cardiac patients:

• Improve functional capacity to perform and enjoy physical activity.
• Develop self-esteem and confidence, qualities frequently weakened by chronic disease.
• Give the child and family knowledge of the patient's physical activity limits.
• Maybe, just maybe, enhance myocardial efficiency through a training effect.

Table 9.1 Pediatric Cardiac Rehabilitation Programs

Reference	N	Controls	Age (yrs)	Frequency (per wk)	Duration (wks)	Location	Diseases	Improvements
Bradley et al. (1985)	9	No	5-13	2	12	Hospital	TOF[a] TGA[b]	$\dot{V}O_2$max Endurance
Goldberg et al. (1981)	26	No	7-18	4	6	Home	VSD[c] TOF	Submax $\dot{V}O_2$ Endurance
Longmuir et al. (1985)	20	Yes	6-12	2	6	Home	Multiple	Performance
Mathews et al. (1983)	4	Yes	12-20	3	52	Gymnasium	Multiple	$\dot{V}O_2$max $\dot{V}_E$max
Ruttenburg et al. (1983)	12	Yes	7-18	3	9	Gymnasium	Multiple	Endurance
Vaccaro et al. (1987)	5	No	5-12	2	12	Hospital	TGA	$\dot{V}O_2$max Endurance

[a]Tetralogy of Fallot
[b]Transposition of great arteries
[c]Ventricular septal defect

"Carefully regulated" is important, because it must be appreciated that exercise programs are not without risk for certain patients. Fortunately, such risk situations, which will be addressed later in this chapter, are few.

Cardiac abnormalities encountered in the pediatric age group are, of course, very different from those observed in adults. Congenital anomalies—mistakes in cardiac organogenesis—constitute the great majority of cases, whereas acquired heart disease is uncommon (particularly given the marked reduction in incidence of rheumatic fever). In particular, ischemic coronary disease and cardiac complications of systemic hypertension, major causes of adult cardiac morbidity and mortality, are exceedingly rare.

Whether exercise performance will be impaired by a particular form of congenital heart anomaly depends on both the type and the severity of the lesion. Only in a minority of cases is diminished exercise capacity clinically evident; most children with congenital abnormalities exercise fully without problems. Anomalies that allow desaturated blood to reach the systemic circulation (right-to-left shunts such as tetralogy of Fallot) produce exercise intolerance by limiting oxygen delivery to peripheral muscle. Left-to-right shunts (ventricular septal defect, patent ductus arteriosus) create a volume overload on the heart and diminish lung compliance. When such communications are large enough, the resulting ventricular overwork reduces cardiac output reserve for exercise. Small shunts, on the other hand, cause no difficulties. Obstructive forms of congenital heart disease (aortic stenosis, pulmonary stenosis) likewise impair exercise performance only when outflow gradients are severe. In these cases physical activity causes inordinate fatigue because of a dampened rise in cardiac output, which may be accompanied by symptoms of chest pain, dizziness, and syncope.

Children with hemodynamically significant congenital heart disease usually undergo corrective surgery in early childhood. In some situations, however, operative intervention is only partially successful in reversing cardiac abnormalities, resulting in significant residual dysfunction that interferes with normal exercise tolerance. This is not to imply that easily becoming fatigued from physical activity is always cardiac-based. Years of limited or restricted exercise prior to surgery may impair peripheral muscular aerobic functions, and the patient's and his or her family's residual fears surrounding the stress that exercise might cause may also play important roles. If the experience with exercise training in children mirrors that of adults, the last two factors can be effectively ameliorated; whether direct effects on cardiac function can be expected is unclear. Rehabilitation programs for children and adolescents have generally centered around postoperative patients who have been left with some degree of impaired myocardial function.

Tetralogy of Fallot

In this anomaly, desaturated blood passes from the right ventricle through a ventricular septal defect to the aorta as an "easier" route than out an obstructed pulmonary outflow tract. Complete surgical repair previously was performed only in older children but is now routinely carried out in early infancy; a successful operation normalizes right-ventricular pressure by widening a hypoplastic pulmonary outflow tract and eliminating interventricular shunting by patch closure of the ventricular septal defect. Postoperative prognosis is excellent, and these patients generally live normally active lifestyles without complaints of exercise intolerance.

In the exercise laboratory, however, postoperative children may still show abnormalities in both right- and left-ventricular function, including diminished ejection fractions and dampened submaximal and maximal heart rate responses to treadmill or cycle testing. These findings are less prominent in patients who have been operated on in the first several years of life and who experienced good anatomical repairs (e.g., producing low right-ventricular pressure and elimination of ventricular septal defect shunt). Several explanations have been offered for residual ventricular dysfunction following tetralogy surgery, including these (Bar-Or, 1983; Graham, 1983):

- Persistent parental overprotection
- Effects of the right-ventriculotomy incision
- Low habitual activity
- Diminished myocardial compliance from previous right-ventricular hypertrophy

Children who have undergone surgical repair of tetralogy of Fallot have been participants in several pediatric rehabilitation programs (Goldberg et al., 1981; Longmuir et al., 1985; Ruttenberg, Adams, Osmond, Conlee, & Fisher, 1983). The numbers of patients involved are too small to allow firm conclusions regarding the effects of this intervention. Reduced $\dot{V}O_2$ requirements at a given submaximal workload were observed by both Ruttenberg et al. (1983) and Goldberg et al. (1981) in 3 and 16 postoperative tetralogy patients, respectively, after an exercise training program (Figure 9.1). In neither study did $\dot{V}O_2$max or peak heart rate change, although the subjects in both reports endured longer on exercise testing.

Transposition of the Great Arteries

The aorta and pulmonary arteries of babies with transposition of the great arteries (TGA) are literally transposed, or interchanged, across the ventricular septum: The right ventricle pumps to the systemic circulation while the left ventricle provides pulmonary blood flow. The result is two independent systemic and pulmonary circulations, a condition that is

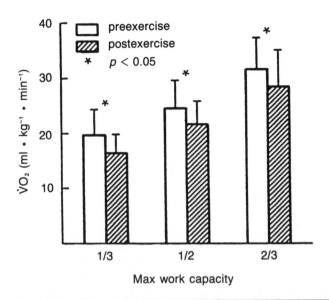

Figure 9.1 Oxygen uptake during submaximal exercise in 16 patients with tetralogy of Fallot before and after exercise training. *Note.* From ''Effect of Physical Training on Exercise Performance of Children Following Surgical Repair of Congenital Heart Disease'' by B. Goldberg, R.R. Fripp, G. Lister, J. Loke, J.A. Nicholas, and N.S. Talner, 1981, *Pediatrics*, **68**, p. 695. Copyright 1981 by the American Academy of Pediatrics. Reprinted by permission of *Pediatrics*.

quickly fatal following delivery unless a communication is created between the two sides of the heart, or—even better—the two great vessels are placed surgically back where they belong. The latter procedure, termed a ''switch'' operation, has grown in popularity in recent years as surgical techniques have improved to provide an optimistic outcome.

The older procedure is to first, in the newborn period, create a defect in the atrial septum with a balloon catheter to allow mixing of systemic and pulmonary circulations. A more definitive operation rerouting arterial blood flow is performed several months later (Mustard or Senning operation). By this technique, systemic venous blood returns to the right atrium, passes across the mitral valve to the left ventricle and out to the pulmonary circulation. Saturated blood arrives in the left atrium, subsequently flowing across the tricuspid valve to the right ventricle and aorta. The basic arrangement is now appropriate, but the right ventricle, originally designed for low-pressure work, serves as the systemic pump, and will be required to do so for life. Although patients generally do well following these procedures, the long-term outlook for right-ventricular and tricuspid valve function is questionable. Moreover these patients often experience supraventricular arrhythmias and a disconcerting trend for progressive sinus node dysfunction even decades after the initial operation. These complications have served as an impetus for development of the conceptually more attractive switch operation.

It is unknown whether children undergoing a successful switch operation for TGA will demonstrate abnormalities with exercise. That question won't be answered for at least a decade, when these infants have grown old enough for exercise testing. In the meantime, significant right-ventricular dysfunction, reduced maximal heart rate, and lower exercise capacity on cycle testing are typically observed following the traditional Mustard or Senning procedures. Resting right-ventricular ejection fraction is reported to average .43 to .47 (normal = .65) in these patients, often with little change following exercise. Patients with this level of ejection fraction usually do not describe fatigue with exercise and do not require medication. Whether future follow-up of these patients into older adulthood will disclose progression to right-sided myocardial failure and tricuspid valve regurgitation is unclear but worrisome (Graham, 1983). Why the right ventricle should function suboptimally following intra-atrial repair of TGA is unknown. High-pressure work pumping into the systemic circulation does not appear to be the answer, because normal ejection fraction is observed in patients with severe valvar pulmonary stenosis.

Vaccaro et al. (1987) described the physiological effects of a 12-week exercise program on five children who had undergone a Mustard operation for TGA 4 to 10 years previously. Three of the patients had pacemakers; two of them were also taking propranolol for dysrhythmias. In this uncontrolled study, $\dot{V}O_2$max increased from 32.9 to 37.8 ml • kg^{-1}min^{-1} with improvement in treadmill endurance time from 10.0 to 13.4 min. Similar changes were reported in three post-Mustard patients following training by Ruttenberg et al. (1983).

Tricuspid Atresia, Single Ventricle (Fontan Operation)

Patients born with a single functioning ventricle (hypoplastic right or left ventricle with atrioventricular valve atresia; single ventricle) have benefited from the Fontan procedure. In this operation the right atrium is anastomosed to the pulmonary artery, and the tricuspid orifice is closed (if not already atretic) and the pulmonary outflow tract obliterated. The right atrium, in effect, becomes the pump for the pulmonary circulation, and the single ventricle provides for systemic flow. Right-atrial pressure is elevated, and pulmonary flow is generally nonpulsatile, but effective cardiac output can be maintained, at least at rest. As might be expected, augmentation of systemic flow with exercise is limited. In nine patients who had undergone a Fontan operation for single ventricle, stroke volume did not rise appreciably with exercise, and $\dot{V}O_2$max was only 56 percent of predicted (Driscoll et al., 1987). Others have confirmed a subnormal cardiac output response to exercise following the Fontan procedure (Ben Shachar, Fuhrman, Wang, Lucas, & Lock, 1982; Hellenbrand, Laks, Kleinman, & Talner, 1981). When postoperative exercise parameters are compared to values *prior to* this procedure, however, significant improvements in $\dot{V}O_2$max, exercise endurance, and ventilatory responses are observed (Driscoll et al., 1986). Although experience of patients with a Fontan procedure following exercise training has not been described, these individuals would appear to be good candidates for rehabilitation programs.

Other Lesions

Residual cardiac dysfunction that may interfere with normal work performance is typical of the defects described, and preliminary information suggests that rehabilitation programs are useful in improving exercise tolerance. In forms of congenital heart disease in which surgery should be expected to "fix" the defect, subtle abnormalities in myocardial function and exercise performance are also sometimes observed. Abnormalities in ventricular size and ejection fraction have been reported following surgical closure of both atrial and ventricular septal defects. This has almost always occurred when the operation was performed during young adulthood; earlier closure of these shunts in infancy and early childhood should not be expected to be associated with residual myocardial disease.

EXERCISE AND VENTRICULAR DYSFUNCTION

The role of exercise training in children with cardiac disease has focused primarily on those with diminished myocardial function, usually following surgery. But what about the risks involved in stressing an already damaged myocardium? After all, *rest* is a hallmark feature of the management of heart failure; common sense dictates that exercise might hasten rather than ameliorate myocardial decompensation as well as increase the chances of life-threatening arrhythmias. Paradoxically, however, investigations in adults with CAD indicate that exercise rehabilitation can be conducted safely with favorable responses in ventricular function (R.S. Williams, 1985).

Endurance exercise performance is related to the capacity to deliver oxygen to exercising muscle ($\dot{V}O_2$max), which in turn is dependent on heart rate, stroke volume, and oxygen extraction by peripheral muscle. Patients with myocardial disease demonstrate limited ventricular contractility, measured by the ejection fraction, which largely determines stroke volume. It is surprising, then, that in adult patients with depressed ventricular function, endurance time during exercise testing (functional fitness) is not related to resting left-ventricular ejection fraction. Instead, the determinants limiting endurance in these subjects are mainly the rise in heart rate and the maximal arteriovenous oxygen uptake. Because endurance exercise training can be expected to improve the latter by increasing aerobic capacity of muscle, there is a rationale for rehabilitation programs for these patients. The experience in adult patients reviewed by R.S. Williams (1985) bears this out. Significant improvements in exercise performance are observed after training, without observed complications. Whether these findings can be translated to all children with ventricular dysfunction from congenital heart disease is unknown. Likewise, the role of rehabilitative exercise in other cardiac anomalies such as aortic insufficiency, rheumatic heart disease, and dilated cardiomyopathies has not been evaluated.

Psychological Gains

The limited experience of rehabilitation programs for children with heart disease indicates that exercise training is useful for improving functional work capacity and social confidence in these patients. Although the evidence is largely anecdotal, the directors of these programs report that their subjects improve in social interaction skills, become more outgoing, and have fewer anxieties surrounding physical activity (Ruttenberg et al., 1983; Tomassoni, Galioto, Vaccaro, Vaccaro, & Howard, 1987). Mathews et al. (1983) described psychological changes observed by interview and testing during a year-long exercise program in adolescents with congenital heart disease. Before the program parents had tried to restrict their children's physical activities from fear that the children could suffer sudden death. Similar fears were expressed by the patients themselves, who viewed themselves as weak and physically inadequate. By the end of the program these maladaptive responses had diminished: Parents were supporting rather than restricting their children's activities, patients' self-confidence and self-images improved, and fears of death lessened.

Program Design

Pediatric exercise rehabilitation programs have been modeled after those devised for adults, and no guidelines have been created specifically for young cardiac patients. As a result, a variety of approaches to location, monitoring, assessment, and design are evident in published descriptions of these programs. Yet the basic concerns are similar.

First, preparticipatory exercise testing is important to assess baseline fitness levels. In most cases this is performed by cycle ergometer or treadmill with measurement of $\dot{V}O_2$max, heart rate, electrocardiogram, endurance time, and often anaerobic threshold. This provides information regarding exercise prescription (target heart rate), aerobic fitness, and risk of dysrhythmias with exercise. Longmuir, Turner, Rowe, and Olley (1985), however, used field tests (such as the shuttle run and sit-ups) to assess their patients before and during a home exercise program. Most authors recommend repeat testing at 3- to 6-month intervals. More frequent testing may not show improvement and may serve as a negative rather than positive reinforcer for continued participation.

Second, patients with the following conditions are at significant risk from exercise and should probably be excluded from rehabilitation programs (Balfour, Drimmer, & Nouri, 1986):

- Severe aortic or pulmonary stenosis
- Less than 6 weeks post–open heart surgery
- Arrhythmia increased by exercise, uncontrolled by medication
- Eisenmenger syndrome
- Hypertrophic obstructive cardiomyopathy
- Acute inflammatory myocardial disease
- Uncontrolled congestive heart failure

Third, a well-rounded exercise program should include activities to increase flexibility and strength as well as endurance. Flexibility is improved by stretching exercises during the 5- to 10-min warm-up and cool-down before and after each session. Resistance and aerobic exercises can be alternated at 5-min intervals during the 20- to 30-min exercise sessions. Resistance exercises should be high-repetition exercises (using hand or wall weights) that can be performed for 5 min without fatigue. The intensity of aerobic activities (e.g., run/walk, cycling, rowing, dancing) should be graded in respect to the fitness state of the participant. A target heart rate of 70 to 85 percent of *measured* maximal heart rate, or the heart rate at anaerobic threshold, have commonly been used to gauge proper intensity. Goforth and James (1985) emphasized that exercise for cardiac patients should be comfortable; exercise beyond that which causes shortness of breath is not necessary for gaining a cardiovascular training effect, is not conducive to compliance, and may be dangerous for some patients. The amount of exertion perceived as comfortable by the subject is a good guide to proper training intensity.

Fourth, the duration of reported programs has ranged from 6 weeks up to 1 year, with frequency from every other day to twice a week.

Fifth, most programs have taken place in hospitals or institutions where full resuscitation equipment and qualified personnel (e.g., physicians, nurses, and exercise physiologists) are on-site. Others have involved only exercise at home, using field-test activities or cycle ergometers. EKG telemetry has not been frequently utilized. Balfour et al. (1986) indicated that telemetry should be reserved for high-risk patients (such as those with "more than mild aortic stenosis," known arrhythmias, or exercise-induced ischemia). In addition, Miller (1985) recommended that adult patients should exercise only in a medically supervised setting if they had cardiomegaly or evidence of heart failure, abnormal blood pressure response to exercise testing, ejection fraction less than 40 percent, gallop rhythm, very low fitness levels, fixed heart rate pacemakers, or prolonged QT interval on the electrocardiogram.

Last, as with adults, compliance is not high in pediatric rehabilitation programs. A number of strategies have been devised to help prevent subject dropout, including giving rewards such as T-shirts, tickets to athletic events, contests, and picnics. In some programs parents and siblings are encouraged to participate.

A summary of specific guidelines for prescribing an exercise program for children with heart disease can be found in the following box.

Exercise Prescription Guidelines for Children With Heart Disease

- Ensure patient safety. Is exercise contraindicated, or is ECG telemetry important?
- Perform preparticipatory exercise testing to examine fitness levels, ECG response, and subject-specific target heart rate. Follow-up testing should be performed at 3- to 6-month intervals.
- Exercise programs should be aimed at well-rounded fitness, including aerobic, flexibility, and strength activities.
- Strategies to ensure compliance are particularly important in this group of subjects, who typically have low initial levels of fitness.
- Utilize the advantages of group sessions to improve social confidence.

ASTHMA

During the 1972 Olympic Games in Munich, swimmer Rick DeMont of the United States took the gold medal in the 400-meter freestyle only to later have his award revoked. DeMont suffered from asthma, and ephedrine, a drug taken to prevent bronchospasm during competition, was detected during a routine urine check. Because ephedrine has adrenalin-like properties that were thought to potentially enhance performance, use of this drug by athletes had been declared illegal by the International Olympic Committee (IOC), and DeMont was unfortunately stripped of his title.

As much as this incident was both a personal and team tragedy, it did serve to focus attention for the first time on the significance of asthma for athletic participation. At the level of world-class competition it forced the IOC and other regulatory bodies to recognize that the use of therapeutic medication for athletes with asthma needed to be legitimized and guidelines for acceptable yet effective drugs created. Even more importantly, this focus on asthma and exercise extended to nonathletic individuals as well. In 1974, a symposium on exercise and asthma in children was held in Seattle to consider the effect of this disease on physical activity and provide guidelines for practicing physicians. Ghory (1975) summarized the conclusions from this meeting:

• The goal of physicians should be to assist the asthmatic child in leading as normal a life as possible.
• Untreated bronchospastic disease may interfere with normal exercise capacity, yet children with asthma benefit from exercise and need regular physical activity.
• With proper medical management most asthmatic children can participate normally in physical education classes as well as competitive sports.
• Children with asthma should not be overprotected from physical activities; instead they need to be encouraged to exercise regularly with the help of appropriate therapy.

The interplay between exercise and asthma is a complex one, with both beneficial and adverse implications for the asthmatic child. Factors interfering with normal lung function will inevitably impair normal oxygen delivery and exercise performance. It should not be unexpected, then, that the bronchospasm, mucosal edema, and increased airway mucus of an asthma attack should limit physical activity. But more important to these patients, exercise itself serves as a potent stimulus for bronchospasm, even in those whose disease is otherwise quiescent or controlled at rest by medications. This *exercised-induced bronchospasm* (EIB) typically occurs during recovery from physical activity of particular variety, intensity, and duration. EIB is evident in almost all subjects with asthma and a large percentage of patients with other atopic disease as well.

Because of such effects, those with asthma have often been restricted from physical activity by parents, teachers, and coaches, and it is not unusual for children to use their asthma as an excuse for not participating in physical education classes. As a consequence—not withstanding some prominent exceptions—children with asthma often demonstrate inferior levels of physical fitness. Exercise training in these individuals, with EIB controlled by medications and proper selection of activities, can improve exercise capacity. Moreover, there is some evidence to suggest that regular exercise may have beneficial effects on reducing EIB itself.

Responses to Exercise in Asthmatic Children

Surprisingly little is known about the acute physiological responses to exercise of children with asthma. In particular, it is not clear how much preexercise pulmonary status affects exercise performance or predisposes to subsequent EIB. Cropp and Tanakawa (1977) performed maximal cycle ergometer tests on children who had been referred to an asthma-treatment center for diagnostic evaluation of EIB. All were taking bronchodilator medications, and 81 percent required oral corticosteroid therapy. No drugs were administered less than 3 hr before exercise testing, however. Immediately before exercise, pulmonary function tests were essentially normal in 6 patients, mildly abnormal in 13, and moderately abnormal in 1. After exercise most patients experienced a deterioration in pulmonary function, and 13 developed EIB. There was, however, no correlation between preexercise pulmonary function findings and the appearance of EIB afterwards. Interestingly, the authors were convinced by physical examination and patients' reports that bronchospasm did not develop *during* exercise and that dyspnea was not a limiting factor to maximal cycle performance.

Compared to a control group of nonallergic, moderately active children, the asthmatic subjects had depressed work capacity and $\dot{V}O_2$max (accompanied by lower peak heart rate and ventilation). Anaerobic threshold was lower in the asthmatic subjects but was similar to controls when expressed as percent $\dot{V}O_2$max. At a given $\dot{V}O_2$ per body weight the asthmatic children had greater $\dot{V}_E$, tidal volume, and end-tidal pO_2 values (with lower end-tidal pCO_2) than the normals. This relative hyperventilation became more marked as exercise progressed. At rest the ratio of inspiratory to expiratory flow rates was equal in the two groups, but as the exercise load progressed children with asthma demonstrated an inability to increase expiratory rates as well as controls. This suggested that in asthmatic subjects expiratory airway obstruction becomes more severe as intensity of exercise increases. The authors felt that all these departures from normal responses to exercise resulted from preexisting functional abnormalities rather than EIB. It may be difficult, however, to separate out some of these findings from those of subjects with particularly sedentary lifestyles.

In contrast to the study described, asthmatic subjects who are in good control of their disease before exercise usually demonstrate normal work capacity, $\dot{V}O_2$max, and ventilatory measurements with exercise (Bevegard, Eriksson, Graff-Lonnevig, Kraepelien, & Saltin, 1976). These limited data indicate that evidence of bronchospasm during exercise and poor endurance fitness in these patients may be due to either insufficient baseline control of asthma or inadequate amounts of regular physical activity. These alternative explanations for inordinate dyspnea, fatigue, and wheezing with exercise need to be kept in mind when assessing the asthmatic child with presumed EIB.

Exercise-Induced Bronchospasm (EIB)

Given activity of sufficient intensity and duration, virtually all patients with asthma will develop evidence of postexercise bronchospasm. Typically, short bursts of activity (1 to 3 min) are well tolerated, because asthmatic subjects, like normal individuals, demonstrate a period of bronchodilatation early in exercise as a result of increased adrenergic activity. But upon completion of more extended activities (6 to 12 min) at work loads eliciting a heart rate over 85 percent maximum, these patients often experience various degrees of wheezing, cough, dyspnea, and constricting chest discomfort. Symptoms usually peak at 5 to 10 min after termination of exercise and may resolve anywhere from minutes to an hour later. EIB does not trigger status asthmaticus, but delayed asthmatic responses have been described that may appear 3 to 6 hr after exercise. By all measures, the pathophysiology of these episodes is indistinguishable from asthma attacks unaccompanied by exercise.

It is important to recognize that EIB is not limited to those with recognized asthma but is common in other individuals with allergic symptoms. Bierman, Kawabori, and Pierson (1975) examined the incidence of EIB in 134 asthmatic, 102 nonasthmatic atopic (allergic rhinitis, atopic dermatitis), and 56 nonatopic children aged 5 to 18 years. The exercise provocation test was vigorous free running for 5 min with pulmonary function tests performed immediately before exercise and at 5-min intervals afterward. Among the asthmatic group 63 percent demonstrated EIB (as defined as a fall in forced 1-sec expiratory volume [FEV_1] over 15 percent) compared to 7 percent of the controls. Importantly, 41 percent of the atopic, nonasthmatic subjects (who had no previous history or clinical evidence of asthma) also had EIB (Figure 9.2).

An understanding of EIB and its management is essential for physicians caring for asthmatic patients, because EIB can be prevented through appropriate use of preexercise bronchodilators and/or selection of activities. The characteristics, etiology, diagnosis, and management of EIB have been reviewed previously (Bar-Or, 1983; Miller, 1987; Neijens, 1985).

Etiology of EIB

Extensive investigation into the etiology of EIB has centered around two lines of inquiry: cooling and drying of the airways and the release of chemical mediators, particularly from mast cells. Presumably the trigger for EIB represents some combination of these factors (Ben-Dov, Bar-Yiskay, & Godfrey, 1982).

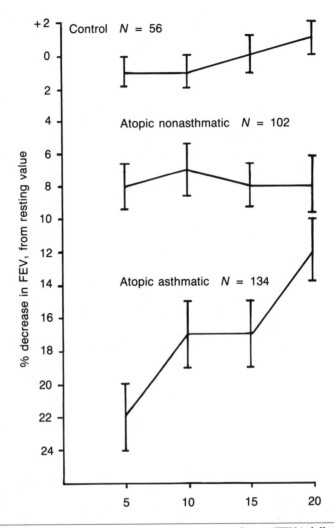

Figure 9.2 Percent fall in forced 1-sec expiratory volume (FEV₁) following exercise in control, atopic nonasthmatic, and atopic asthmatic subjects. *Note.* From "Incidence of Exercise-Induced Asthma in Children" by C.W. Bierman, I. Kawaabori, and W.E. Pierson, 1975, *Pediatrics*, **56**, p. 848. Copyright 1975 by the American Academy of Pediatrics. Reprinted by permission of *Pediatrics*.

During exercise the airways are responsible for both humidifying and warming inspired air. This function is an efficient one, as a mean air temperature of 27 °C in the right lower lobe can be maintained even when inspiring air as cold as −17 °C with moderate hyperventilation (Deal,

McFadden, Ingram, & Jaeger, 1979). As heat and water are transferred from the mucosal surface, the airway lining is cooled and dried, an effect that is directly proportional to the extent of EIB. The amount of ventilation as well as the temperature and humidity of inspired air are therefore important determinants of exercise-induced asthma. When warm, saturated air is provided to exercising asthmatic subjects during laboratory testing, EIB does not occur; conversely, cooling and drying of inspired air increases EIB (Anderson, Silverman, Konig, & Godfrey, 1975). This phenomenon helps explain why swimming in warm, humid pool conditions is much more easily tolerated by asthmatic subjects than such sports as distance running and cycling. No difference in airway cooling is observed between asthmatic and nonasthmatic subjects, indicating that the airways of the former are hyper-reactive to decreased temperature (Deal, McFadden, Ingram, Breslin, & Jaeger, 1980).

When exercise bouts of 5 to 10 minutes are repeated several times within a short time of each other, the degree of EIB is blunted. After a 2-hr rest interval, however, full postexercise symptoms are usually again observed (Edmunds, Tooley, & Godfrey, 1978; James, Faciane, & Sly, 1976). This strongly suggests that EIB is associated with depletion of chemical mediators, which are restored during the "refractory period" after exercise. The ability of disodium cromoglycate (cromolyn), a drug that blocks mast-cell release of allergic mediators, to prevent EIB is further evidence of the importance of these agents in exercise-induced asthma.

Type, Intensity, and Duration of Exercise

For most patients 5 or 6 minutes of continuous exercise are necessary to trigger EIB. Longer exercise may actually diminish bronchospasm, explaining why some subjects are capable of "running through their asthma." The greater the exercise intensity, the more EIB can be expected, at least up to 60 to 85 percent of maximal work capacity, when EIB tends to plateau (Silverman & Anderson, 1972). For most subjects this means that the intensity of activity must be sufficient to raise the heart rate to 85 percent of maximum (for most children approximately 170 bpm). Repetitive bouts of short-burst exercise lasting 1 to 2 minutes interrupted by rest periods will not typically provoke asthma.

Anderson et al. (1975) found that free running produced the greatest degree of EIB, followed in order of bronchospasm effect by treadmill running, cycling, treadmill walking, and swimming in an indoor heated pool (Figure 9.3). Other studies examining these activities in the same humidity and thermal environment have explained these findings by differences in ventilation rates and inspired air conditions.

Based on such findings, proper selection of sport activities may help prevent EIB in asthmatic children. Swimming, wrestling, sprinting, and team sports such as football and baseball may be well-tolerated. Other

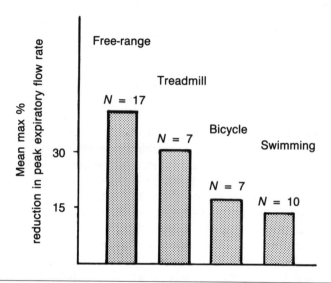

Figure 9.3 Differences in reduction in peak expiratory flow rate (PEFR) induced by various forms of exercise in subjects with exercise-induced bronchospasm. *Note.* From "Comparative Aspects of Available Exercise Systems" by K.D. Fitch, 1975, *Pediatrics, 56,* p. 966. Copyright 1975 by the American Academy of Pediatrics. Reprinted by permission of *Pediatrics.*

activities are associated with a high incidence of EIB, particularly cold-weather sports (except downhill skiing) and those involving prolonged running (e.g., cross-country and basketball). Even in these activities, however, full participation is usually possible with the use of prophylactic bronchodilators.

Diagnosis

The diagnosis of EIB can often be made from a typical history of cough, dyspnea, and wheezing following exercise in an allergic individual. It is important to realize that not all subjects present with these typical features, however. Some might experience principally shortness of breath; in fact, this could be interpreted as a normal response by the affected individual, and EIB may go unsuspected. Chest pain from EIB is probably the most common cause of chest discomfort triggered by exercise in the pediatric age group (Nudel et al., 1987). Cough, abdominal pain, and headache accompanying exercise have each been described as isolated indicators of EIB (Round Table, 1984).

In uncertain cases, pulmonary function tests before and after standardized exercise provocation can be performed. Forced expiratory volume in 1 sec (FEV_1) or the peak expiratory flow rate (PEFR), determined before and at 5-min intervals after exercise, have been used most commonly because of their ease of measurement. It should be noted, however, that not all cases of EIB are detected by these two tests (Rice, Bierman, Shapiro, Furukawa & Pierson, 1985). The severity of EIB is described as the difference between initial and postexercise values expressed as a percentage of the initial value.

In nonasthmatic individuals, running causes an average decrease in PEFR of 2.5 to 3.5 percent, and a fall more than 15 percent is greater than 2 standard deviations from normal (Burr, Eldridge, & Borysiewicz, 1974). The diagnosis of EIB has therefore generally been considered established by a reduction in FEV_1, or PEFR of 15 to 20 percent following exercise (Fitch, 1975a).

Several forms of exercise tests have been used to assess bronchospasm with physical activity. Pierson and Bierman (1975) described a free-running test for EIB that involved a 200-ft concrete runway on a 3 percent grade. Subjects ran as fast as they could for 5 min up and down the ramp, which resulted in a heart rate greater than 180 bpm after the first minute of exercise. In their report, 103 of 198 allergic subjects demonstrated at least a 15 percent drop of FEV_1 during 20 min of postexercise testing. This method has advantages of simulating normal activity, avoiding complicated instrumentation, and being applicable to the clinical setting.

Treadmill running, on the other hand, is easier to standardize and is more reproducible (Godfrey, Silverman, & Anderson, 1975). In this test children are asked to run (not walk) continuously at a comfortable running speed at a slope of 10 percent for 6 min (heart rate should reach 170 bpm). Silverman and Anderson (1972) described EIB in 75 percent of 97 asthmatic children using this method.

Cycle ergometry possesses the advantages of portability, low cost, and ease of monitoring, but the bronchospastic response to exercise may be lower using this method (Eggleston, 1975). The load required to achieve a target heart rate of 85 percent maximum is not known on a subject's initial test and will require adjustment in the early stages of exercise. More complete details regarding standardization of exercise tests for eliciting EIB have been provided by Bar-Or (1983).

EIB and the Athlete

Given proper management, the child with asthma should not be excluded from any form of sport participation. In a survey of 597 participants in the 1984 Summer Olympic Games in Los Angeles, 67 (11 percent) had exercise-induced bronchospasm. During the Games, 41 of those athletes won medals, including 15 golds, in sport events as diverse as basketball, cycling, rowing, swimming, track and field, and wrestling (Voy, 1986). Appropriate use of preexercise bronchodilators is largely responsible for avoidance of EIB in these successful athletes, many of whom were involved in sports that are particularly prone to inducing asthma. There is also subjective information that EIB may be diminished in the competitive setting (Fitch, 1975b). This may occur because of the large production of endogenous catecholamines that accompanies these events.

It may be difficult to judge the success of medical intervention with prophylactic bronchodilators in athletes who typically experience respiratory fatigue and dyspnea with the completion of an exhaustive competitive effort. Ongoing measurements of PEFR before and after athletic participation in the field can be useful in this assessment.

Many athletes with asthma have found an adequate warm-up period to be a valuable means of decreasing EIB during competition or training. Based on observational experience, Fitch (1975a) concluded that intense exercise (at greater than 75 percent $\dot{V}O_2max$) was more likely to stimulate EIB when not preceded by warm-up exercises.

Prevention of EIB

Although prophylactic bronchodilator therapy is an effective means of preventing or blunting EIB for most individuals, nonpharmacological methods, summarized in the following box, may play an important role as well (Katz, 1986). As noted, selection of proper activities may avert EIB altogether. Swimming is the best sport for asthmatic subjects, as are other activities, such as sprints, gymnastics, and wrestling, that avoid prolonged exercise. Endurance events, or those occurring in a dry, cold environment are more likely to evoke EIB. Warm-up exercises within 1 hr of activity are also helpful in diminishing postexercise bronchospasm.

Preventive Measures
Against Exercise-Induced Bronchospasm (EIB)

- Long warm-up; increase exercise gradually
- Proper sports selection: Swimming, sprints trigger less EIB than endurance activities
- Nasal breathing
- Mouth mask
- Bronchodilators

Because EIB generally occurs only after at least 5 min of high-intensity exercise, bronchospasm can be prevented by intermittent, shorter bouts of activity. Circuit training, involving exercise of several minutes interspersed by short rest periods, is a useful pattern of physical activity for asthmatic patients. Whether physical training itself diminishes EIB is controversial (see page 202).

Breathing through the nose may help prevent EIB. The nose is a more efficient heat exchanger than the mouth, and nasal breathing diminishes lower airway cooling and drying. Nasal breathing allows only limited ventilation, however, and cannot be expected to be a practical means of preventing EIB with high-intensity activities. Warming and humidifying inspired air by using a mask or scarf about the mouth may help decrease EIB when exercising in cold weather.

Several classes of medications administered before exercise can block the development of EIB (Table 9.2). In many cases these must be given as supplements to the asthmatic child's usual drug regimen, which may eliminate wheezing at rest but will not block bronchospasm provoked by exercise. As noted previously, however, inadequate baseline control of asthma can result in increased wheezing and dyspnea with exercise, which signal a need for more manipulation of maintenance medications.

Table 9.2 Drugs Useful in Prevention of EIB

Drug	Route
Sympathomimetic amines (beta$_2$ agonists)	
Albuterol	Aerosol
Metaproterenol	Aerosol
Terbutaline	Aerosol
Sodium cromoglycate	Aerosol
Theophylline	Oral

Inhaled beta$_2$-adrenergic bronchodilators (e.g., albuterol, metaproterenol, and terbutaline) have become the most popular agents for prevention (and treatment) of EIB. Administered as 1 or 2 puffs 10 to 15 min before exercise, these aerosols provide protection for up to 4 to 6 hr with minimal cardiovascular side effects. They also effectively reverse EIB once it occurs. These drugs, which are approved for use in world-class competition, can also be given orally, 30 to 60 min before exercise, but are less effective in preventing EIB by this route in most patients.

Cromolyn is not a bronchodilator, but it is useful in preventing EIB, presumably due to inhibition of mediator release from mast cells. Approximately 70 percent of asthmatic patients will experience improvement in EIB after administration of cromolyn, which appears to be more effective in children than in adults (Fitch, 1986). Cromolyn has no effect on the cardiovascular system and is useful in preventing delayed postexercise bronchospasm. It is not effective in treating EIB once it occurs, however. Cromolyn is administered by inhaler, 20 to 40 mg, no more than 1 hr before exercise.

Oral theophylline, one of the mainstays of asthma management, is useful in modifying EIB but only when serum concentrations are high. Its efficacy is similar to that of cromolyn. Increasing the usual dose 1 to 3 hr before exercise may be a simple way of blocking EIB for the asthmatic patient. But for many, the gastrointestinal upset and jitteriness associated with this approach may preclude its use.

Belladonna alkaloids (ipatropium bromide) are of questionable utility in preventing EIB (Fitch, 1986), and glucocorticoids, either inhaled or oral, have no clear-cut effectiveness for blocking EIB. Among the sympathomimetic amines, ephedrine has a moderate effect in preventing EIB, while isoproterenol inhalation is more effective but only for a short period of time. Both of these agents have prominent cardiac side effects (tremor, insomnia, risk of arrhythmias) and are banned by the IOC as doping agents.

In order of preference, then, initial prophylactic therapy with a beta$_2$-adrenergic agent by inhalation is the drug of choice. If the child is already taking an oral form of this medication, cromolyn would be an appropriate alternative to prevent EIB. Incomplete control of EIB with beta$_2$-adrenergic drugs should lead to addition of cromolyn to the treatment regimen. Increased oral theophylline dosage prior to exercise would be an appropriate step if cromolyn and beta$_2$-adrenergic agents together fail to satisfactorily prevent EIB.

It is important, when evaluating these drugs, to recognize the potential for a strong placebo effect. In a study evaluating the side effects of various bronchodilators on preventing EIB, for instance, Godfrey and Konig (1975) showed that aerosol or intravenous saline could reduce the amount of postexercise bronchospasm by one third to one half.

Effects of Physical Training

Children with asthma who participate in a program of regular physical activity typically improve their levels of physical fitness. In the process these patients appear to gain improved social confidence and self-esteem, as do children with other chronic diseases (Fitch, Blitvich, & Morton, 1986). Whether physical training reduces the severity of EIB is controversial; it does appear, however, that regular exercise cannot be expected to improve baseline asthma disease.

Improved Aerobic Fitness

Most studies have shown increased levels of physical fitness in asthmatic children after training, whether measured as $\dot{V}O_2$max, distance run in 12 min, cycle endurance time, or submaximal heart rate response to exercise (Table 9.3). In many cases these reports involved subjects who had very limited physical capabilities before training, partly as a result of habitually sedentary lifestyle.

Table 9.3 Training Studies With Asthmatic Children

Reference	N	Duration (months)	Age (yrs)	Activities	Weekly frequency	$\dot{V}O_2$ and/or work capacity cardiovascular fitness	Improved asthma	Decreased EIB
Graff-Lonnevig et al. (1980)	11	20	11.2	Circuit	2	0	0	—
Fitch et al. (1986)	10	3	10-14	Running games	4	0	?	0
Orenstein et al. (1985)	20	4	6-16	Walk/run	3	+	0	0
Henriksen & Nielsen (1983)	28	1.5	11	Running, gymnastics, circuit	2	+	0	+
Svenonius et al. (1983)	50	3-4	9-16	Running, skipping rope	2	+	?	+
Ludwick et al. (1986)	65	?	12	Cycling	5	+	—	—
Nickerson et al. (1983)	15	1.5	7-14	Running	4	+	0	0
Fitch et al. (1976)	46	5	12	Swimming	3-5	+	+	0

Note. + = training effect, 0 = no training effect, — = not evaluated.

How such training programs should be designed is not at all clear from the available reports, however. Graff-Lonnevig, Bevegard, Eriksson, Kraepelien, and Saltin (1980) described a 20-month training program for asthmatic children that was specifically designed to avoid triggering EIB. This included a low-intensity warm-up and circuit activities of high intensity for short periods. Although these programs were successful from the standpoint of subject enjoyment and compliance, no improvements were noted in maximal respiratory and circulatory function over that expected from growth alone.

Other authors have reported significant improvements in $\dot{V}O_2max$ and functional fitness using protocols similar to those employed with nonasthmatic subjects. These have involved continuous running or cycling at high heart rates that would have triggered EIB if prophylactic medications were not used (Ludwick, Jones, Jones, Fukuhara, & Strunk, 1986; Orenstein, Reed, Grogan, & Crawford, 1985). Whether training intensities sufficient to induce EIB are *necessary* to improve work capacity in poorly fit asthmatic patients is an important but unanswered question.

Changes in Baseline Asthma

Physical training might theoretically help children with asthma by improving respiratory muscle function, increasing mucus clearance, or providing catecholamine-induced bronchodilatation. Measurement of resting pulmonary function before and after training have failed to demonstrate such an effect, however. Subjective reports from exercising patients did indicate improvements in baseline asthma symptoms in two programs (Fitch et al., 1986; Svenonius, Kautto, & Arborelius, 1983). Fitch, Morton, and Blanksky (1976) recorded asthma scores before and after swim training based on daily wheezing, cough and sputum production, and need for medication. The average asthma and medication scores declined during the 5-month study, an effect the authors conceded could have been related to seasonal variation of pollen counts and other allergens.

Decreased Exercise-Induced Bronchospasm

No definite conclusions can be drawn from available data on the use of exercise training to decrease the severity of EIB. Certainly this does not appear to be a predictable outcome of such programs, because most have demonstrated no effect on postexercise pulmonary-function tests. However, Henriksen and Nielsen (1983) demonstrated a reduction in percentage fall of PEFR from 44 to 30 percent after training, using a variety of activities preceded by prophylactic bronchodilators. Similar findings were reported by Svenonius et al. (1983) employing a regular program of interval exercises (alternating 2 min of high-intensity exercise and rest).

Responsibilities of the Physician

Asthma should not interfere with normal childhood exercise activities. The fear of EIB often leads parents and teachers to overprotect asthmatic children and causes patients to be hesitant about exercising. These youngsters, who are already set apart as "different" by their peers, withdraw from sport activities at a time when the physical, psychological, and social benefits of exercise are critically important. Through the approach to EIB management outlined in this chapter, physicians have an opportunity to encourage these patients to take part in regular physical activity.

EIB should be assumed present to some degree in all patients with asthma. Empirical therapeutic trials or free-running testing in the office may be sufficient diagnostic approaches in some cases, but often a standardized cycle or treadmill provocation test is necessary to assess severity of EIB and subsequent response to treatment. This is particularly true for athletes who need to be clear of bronchospasm during competition.

Asthmatic children who seldom exercise and have low fitness levels should be introduced to a program of regular physical activity (you can find exercise prescription guidelines for asthmatic children in the box that follows). This is best provided in a group setting, which is often available through local agencies (e.g., the American Lung Association or YMCA). These programs have typically emphasized swimming, circuit

---

Exercise Prescription Guidelines for Children With Asthma

- Adapt the exercise program to the patient's level of fitness. Initial formal exercise testing is useful for determining this information as well as for documenting severity of exercise-induced bronchospasm (EIB) and establishing target heart rates.
- Emphasize activities that are usually tolerated by children with asthma: swimming, relay races, circuit exercises, and ball games.
- Patients should prepare for exercise with bronchodilator prophylaxis for EIB. A long warm-up of mild intensity may be useful in minimizing EIB.
- Encourage group activities as a means of improving emotional well-being.
- Utilize exercise sessions for patient educational experiences regarding asthma and its control.

training, ball games, and relay races as forms of exercise particularly tolerated by children with asthma. The exercise program needs to be adapted
to the individual's preexisting fitness level. Exercise should be preceded
by prophylactic medication (as necessary) and a long warm-up of mild
intensity (to perhaps deplete mediators that trigger EIB). These programs
increase the child's self-confidence by participation in peer-group activities. They also serve as an educational tool for increasing the patient's
knowledge about his or her disease and how it affects exercise capabilities.

CYSTIC FIBROSIS

The long-term outlook for patients with cystic fibrosis has improved
dramatically over the past 2 decades. Severe incapacity and death during
childhood from this disease were once common, but now most patients
can expect to live reasonably comfortable lives to the young adult years.
Thanks to early diagnosis and aggressive therapy, up to 80 percent may
currently survive to at least 20 years of age (Phelan and Hey, 1984). Still,
this disease is marked by relentless deterioration of pulmonary function,
with complications of pneumonia, hypoxemia, and secondary cardiac
involvement that seriously impair quality of life. The thick, tenacious
mucus typical of cystic fibrosis obstructs airways and leads to progressive emphysema, atelectasis, bronchiectasis, and secondary infections;
in 90 percent of cases, lung involvement is the cause of death (Wood,
Boat, & Doershuk, 1976).

As might be expected, exercise intolerance is common in these patients
and generally varies in proportion to the severity of the disease (Canny
& Levison, 1987). The ability to engage in physical activities thus
varies widely, from those markedly restricted in exercise to champion athletes, including marathon runners (Orenstein, Henke, & Cerny, 1983;
Stanghelle & Skyberg, 1983). Eventually, though, exercise tolerance
declines as the natural course of the disease progresses, leading to marked
disability in its terminal phases.

Exercise for patients with cystic fibrosis has long been considered beneficial, and recent studies have begun to place earlier subjective observations on firmer scientific grounds (Stanghelle, 1988). These findings have
provided an impetus for programs of regular physical activity for patients
with cystic fibrosis as well as other forms of chronic lung disease. They
have also, in the process, provided an improved understanding of the
pathogenic mechanisms that limit exercise in this disease.

Mechanisms Inhibiting Exercise Tolerance

In the normal individual, the maximum delivery of oxygen to muscle—a
major determinant of exercise endurance—is limited by cardiac and

peripheral muscular aerobic capacity. The healthy lung has been traditionally considered a strong link in the oxygen delivery chain, because respiratory function at $\dot{V}O_2$max is only approximately 70 percent of peak lung capacity (Godfrey & Mearns, 1971). In individuals with cystic fibrosis, however, ventilatory factors figure prominently in the limitation of exercise endurance.

Several aspects of pulmonary function combine to define these limits. Maximal work capacity is closely related to the degree of airway obstruction, which must be overcome by raising minute ventilation. Ventilatory requirements are also increased in patients with cystic fibrosis from mismatches of ventilation and perfusion that create hypoxemia and enlarge physiological dead space, sometimes by as much as 300 percent of normal values (Godfrey & Mearns, 1971).

During exercise, then, these patients demonstrate compensatory increases in minute ventilation compared to normal subjects at a given workload and often at maximal effort as well. As shown in Figure 9.4, the greater the degree of resting impairment in pulmonary function, the more exaggerated is the rise of $\dot{V}_E$ with exercise (Cerny, Pullano, & Cropp, 1982). This is, in fact, accomplished effectively, as there is no loss of respiratory drive, even when the disease is severe (Bureau, Lupien, & Begin, 1981). This compensation requires increased breathing work and stresses the ventilatory muscles. Respiratory muscle fatigue may therefore further limit exercise endurance. Interestingly, patients with cystic fibrosis appear to have greater ventilatory muscle endurance than normal individuals (Keens et al., 1977). This presumably reflects a training effect of respiratory muscles in response to the chronic stress of breathing against flow-resistive loads.

Because pancreatic enzyme secretion is blocked, patients with cystic fibrosis suffer malabsorption and failure to thrive unless supplementary enzymes are provided. Even so, older individuals with this disease often demonstrate various degrees of undernutrition that may contribute to depressed exercise capacity (Coates, Boyce, Muller, Mearns, & Godfrey, 1980). This could be manifested by loss of leg-muscle mass or impaired respiratory-muscle strength. Marked increases in maximal exercise capacity have been described following improvement of nutritional status in these patients (Skeie et al., 1987).

Evidence indicates that impaired cardiac stroke volume may depress exercise tolerance in some adults with chronic obstructive pulmonary disease. This does not appear to be a significant factor for those with cystic fibrosis, however. Marcotte, Grisdale, Levison, Coates, and Canny (1986) studied determinants of exercise capacity in patients with a wide range of resting pulmonary function. Multiple regression analysis revealed that maximal voluntary ventilation accounted for 71 percent of the variance in maximal work capacity. Submaximal stroke volume and cardiac output measured by the CO_2 rebreathing method at 50 percent $\dot{V}O_2$max did not

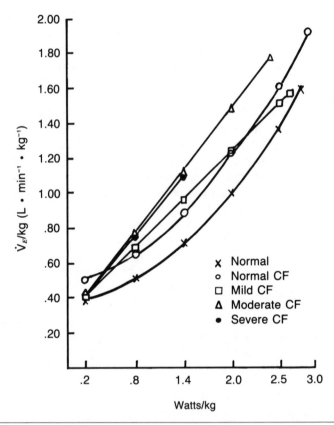

Figure 9.4 Minute ventilation plotted against cycle-exercise work load in normal children and four groups of patients with cystic fibrosis of varying severity. *Note.* From "Cardiorespiratory Adaptations to Exercise in Cystic Fibrosis" by F.J. Cerny, T.P. Pullano, and G.J.A. Cropp, 1982, *American Review of Respiratory Disease,* **126**, p. 218. Copyright 1982 by the American Lung Association. Reprinted by permission.

make any further significant contribution to the prediction of exercise tolerance.

Hypoxemia develops with exercise only in patients with severe disease (Cropp, Pullano, Cerny, & Nathanson, 1982). This may be a consequence of increased ventilation–perfusion mismatch or alveolar hypoventilation—because these patients, despite increased $\dot{V}_E$, fail to prevent alveolar hypoventilation with rise in end-tidal pCO_2 as exercise progresses. Although oxygen saturation remains normal during exercise testing in those with mild to moderate disease, patients with severe cystic fibrosis (resting FEV_1 30 to 50 percent predicted) may demonstrate declines of as much as 12 to 14 percent. Conversely, in the patients described by Marcotte et al. (1986), none with an FEV_1 of 60 percent predicted at rest demonstrated a fall in oxygen saturation over 5 percent with exercise.

$\dot{V}O_2$max values vary widely in patients with this disease but tend to average at the low end of normal (Marcotte et al., 1986). Maximal heart rates are typically less than predicted (Cropp et al., 1982). This suggests that ventilatory factors limit exercise before cardiac limits are reached. Patients with cystic fibrosis do not usually develop bronchoconstriction with exercise. Therefore, prophylactic bronchodilators are typically of no value in improving tolerance to physical activity.

Cystic fibrosis is characterized by an increased concentration of sodium and chloride in sweat, which may predispose patients to a greater risk for heat injury. It does not, however, appear to increase the chances of hyperthermia with exercise. Orenstein, Germann, and Costill (1981) showed that rectal temperatures in subjects with cystic fibrosis were no different from those of control subjects when exercising at 50 percent $\dot{V}O_2$max in 100 °F conditions. In this study, however, serum chloride concentrations dropped significantly. Stanghelle (1988) followed serum electrolytes in patients with cystic fibrosis running a marathon race in 28 °C temperature and high humidity. Only a slight decrease in sodium concentration was observed to the low range of normal. The author concluded that salt depletion was not a major problem for these individuals, who may compensate for increased sweat salt loss by decreasing excretion of salt in urine. It is generally recommended, however, that individuals with cystic fibrosis be particularly careful to replace fluid and salt when exercising in warm environments.

Effects of Physical Training

Historically, physicians have encouraged their patients with cystic fibrosis to exercise regularly. Exercise was felt intuitively to be useful for stimulating deep breathing, coughing, and sputum production, as well as for improving morale and feelings of independence and self-confidence. Current research has borne out these subjective impressions: Exercise provides benefits for most patients with this disease (Canny & Levison, 1987; Keens, 1979). There is still no good evidence that the disease process itself is retarded, or that the natural course is impeded, by a program of physical activity. But individuals with cystic fibrosis who exercise regularly enjoy an improved physical and psychological quality of life that justifies the promotion of exercise for these patients.

The most immediate benefit from exercise training in these patients is the improved ability to tolerate physical activity. Daily functions can be conducted with less fatigue, and these individuals are able to enjoy the company of others in more physically taxing activities. Orenstein, Franklin, Doershuk, Hellerstein, and Germann (1981) conducted a 3-month conditioning program of walking and running in 21 patients with cystic fibrosis. The exercising subjects improved $\dot{V}O_2$max and exercise tolerance compared to a control group, although no changes in pulmonary function were noted (Figure 9.5). Similar results have been reported following swimming training (Edlund, French, Herbst, Ruttenberg, & Ruhling, 1986) and trampoline exercise (Stanghelle, Hjeltnes, Bangstad, & Michalsen, 1988).

Zach, Purrer, and Oberwaldner (1981), moreover, were able to show beneficial changes on the pulmonary status of children with cystic fibrosis after a swimming program. Ten patients participated in 17 sessions over a 7-1/2 week period. In this uncontrolled study, the group mean values

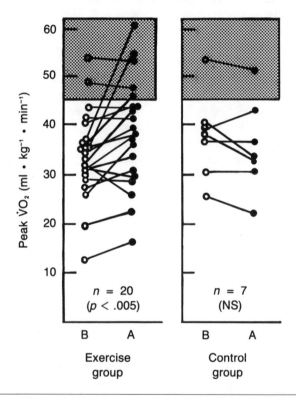

Figure 9.5 Effects of a 3-month physical training program on maximal aerobic power in subjects with cystic fibrosis compared to nontraining controls. *Note.* From "Exercise Conditioning and Cardiopulmonary Fitness in Cystic Fibrosis" by D.M. Orenstein, B.A. Franklin, C.F. Doershuk, H.K. Hellerstein, and K.J. Germann, 1981, *Chest,* **80,** p. 394. Copyright 1981 by the American College of Chest Physicians. Reprinted by permission.

for FEV$_1$ and PEFR improved significantly during the course of the program.

Keens (1979) proposed that exercise proves beneficial to patients with cystic fibrosis by improving respiratory muscle endurance. Therapeutic interventions do little to change the basic pathophysiology of the disease, but strengthening compensatory mechanisms might be a useful alternative. Ventilatory muscle, like skeletal muscle, improves its functional reserve with training, and in patients with cystic fibrosis the increased demands placed on ventilation may be better met by a "fit" respiratory machine.

Keens et al. (1977) showed that 25 min daily of maximal normocapnic hyperpnea performed 5 days a week for 4 weeks improved ventilatory muscle endurance in both normal subjects and those with cystic fibrosis. Fortunately, the same result was observed following more pleasurable activities (swimming, canoeing). Orenstein et al. (1981) demonstrated that a running program also produced the same effect. Whether improved respiratory muscle endurance has clinical significance for the patient with cystic fibrosis remains to be seen. It does appear that these training effects rapidly disappear if exercise is not continued. Once stopped, half of the observed improvement was gone by 10 weeks (Keens et al., 1977).

Can exercise improve the mobilization of airway mucus in these patients? The coughing and increased sputum production observed during physical activity is an effect that could decrease the need for—or replace—routine chest physical therapy. In the swimming program of Zach et al. (1981) sputum production was greater on swimming days. Andreasson, Jonson, Kornfaldt, Nordmark, and Sandstrom (1987) described the response of 7 patients with cystic fibrosis to a 30-month program of daily exercise. After 12 months, chest physical therapy was withdrawn without significant change in pulmonary function tests. Orenstein et al. (1983) reported two preliminary studies that indicated that exercise may be as beneficial as traditional postural drainage and clapping in sustaining pulmonary function.

Exercise training has long been considered important in improving the psychological well-being of patients with cystic fibrosis. Andreasson et al. (1987) evaluated the responses of their 7 subjects to a 30-month program by questionnaire. Most reported "enjoying the physical training and especially the possibility of exercising together with friends. The therapy contributed to the independence of the patient, according to the parents of five patients" (p. 72).

Experience with cystic fibrosis patients in exercise training has demonstrated that these programs can be conducted without risk of complications. Fears of salt depletion, pneumothorax, hemoptysis, and exacerbation of their disease have not been supported. Still, activities should be carefully supervised for those with desaturation, extensive bronchiectasis, or pneumatoceles. Esophageal varices associated with cirrhosis of the liver preclude exercise activities (Stanghelle, 1988).

Exercise Programs

Most patients with cystic fibrosis can be expected to respond to a program of physical activity in the following ways:

- Increased exercise tolerance
- Improved ventilatory muscle endurance
- Augmented sputum clearance
- Feelings of psychological well-being

Exercise may be integrated into their daily lifestyle, but the support and guidance necessary for motivating patients into regular activities is best scheduled through a structured, supervised exercise program. In most situations, it is prudent to give a treadmill or cycle stress test before beginning these programs. Findings allow the physician to appreciate the baseline fitness level of the patient and establish target training heart rates based on a percentage of that individual's maximal rate. Target rates based on predicted peak heart rate frequently prove overly intense for patients with chronic lung disease and can discourage patients, leading them to drop out from the program. Further exercise prescription guidelines for children with cystic fibrosis can be found in the box that follows.

Exercise Prescription Guidelines for Children With Cystic Fibrosis

- A structured, supervised exercise program can be effectively combined with instructions for increasing daily activity levels.
- Preparticipation exercise testing should include oximetry measurements in patients with advanced disease. A significant fall in saturation with exercise (more than 5 percent) may call for limitation of activities.
- Although a well-rounded exercise program is important, emphasis should be placed on aerobic activities that stimulate mild respiratory effort.
- Social benefits of a structured program can provide valuable psychosocial support.
- Exercise programs for patients with cystic fibrosis can include an educational component of nutrition, activity, and lifestyle counseling.

Patients with severe disease (resting FEV_1 50 percent of predicted) should have oximetry performed during stress testing. Cropp et al. (1982) suggested that exercise in this group should be limited to the extent that will cause a drop in arterial saturation of no more than 5 percent or an absolute saturation of no less than 80 percent. Although the authors confessed the arbitrary nature of such guidelines, concern was raised that exercise-induced desaturation beyond these limits might contribute to pulmonary hypertension, right-ventricular hypertrophy, and cardiac arrhythmias.

The basic structure of exercise programs for patients with cystic fibrosis should follow that of other programs designed to improve tolerance for exercise. Exercise should be principally aerobic (running, walking, cycling, swimming) with care taken to adjust the intensity to each subject's pre-existing fitness level. Activity that will create a heart rate of 70 to 85 percent of the individual's maximum heart rate is an appropriate target. Self-selected levels of exercise that do not produce dyspnea or inordinate muscle soreness the day after are a good starting point. Exercise may begin in sessions of 5 to 10 min for unfit subjects but should progress to 30 min at least three times a week. Each session should be preceded and followed by a 5- to 10-min period of stretching and calisthenics.

Motivating patients with cystic fibrosis to exercise may not be as difficult as with other groups. These children and adolescents suffer from a disease characterized by a relentless progression of recurrent lung infections, sputum production, and fatigue. Interventions that are effective in improving their well-being—and that are under their control—can provide a valuable degree of positive feedback. Allowing patients the benefits of exercising in social situations, seeing levels of fitness improve, and "feeling better" after physical activity are all powerful motivating factors for sustaining participation in these programs.

SUMMARY

This chapter took a look at the role of exercise in the lives of children with cardiac dysfunctions, asthma, and cystic fibrosis. Several recommendations were given for including exercise as part of the treatment of these patients.

- It is important to determine baseline fitness levels in cardiac patients before they begin an exercise program, because there are some categories of patients for whom involvement is unwise. A good fitness program should increase flexibility and strength, as well as improve endurance. Achieving compliance in children is often a problem, and rewards may be appropriate for increasing motivation.

- Parents and children should be taught to realize that asthma need not interfere with sport participation. In fact, a program of regular physical activity benefits these children if the exercise is adapted to their fitness levels and is preceded by prophylactic medication.
- Patients with cystic fibrosis are probably best served by a structured and supervised exercise program focused on improved exercise tolerance. This group is more motivated than most others to maintain a program, because these patients typically feel better after physical activity.

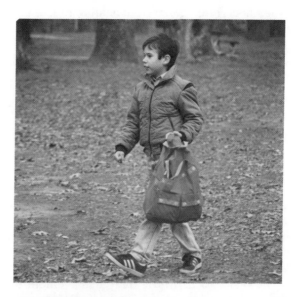

CHAPTER 10

Physical Activity and Diabetes Mellitus

Over a half century has elapsed since insulin first became available for the treatment of diabetes mellitus, yet this disease remains a serious health problem. Significant morbidity and early mortality will befall most of the 5 to 10 million persons with diabetes in the United States. Diabetes is described as the sixth leading cause of death in this country, which is almost certainly an underestimate because many cardiovascular-related deaths in these patients are categorized not as deaths due to diabetes but under other labels (e.g., congestive heart failure or stroke). Although type I (or juvenile-onset) diabetes represents a minority of these cases, this chapter deals exclusively with this group because it encompasses virtually all young people with diabetes.

TYPE I DIABETES

Type I diabetes is characterized by inadequate pancreatic secretion of insulin and the subsequent need for daily replacement of this hormone by subcutaneous injection. In the absence of exogenous insulin, the transport of glucose into cells is impaired, resulting in progressive hyperglycemia and ketoacidosis. Individuals with type II (or adult-onset) diabetes mellitus are generally over 45 years of age and typically suffer from insulin resistance rather than quantitative insufficiency. Oral medications and weight loss are usually capable of controlling hyperglycemia in type II diabetes, without need for insulin injections.

The major focus in the daily management of the patient with type I diabetes is maintaining a state of euglycemia—preventing hyper- and hypoglycemia—by balancing the influences of diet, exercise, and insulin on blood glucose levels. The ultimate morbidity and mortality of this disease, however, relates to progressive vascular and neurological complications that typically become clinically manifest in young adulthood, including these (Figure 10.1):

- A generalized thickening of capillary basement membranes (microangiopathy) that affects many organs, most prominently the eye (diabetic retinopathy) and kidneys (diabetic nephropathy)
- Accelerated atherosclerotic vascular disease (macroangiopathy) presenting as early coronary artery disease (CAD) and stroke
- A peripheral neuropathy affecting sensory, motor, and autonomic function

The relationship between insulin deficiency and these chronic complications of diabetes is not clear. More specifically, whether close control of blood sugar levels will favorably influence the natural course of neurovascular manifestations of diabetes is not known (The DCCT Research Group, 1988). Still, avoiding fluctuations of glucose concentrations outside the normal range is considered an important goal by most physicians caring for these patients.

The observation by McMillan (1979) that physical activity has been advocated for the treatment of diabetes mellitus since "time immemorial" is hardly an overstatement. Historians have traced the exercise–diabetes connection as far back as 600 B.C., when the Indian physician Sushruta prescribed exercise for patients with this disease. His successors, who

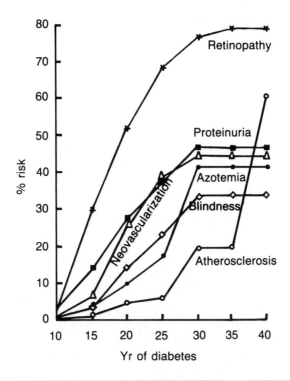

Figure 10.1 Natural history of end-organ complications of diabetes mellitus. *Note.* From "Juvenile Diabetes and the Heart" by R.S. Cooper, 1984, *Pediatric Clinics of North America*, **31**, p. 654. Copyright 1984 by W.B. Saunders Co. Reprinted by permission.

were also convinced of the benefit of regular exercise for diabetes, included the Roman Celsus and the prominent Chinese doctor Chao Yuan-Fang, who practiced during the Sui dynasty in 600 A.D. What these physicians witnessed was an improved sense of well-being in patients with diabetes, and the subsequent demonstration that physical activity could lower blood glucose levels in this disease suggested an added rationale for including exercise in its treatment. By the time Lawrence (1926) showed that physical activity enhances the hypoglycemic effect of administered insulin, regular exercise had become established as a key element in the triad in diabetes management—insulin, exercise, and diet (Joslin, 1959).

This enthusiasm for exercise was based on the premise that the glucose-lowering effects of physical activity would improve metabolic control while improving the quality of life for patients with diabetes. A close scientific scrutiny of the relationship between exercise and diabetes over the past 2 decades has substantiated only a portion of such hopes, but in the overall analysis regular exercise continues to play an important role in the health of these children and adolescents.

Quite apart from any specific effects of exercise on the diabetic state, children with this disease deserve to enjoy the same health and social benefits of regular physical activity as do nondiabetic youngsters. Yet fear of metabolic changes during exercise that may precipitate hypo- or hyperglycemia cause many children with diabetes to shun physical activities. Physicians have the opportunity to contribute to the well-being of these patients by helping them to adapt their diabetes management to allow safe participation in sport events.

ACUTE METABOLIC EFFECTS OF EXERCISE

The child with diabetes encounters a particular problem regulating blood glucose during exercise, best understood relative to the normal metabolic responses to physical activity in nondiabetic individuals (Kemmer & Berger, 1983; Larsson, 1984; Vranic & Berger, 1979). During acute bouts of exercise, the energy demands of increased muscle contraction are met through an augmented oxygen supply (rise in ventilation, cardiac output) and enhanced source of fuels (glucose, fatty acids). When exercise begins, glucose derived from glycogen stored within the muscle cell serves as the major fuel supply. This source becomes depleted with increasing exercise intensity, and the muscle turns to circulating blood glucose and fatty acids.

At high exercise work loads, energy requirements reach 10 to 20 times that at rest, and this high rate of glucose uptake from the blood would rapidly result in hypoglycemia were it not for a constant replenishment of circulating glucose by the liver. This is critical, because maintenance of normal blood-glucose levels are essential during exercise for normal brain function as well as muscular energy substrate. The liver serves as the supply line for the glucose necessary for prolonged exercise, with production closely matching utilization through the breakdown of liver glycogen (glycogenolysis) and the creation of glucose by conversion from protein (gluconeogenesis). Failure of hepatic glucose production during exercise results in hypoglycemia and exhaustion.

This sequence of events is mediated by a complex hormonal interplay that involves a reduction of serum insulin and increase in counterregulatory hormones (catecholamines, cortisol, glucagon). The fall in insulin levels with acute exercise increases the release of fatty acids from peripheral depots and stimulates hepatic glycogenolysis and gluconeogenesis. High glucose uptake by the muscle is evident despite these low insulin levels, a phenomenon perhaps explained by increasing sensitivity of muscle cells to insulin during exercise.

These metabolic events are not so neatly orchestrated for the diabetic patient. In these individuals, insulin levels are determined not by physiological responses to exercise but instead by the timing and amount of the daily injected dose. As a result exercising diabetic subjects do not experience stable blood glucose levels; their levels vary according to serum insulin concentration, duration and intensity of exercise, site of injection, diet, and other factors.

Optimal Metabolic Control

The person with diabetes who exercises in a state of good metabolic control (adequate insulin levels and normal blood-glucose concentration) typically demonstrates a gradual fall in serum glucose with prolonged exercise, which can eventuate in symptomatic hypoglycemia. Glucose uptake by muscle is appropriately increased in this situation, but blood sugar levels decline because the absence of an exercise-induced decrease in serum insulin inhibits hepatic glucose production (glycogenolysis, gluconeogenesis) as well as fatty-acid mobilization from lipid stores. That is, the exercise machinery functions normally, but the energy supply line is shut off.

Several factors determine the extent of fall in blood glucose and risk of hypoglycemia. The drop in blood sugar is more precipitous if exercise takes place at the time of peak action of injected insulin. That occurs 2 to 4 hours after injection of regular insulin, and vigorous exercise is more likely to trigger hypoglycemia at that time. As shown in Figure 10.2, there is some evidence that the rate of insulin absorption is magnified, and the rate of blood glucose declines are greater, if the injection is made into the exercising limb (Koivisto & Felig, 1978). It may be recommended, for instance, that runners inject insulin into abdominal sites prior to exercise rather than into the thigh. The longer exercise takes place after an injection, the less likely it is that this effect will occur. The child with diabetes also needs to be aware that decreasing glycemia is exaggerated in exercise of longer duration and greater severity (Hagan, Marks, & Warren, 1979).

In conditions of adequate insulin, the degree of fall in blood sugar with exercise is also dependent on the initial glucose level. Higher concentrations predispose to a greater decline in glucose with physical activity, an effect that can be viewed as beneficial to diabetic control (Persson & Thoren, 1980). Extended exercise can still lead to hypoglycemia, however, with excessive fatigue, dizziness, disorientation, syncope, and seizures. Moreover, in some patients low blood-glucose levels can occur up to 15 hr *after* exercise is completed, an effect of continued glucose uptake by the exercised muscle cells as they rebuild intracellular glycogen stores (MacDonald, 1987). Each diabetic patient needs to learn his or her

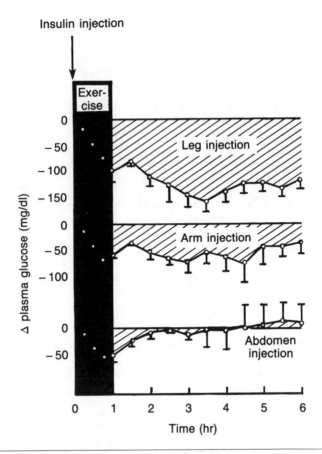

Figure 10.2 Fall in plasma glucose (shaded areas) in response to exercise with injection of insulin into exercising leg, arm, and abdomen. *Note.* From "Physical Training in Juvenile Diabetes" by V.A. Koivisto and L. Groop, 1982, *Annals of Clinical Research*, **14**, p. 77. Copyright 1982 by the Finnish Medical Society. Reprinted by permission.

own personal responses to exercise through blood-glucose monitoring, because the risk of hypoglycemia with exercise may vary markedly from one person to the next. Based on this information, strategies for increasing carbohydrate intake and adjusting insulin doses can be created that should permit full participation in sport activities. These tactics are reviewed later in this section.

Poor Metabolic Control

When the diabetic child exercises under conditions of poor metabolic control, with insulin deficiency and hyperglycemia, the metabolic responses to and risks of exercise are entirely different (Horton, 1988) (Figure 10.3). The low insulin levels permit increased hepatic glycogen breakdown to glucose and the mobilization of free fatty acids, but the peripheral uptake of glucose by exercising muscle is impaired. Hyperglycemia worsens and ketoacidosis supervenes; that is, exercise exacerbates poor metabolic control. Now the supply line is working fine, but energy substrate cannot enter the exercising muscle cell. Vigorous exercise is contraindicated in this state, and when blood-glucose levels exceed 250 to 300 mg/dl diabetic control needs to be improved by additional insulin before sport participation. The diabetic patient, therefore, needs to be aware of his or her metabolic control prior to vigorous physical activity.

Status of plasma insulin	Hepatic glucose production	Muscle glucose utilization	Blood glucose
Normal or slightly diminished	⬆	⬆	→
Markedly diminished	⬆	↑	↑
Increased	↑	⬆	↓

Figure 10.3 Effect of insulin sufficiency on metabolic responses to exercise. *Note.* From "Diabetes and Exercise" by E.A. Richter, N.B. Ruderman, and S.H. Schneider, 1981, *The American Journal of Medicine*, 70, p. 205. Copyright 1981 by Cahners Publishing Co. Reprinted by permission.

PHYSICAL TRAINING AND DIABETIC CONTROL

The discovery that acute exercise could lower blood glucose in diabetic subjects led to the hope that regular physical activity, or training, could help normalize glycemia and reduce insulin requirements on a chronic basis. This in turn might be expected to reduce the long-term complications of diabetes. Results of studies examining this possibility are summarized in Table 10.1 and discussed in the following sections.

Research

Early observations of children attending diabetic camp supported this idea (Gabriele & Marble, 1949). Sterky (1970) reported that juvenile diabetics experienced decreased glycosuria in this high-activity setting, and Kinsell (1955) described a 40 percent reduction in insulin dose in diabetic children

Table 10.1 Physical Training in Type I Diabetes Mellitus

Reference	N	Age (yrs)	Duration (wks)	Frequency (per wk)	Exercise	Results
Baevre et al. (1985)	6	14-17	24	2	?	Increased $\dot{V}O_2$max 19% No change in HbA_1[a]
Campaigne et al. (1985)	14	12-19	12	3	Aerobics to music	Increased $\dot{V}O_2$max 8% No change in HbA_1
Costill et al. (1979)	12	21	10	5	Running	Increased $\dot{V}O_2$max 11%
Dahl-Jorgensen et al. (1980)	8	9-13	20	2	?	No change in $\dot{V}O_2$max Decreased HbA_1
Larsson et al. (1962)	6	13-18	8	2	Gymnastics	Increased physical work capacity (PWC)
Larsson, Persson, & Sterky (1964)	6	15-19	20	1	Swim/run	Increased PWC 30%
Rowland et al. (1985)	14	9-14	12	3	Run/walk	Increased $\dot{V}O_2$max 9% No change in HbA_1
Stratton et al. (1987)	8	15	8	3	Aerobic activities	Increased endurance Decreased submaximal heart rate No change in HbA_1 Decreased glycosylated serum albumin
Wallberg-Henriksson et al. (1982)	9	35	16	3	Aerobic activities	Increased $\dot{V}O_2$max 8% No change in HbA_1

[a]HbA_1 = glycosylated hemoglobin

at camp, which he attributed to physical exercise. These reports may have been confounded by the accompanying regimentation of both dietary control and insulin administration, but early studies indicating improvement in metabolic control after physical training supported their conclusions. Engerbretson (1965) described reduced urinary glucose excretion, decreased blood glucose levels, and lowered insulin doses in five diabetics after 6 weeks of interval training. Ludvigsson (1980) administered an exercise questionnaire to 143 children and adolescents with diabetes and found a positive correlation between habitual physical activity and metabolic control (proportion of daily tests without glycosuria). When Larsson, Persson, and Sterky (1964) put six diabetic boys through a 5-month, 1-hr-per-week exercise program, however, no changes were observed in urinary glucose spillage. What was missing from these studies, besides a sufficient number of subjects and adequate exercise regimen, was a satisfactory means of measuring metabolic control over an extended period of training time.

In 1980 Dahl-Jorgensen, Meen, Hanssen, and Aagenaes first reported the use of glycosylated hemoglobin (HbA_1) levels to assess the effect of physical training on diabetic children. Glycosylated hemoglobin is that portion of total hemoglobin that is bound with a glucose molecule, and the concentration of HbA_1 in the circulation is a reflection of blood glucose levels over the life span of the red blood cell. Expressed as a percentage of total hemoglobin, HbA_1, therefore, serves as a valuable marker of glycemic control over the 4 to 6 weeks prior to its determination. HbA_1 levels have subsequently become a valuable means for diabetologists to monitor control of their patients.

Dahl-Jorgensen et al. (1980) studied the effects of a 5-month exercise program on HbA_1 levels in 14 diabetic children ages 9 to 15 years. Although HbA_1 levels fell during training, results were weakened by several methodological problems. $\dot{V}O_2$max did not increase at the end of the program, suggesting low-intensity exercise. Blood samples were frozen, and HbA_1 levels were determined 5 months after the study ended. In 7 of 8 control subjects, HbA_1 also fell, and the level of habitual physical activity in this group was not evaluated.

A beneficial effect of regular exercise on metabolic control was described in nine diabetic children 5 to 11 years old by Campaigne, Gilliam, Spencer, Lampman, and Schork (1984). HbA_1 and fasting blood-glucose levels fell significantly in these children after a 12-week exercise training program. In a second training study of 14 adolescents with juvenile diabetes, however, no improvements in control were observed (Campaigne et al., 1985). Mean HbA_1 levels remained unchanged at 12 percent (normal 7.1 ± .11 percent) after a 3-month program of aerobic exercise three times weekly.

Similar findings were reported by Rowland, Swadba, Biggs, Burke, and Reiter (1985) in 14 children ages 9 to 14 years (average duration of diabetes was 4.2 years). No significant changes in HbA_1 levels were seen after a 12-week aerobic exercise program despite increases in $\dot{V}O_2$max. Pretraining HbA_1 was 9.9 percent, indicating a reasonably well-controlled group of subjects. No significant changes in insulin dose (based on home glucose monitoring) were observed during the program.

Baevre, Sovik, Wisnes, and Heiervang (1985) could find no changes in HbA_1 after a 6-month, twice-weekly exercise program for a small group of 16-year-olds with diabetes. Stratton, Wilson, Endres, and Goldstein (1987) measured metabolic responses of eight insulin-dependent adolescents to an 8-week program of supervised exercise. HbA_1 values did not fall, but a significant reduction was observed in glycosylated serum albumin, considered by the authors to be a more sensitive index of glycemic control.

Results of these types of studies are mixed in adults as well. Peterson, Jones, Esterly, Wantz, and Jackson (1980) reported a reduction in HbA_1 after aerobic training in 10 adult subjects with type I diabetes (average age 25 years). In this study, however, improved metabolic control could have resulted from the concomitant introduction of home blood-glucose monitoring. Zinman, Zuniga-Guajardo, and Kelly (1984) could demonstrate no changes in HbA_1 after a 12-week bicycle exercise program in 13 adults with insulin-dependent diabetes. Likewise, Wallberg-Henriksson et al. (1982) described no changes in HbA_1, 24-hr urinary glucose excretion, or home-monitored urine tests in nine adults following a 16-week training program.

Increased insulin sensitivity has been reported following exercise training in both diabetic and nondiabetic individuals. This response does not appear to alter insulin requirements or other markers of metabolic control, however (Baevre et al., 1985; Wallberg-Henriksson et al., 1982).

Failure of Exercise to Control Diabetes

In summary, although much data are conflicting, there is no convincing evidence at present that regular physical activity will improve diabetic control beyond the hypoglycemic effect observed with acute exercise. As Kemmer and Berger (1983) noted,

> To use exercise as a therapeutic tool for long term improvement of glycemic control in [type I] diabetes, the patient would have to exercise every day on a regular schedule for a defined period at a defined workload with doubtful prospects as to the success. . . . The use of physical exercise as a tool to improve metabolic control in type I diabetes appears to be impractical.

It would seem that any effects of regular exercise specifically beneficial for diabetic patients must be directed toward other goals.

DIABETES, EXERCISE, AND ATHEROSCLEROSIS

Premature death from atherosclerotic vascular disease (myocardial infarction, stroke) is the greatest health hazard for diabetics. CAD is the underlying cause of death in approximately 40 percent of individuals with diabetes, a frequency twice that expected in the nondiabetic population. Diabetic patients are less likely to survive a myocardial infarction, and those that do have a poorer prognosis than nondiabetics (Bennet, 1981).

Why both individuals with type I and individuals with type II disease possess this tendency for atherosclerosis is not clear. CAD risk factors may cluster in diabetes (particularly those with type II); alternatively, the intrinsic metabolic derangements of the diabetic state itself may play a role. As outlined in chapter 6, there is sufficient available information to encourage exercise as a means of preventing ischemic heart disease in adulthood. It follows, then, that regular physical activity should be a particularly important part of the daily lives of diabetic patients.

Blood Lipid Levels

When diabetic children receive appropriate insulin therapy, their average blood lipid levels are typically within the normal range for age (Sterky, Larsson, & Persson, 1963). Campaigne et al. (1985) followed blood lipid profiles of 14 adolescent diabetics during the course of a 12-week exercise program. A significant decrease in mean LDL-cholesterol level was apparently related to a training effect, because $\dot{V}O_2$max increased, and other factors that affect blood lipids (e.g., diet and weight) were not contributory. In that study, there were no changes observed in triglycerides, total cholesterol, or HDL-cholesterol. Older diabetic subjects (mean age 35 years) studied by Wallberg-Henriksson et al. (1982) likewise experienced no changes in HDL-cholesterol during a 16-week training period, but serum cholesterol fell 14 percent.

Triglycerides

Elevated triglyceride levels are generally not considered a strong risk factor for CAD but may play a more significant role in promoting atherosclerosis in diabetic subjects. Serum triglyceride levels rise in an insulin-deficient state because enhanced lipolysis stimulates hepatic triglyceride secretion rates. In an early study, Larsson, Persson, and Sterky (1964) showed a significant fall in triglycerides in six adolescent diabetic boys after 5 months of gymnastics, 1 hr per week. The same effect was demonstrated in insulin-dependent diabetic adults by Costill, Cleary, and Fink (1979). Triglyceride and total cholesterol levels decreased 18 and 10 percent, respectively, during a 10-week aerobic exercise program.

Fibrinolytic Activity

Deficiencies of serum fibrinolytic activity may contribute to the pathogenesis of CAD and its complications. This poses a potential risk for diabetic patients, who possess a tendency for elevated fibrinogen levels and blood viscosity as well as depressed fibrinolytic activity (Jarrett, Keen, & Chakrabarti, 1982). Exercise training has been demonstrated to enhance fibrinolytic responses and lower blood viscosity by increasing plasma volume in nondiabetic subjects (Koch & Rocker, 1980; Williams et al., 1980). Similar studies have not yet been performed with diabetic individuals, but it has been suggested that regular exercise may reduce platelet adhesiveness in this group (Gonzalez, 1979).

Role of Exercise

The implications for the role of exercise in preventive cardiology are especially pertinent for children and adolescents with diabetes. More information is needed to assess the response of coronary risk factors to physical activity in these patients, but it can be reasonably assumed that a sedentary life poses as much increased a risk of CAD for diabetic patients as it does for the nondiabetic population.

EXERCISE AND DIABETIC MICROVASCULAR DISEASE

Diabetic patients suffer a generalized, progressive microvascular disease that produces its most devastating effects on the eyes and kidneys. This diffuse thickening of capillary basement membranes often induces progressive blindness and renal failure in mid-adulthood (McMillan, 1975). Children were initially felt to be spared diabetic microvascular changes, but increasing evidence indicates that this process begins during the pediatric years. Forty percent of diabetic children between the ages of 6 and 20 years have an increased quadriceps muscle capillary basement membrane width (Raskin, Marks, Burns, Plumer, & Siperstein, 1975), and renal vascular abnormalities can be detected in 75 percent of diabetics in the same age group (Malone, Cader, & Edwards, 1977). When diabetic children exercise they increase urine albumin excretion, presumably reflecting early renal microvascular changes (Morgensen & Vittinghaus, 1975).

Improvement Through Exercise?

In 1980 Larsson proposed that "it is probable that regular exercise may postpone the appearance of diabetic microangiopathy by means of increasing circulatory dimensions and improving blood flow and oxygen transport" (p. 122). Is there any evidence this is true? Very few studies have addressed this issue. Peterson et al. (1980) reported a decrease in skeletal muscle membrane thickening in 6 of 10 adult diabetic subjects after instituting a combined program of endurance exercise and home glucose monitoring.

LaPorte et al. (1986) evaluated the association of physical activity and long-term microvascular complications in 696 type I diabetic adults. Using participation on high school or college athletic teams as a marker of activity, they showed no relationship between early regular exercise and severe retinopathy or blindness later in life (most with duration of diabetes over 20 years). Participation on sports teams was, however, negatively associated with macrovascular complications (stroke, myocardial infarction, claudication), although only in male subjects.

Worsening Through Exercise?

This study is also important from another standpoint. It has been suggested that exercise might *exacerbate* microangiopathic damage by raising blood pressure, increasing glomerular albumin leakage, and causing surges in growth hormone (McMillan, 1979; Morgensen & Vittinghaus, 1975). Ocular hemorrhages have been described following exercise in subjects with diabetic retinopathy (Anderson, 1980). Although the report by LaPorte et al. (1986) is weakened by its narrow retrospective definition of exercise, it did fail to demonstrate any evidence that vigorous sport participation aggravates ophthalmological manifestations of diabetic microangiopathy.

PSYCHOLOGICAL BENEFITS

No one has yet published a systematic evaluation of the psychosocial benefits of exercise in children with diabetes. It would seem, though, that the emotional gains associated with regular physical activity reviewed in chapter 8 are particularly relevant to this group of patients. Anecdotally, those who work with young diabetic patients have been impressed with improvements in their emotional well-being during participation in group physical activities (Riley & Rosebloom, 1980; Rowland, 1986). The increased self-confidence and optimism gained in such programs may also help improve compliance in all aspects of diabetic care.

Diabetes mellitus presents the patient and her or his family with particularly difficult issues in psychological adjustment. This is a disease of unknown cause and pessimistic long-term outlook, with no guarantee that careful management will truly affect its ultimate outcomes. The patient is required to regulate diet, administer insulin doses, monitor blood-glucose levels, and adjust exercise habits, all of which reinforce the stereotype of a handicapped, disabled individual. It is no surprise that loss of self-esteem, impaired interpersonal relationships, and non-compliance are all characteristics frequently observed in diabetic children (Johnson & Rosenbloom, 1982).

Regular exercise has the potential for reversing many of these emotional reactions. Improved self-image, sense of self-mastery, social confidence, and energy for school and recreational activities are all changes that have been attributed to increased physical activity. In short, exercise programs can make these youngsters with chronic disease feel good about themselves. This alone justifies an emphasis on exercise as a vital part of diabetic management.

DOES DIABETES LIMIT PHYSICAL FITNESS?

Depressed levels of physical fitness have been repeatedly demonstrated in diabetic subjects compared to nondiabetic controls. The following characteristics are reported in children with diabetes:

- Higher heart rate at a given exercise work load (Larsson, Sterky, Ekengren, & Moeller, 1962; Sterky, 1963)
- Lower maximal heart rate (Rubler & Arvan, 1975)
- Diminished exercise tolerance
- Decreased $\dot{V}O_2max$ (Larsson, Persson, Sterky, & Thoren, 1964)

A wide range of fitness exists among diabetic subjects, however, and some have become world-class amateur and professional athletes. This may explain why other studies have failed to reveal deviations from normal levels of physical fitness in diabetic children (Hagan et al., 1979; Larsson et al., 1962; Olavi, Hirvonen, Peltonen, & Valimaki, 1965). Because fitness depends on selection of subjects and controls, it is difficult to conclude for certain that a given diabetic patient is truly impaired in exercise capacity, or, if so, whether this is due to influences of the diabetic state on physiological function or simply the tendency of diabetic children to assume a more sedentary lifestyle (Ludvigsson, 1980).

Some insight into this question was provided by a study examining the relationship of degree of metabolic control (HbA$_1$ levels) and physical fitness (maximal cycle testing) in adolescent diabetics (Poortmans, Saerens, Edelman, Vertongen, & Dorchy, 1986). Maximal work load and $\dot{V}O_2max$ were significantly lower in the group of diabetic subjects than in controls, both of which were described as sedentary. In addition, an inverse relationship was observed between HbA$_1$ level and maximal work load.

Limiting Factors of Performance

Diabetic subjects have several physiological and biochemical characteristics that could account for impaired exercise performance. These have been identified principally in adult patients but may have their inception during childhood.

Cardiac Dysfunction

Studies in adult diabetics utilizing cardiac catheterization, systolic time intervals, and radionuclide angiography have disclosed a high incidence of cardiac dysfunction with exercise that is apparently independent of atherosclerotic disease (Cooper, 1984). Histological findings of endothelial proliferation, myocardial fibrosis, and capillary basement thickening further support the existence of a distinct diabetic cardiomyopathy (Fein & Sonnenblick, 1985).

The degree of ventricular dysfunction generally parallels the duration of diabetes, and children had previously been considered exempt from cardiac involvement. Recent echocardiographic studies have suggested, however, that changes in heart function can be observed at an early age. Friedman, Levitsky, and Edidin (1982) demonstrated an increased end-systolic left-ventricular volume, diminished ejection fraction, and lower velocity of circumferential fiber shortening in 33 diabetic children at rest. Lababidi and Goldstein (1983) performed a similar study in 107 subjects aged 2 to 24 years and reported age-related abnormalities in the dimensions of the left atrium, right ventricle, and left ventricle as well as flattened ventricular septal motion.

Baum, Levitsky, and Englander (1987) evaluated cardiac function immediately following exercise in 30 insulin-dependent diabetic patients aged 10 to 19 years. Abnormalities in fractional shortening and velocity of circumferential fiber shortening were observed when echocardiograms were measured within 3 min after maximal exercise on a supine bicycle ergometer. These findings suggested to the authors that "myocardial dysfunction [during childhood and adolescence] may be the harbinger of the severe cardiomyopathy of long-term diabetes" (p. 322).

Noncardiac Factors

Noncardiac factors may also be responsible for limiting exercise capacity in diabetic subjects. McMillan (1978) commented that "the basement membrane is the structure across which all oxygen molecules have to pass to enter muscle. It is not illogical to believe that the thickening could impair oxygenation during exercise" (p. 402). Basement membrane thickening is commonly observed in the skeletal muscle of diabetic subjects, but there is as yet no experimental proof that this limits oxygen delivery to muscle.

Changes in hemoglobin–oxygen affinity may affect oxygen transport in diabetic subjects. When attached to glucose as HbA_1, hemoglobin binds more poorly with 2,3 diphosphoglycerate (2,3 DPG), a compound important in promoting unloading of oxygen at the tissue level. In poorly controlled diabetic individuals with elevated HbA_1, the resulting increase in hemoglobin–oxygen affinity might interfere with oxygen delivery to muscle.

Ditzel, Kawahava, and Mourits-Andersen (1981) evaluated a group of diabetic children to determine whether these differences had any functional significance. Hemoglobin, HbA_1, and 2,3 DPG concentrations were all higher in diabetic subjects than in nondiabetic controls, but the hemoglobin–oxygen affinity was identical. The authors interpreted these findings as indicating that any decrease in oxygen delivery was compensated by the increased DPG levels. The elevated hematocrit levels, which correlated with both 2,3 DPG and percent HbA_1, indicated the possibility of relative tissue hypoxia in diabetic individuals.

The muscle biopsy study by Saltin, Houston, and Nygaard (1979) in adult diabetic men suggested that peripheral capillary density and oxidative enzyme concentrations might be less in this disease. Costill et al. (1979), however, could not substantiate these findings, either before or after exercise training. Another potential factor that could limit exercise in diabetic subjects is the influence of HbA_1 on reducing deformability of red blood cells (McMillan, Utterback, & LaPuma, 1978). This effect would increase blood viscosity and impede blood flow with exercise.

Regardless of any impairments in aerobic fitness, individuals with diabetes respond normally to endurance training (refer back to Table 10.1). Maximum oxygen consumption, physical work capacity (work load at a heart rate of 170 bpm), and submaximal heart rates improve in these programs in parallel with changes observed in nondiabetic subjects.

RECOMMENDATIONS FOR EXERCISE

Diabetic children should be encouraged to participate in physical activities for the same reasons as nondiabetic subjects—adding zest to life, feeling good about oneself, controlling obesity, improving work capacity, and lessening the risks of adult cardiovascular disease. From the foregoing discussion it is evident that, in fact, these benefits may have even more relevance for diabetic subjects. At the same time, many children and adolescents with diabetes, a group at particular risk from a sedentary lifestyle, are reluctant to participate in vigorous activities for fear of exercise-induced hypoglycemia. The role here for physicians is twofold: These patients need to be motivated to join in regular sport and fitness activities, and at the same time they need to be educated in the ways to make this participation safe. The strategies for achieving the former will be addressed in Part III; accomplishing the latter requires that the diabetic patient have a clear understanding of the relationships between insulin, diet, and exercise.

The task of helping the diabetic child adjust insulin and diet to physical activity would be simpler if exercise activities were regular, planned events (like meals). Life for diabetic patients would also be easier if their metabolic responses to a given exercise were predictably similar. In the absence of such good fortune, adjustment of diet and insulin to exercise for a given child requires a trial-and-error approach with careful blood-glucose monitoring before, during, and after exercise. Experience will educate each patient as to what metabolic responses he or she can expect to exercise of various intensities and duration. The guidelines summarized in the box and explained fully in the following text can be used during this learning process.

Exercise Prescription Guidelines for Children With Diabetes Mellitus

- All children with diabetes should be encouraged to participate in regular exercise, preferably aerobic (running, swimming, cycling).
- Means of adjusting carbohydrate intake and insulin dose to prevent hypoglycemia during exercise need to be individualized for each patient.
- Children with diabetes need to be aware that carbohydrate intake prior to physical activity is dictated by preexercise serum glucose levels.
- Insulin should be injected into a nonexercising site.
- Children with diabetes should always exercise with individuals who know about their disease. A source of rapidly absorbed carbohydrate should be immediately available.

Activity

No form of physical activity is contraindicated for diabetic patients. However, these children should always exercise with someone who knows that they have diabetes and what to do in an emergency. Extensive exercise should be avoided during periods of peak insulin activity, particularly 2 to 4 hr after an injection of regular insulin or 7 to 10 hr after administration of intermediate-acting insulin. Instead, exercise is best undertaken within 2 hr of eating a meal. Patients should not exercise after a prolonged fast.

Carbohydrate Coverage

The idea is to exercise with a little extra fuel on board to prevent any blood-sugar decline during exercise from reaching hypoglycemic levels. How much this "extra" needs to be depends on the initial blood-glucose level, intensity and duration of exercise, temporal relationship to insulin dose and meals, and, again, a good deal of individual variation.

Carbohydrate Prescriptions

- If **preexercise blood glucose** is under 100 mg percent, coverage with 10 to 15 g of rapidly absorbed carbohydrate for a child or 25 to 50 g for an adolescent will almost certainly be necessary. This can be provided by a fruit or bread exchange, taken 20 to 30 min before exercise. Many patients require similar extra carbohydrate when glucose concentrations are between 100 and 180 mg percent.
- If **initial blood-glucose level** is between 180 and 250 mg percent, no extra carbohydrate is usually necessary.
- If **prolonged exercise** (such as a day-long hike) is planned, approximately 1 g of carbohydrate for each minute of exercise should be taken at 30- to 60-min intervals. Fruit juice suffices well in this situation by providing fluids as well as sugar.

Insulin Dose

Changes in insulin dose are generally not required unless exercise is prolonged. A minimum of 20 percent reduction in daily dose (plus carbohydrates) may, however, be needed to maintain normal blood-glucose levels during activities involving many hours. Insulin injections prior to physical activities should be administered in a nonexercising extremity (abdominal site for running and biking, thigh for canoeing), particularly if the activity is performed within a few hours of the insulin injection.

Avoiding Ketoacidosis

Metabolic status should be recognized before sport activities. Exercise should be postponed if blood sugar is over 250 to 300 mg percent or if there is ketonuria, until improved control is established.

Safety

Diabetic children need to carry some form of carbohydrate (e.g., dextrose tablets, regular soda), or have it immediately available, during exercise. They should be prepared for postexercise hypoglycemia, which can occur hours after physical activity. Drinking plenty of fluids is important before, during, and after exercise. Patients should try to exercise according to a regular routine if possible, at least 1/2 hr four times a week.

The following box summarizes some exercise prescription guidelines for children with diabetes mellitus.

SUMMARY

Juvenile or type I diabetes mellitus is characterized by acute metabolic changes in response to relative insulin deficiency and chronic micro- and macrovascular alterations that affect principally renal, cardiovascular, ophthalmological, and neurological function. It is important that clinicians understand the relationship between diabetes and exercise, for these reasons:

- Acute bouts of exercise may provoke hypoglycemia or ketoacidosis, depending on the state of insulin sufficiency. Patients can be protected from these effects by proper diabetic monitoring and management.
- Fear of these complications causes many diabetic patients to avoid strenuous physical activity. Possible effects of their disease on cardiovascular function may therefore be compounded by a sedentary lifestyle.
- Although regular exercise does not appear to affect diabetic control, physical activity should be promoted in patients with diabetes as a preventive measure against the long-term cardiovascular complications of this disease.
- The diabetic state itself may limit physical fitness by interfering with oxygen delivery mechanisms.
- Participation in regular exercise is important for countering the negative emotional effects of diabetes through improvement in self-image and social confidence.

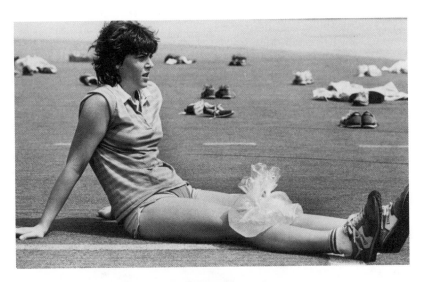

CHAPTER 11

Risks of Sport Participation During Childhood

Should the 8-year-old boy be allowed to go jogging with his father? Is it safe for prepubertal girls to play vigorous sports? Should the organizer of a 2-mi road race for children be spared public condemnation? For almost all children the answers are "Yes"—these are healthful activities that pose no real health danger to growing children.

The amount of exercise important for healthy living does not create any significant risks for the normal child. Still, both the lay press and medical authorities have raised concern over possible risks faced by prepubertal athletes who are involved in intense training regimens. Fortunately, these concerns do not have any bearing on the promotion of physical activity for the great majority of children. Physicians can help youngsters and their families understand that regular exercise during the growing years is not only safe but necessary, and that any serious risks of sport participation are confined, in general, to elite child athletes.

This is, however, an important chapter. Physicians need to be aware of current knowledge concerning the limits of safe activity, both for safeguarding the health of child athletes and for reassuring their patients in more recreational pursuits. The potential risks for children involved in sports concern principally these systems:

- Cardiac
- Musculoskeletal (including sport injuries)
- Neurological/psychological
- Endocrine/reproductive

The possible responses of each of these organ systems to exercise in the growing child is addressed in the following sections.

SUDDEN DEATH AND CARDIAC DISEASE

Heart disease is not common in children, affecting only about 0.5 percent of school-aged youngsters. Moreover, children's cardiac disorders are seldom occult and are usually easily recognized by abnormal findings on physical examination, and they rarely predispose to sudden death, with or without athletic activity (Lambert, Menon, Wagner, & Vlad, 1974). The chances of a child or adolescent athlete dying unexpectedly during training or competition from previously unrecognized heart disease is extremely small, estimated to be no greater than 1 in every 200,000 participants (Epstein & Maron, 1986). The chance might be lowered by effective preparticipation screening, although certain conditions (fortunately extremely rare) will be missed by routine clinical evaluation. The following four cardiac anomalies deserve particular attention:

- Hypertrophic cardiomyopathy
- Marfan syndrome
- Coronary artery anomalies
- Aortic stenosis

Hypertrophic Cardiomyopathy (Idiopathic Hypertrophic Subaortic Stenosis [IHSS])

Idiopathic hypertrophic subaortic stenosis (IHSS) is characterized by idiopathic hypertrophy of the left-ventricular myocardium with exaggerated involvement of the ventricular septum, sometimes to dramatic proportions. The risk of sudden death in this condition is high (2 to 4 percent per year) and probably relates to arrhythmias associated with diastolic dysfunction of poorly compliant ventricular walls (Maron, Bonow, Cannon, Leon, & Epstein, 1987). Although sudden death usually occurs at rest or with mild activity, a large percentage of these catastrophies accompany vigorous exercise. Of 78 adult patients with hypertrophic cardiomyopathy who died suddenly, 39 percent were reported to have been participating in moderate to severe exertion (such as running, lifting, horseback riding) at the time (Maron, Roberts, & Epstein, 1982).

Approximately 60 percent of patients with IHSS report symptoms of dyspnea on exertion, angina, or syncope, and the family history is positive for the disease in 20 percent. The medical history therefore represents an important screening mechanism (Fiddler et al., 1978; Maron et al., 1976).

Physical examination is unfortunately often deceptively benign. One fourth have either a faint or no murmur. Even those with loud murmurs along the mid-left sternal border may be felt to have either a functional murmur or ventricular septal defect. Additional clues may be helpful: The murmur of IHSS may become louder in the sitting position or with a Valsalva maneuver, the pulse may be bifid, and a separate murmur of mitral insufficiency may be audible. The electrocardiogram is frequently abnormal, and up to 90 percent will demonstrate left-ventricular hypertrophy, deep Q waves over the left precordial leads, or ischemic ST changes. The best test for identification of IHSS is the echocardiogram, which reveals asymmetric ventricular septal hypertrophy. Table 11.1 summarizes these methods of identification. Patients with IHSS should be

Table 11.1 Identification of Hypertrophic Cardiomyopathy

Diagnostic tool	Manifestation
Family history	
Symptoms	Angina
	Syncope
	Exercise intolerance
Physical examination	Bifid pulse
	Fourth heart sound
	Systolic murmur (louder when sitting)
	Mitral insufficiency
Electrocardiogram	Left-ventricular hypertrophy
	Ischemic ST changes
Echocardiogram	Asymmetric septal hypertrophy

limited in their activities and not be allowed to participate in competitive athletics.

Marfan Syndrome

This hereditary disease in tall individuals with long extremities presents with manifestations of weakened connective tissue: hyperextensible joints, ectopia lentis, kyphoscoliosis, and cardiovascular disease (Pyeritz & McKusick, 1979). The media of the aorta is abnormally distensible, leading to progressive dilatation and risk of aneurysm rupture. Aortic valve insufficiency is typically observed in the adult years; clinical evidence of mitral valve prolapse (apical midsystolic click, sometimes with a late systolic murmur) is usually the initial cardiac finding in children (Geva, Hegesh, & Frand, 1987).

It is assumed that athletic participation can accelerate these cardiac findings and predispose to sudden death from aortic rupture, although the influence of exercise on the progression of cardiac disease in Marfan syndrome has never been evaluated. Still, it is considered prudent to restrict these patients from certain activities—resistance exercise, collision sports, and intensive endurance training—to prevent cardiovascular catastrophies (Cantwell, 1986; Pyeritz & McKusick, 1979).

Marfan syndrome should be suspected by the typical physical features and positive family history. Echocardiographic examination revealing dilatation of the aortic root and mitral valve prolapse is particularly useful in confirming the diagnosis.

Congenital Coronary Artery Anomalies

Abnormal origin of the coronary arteries is an extremely rare cause of sudden death in athletes. Myocardial ischemia may result when the left coronary artery arises from the pulmonary artery or when it originates from the right sinus of Valsalva (Maron, Epstein, & Roberts, 1986). Sudden death has occurred in a professional athlete with a single right coronary artery system and distal branch stenosis (Van Camp & Choi, 1988). Physical examination may be normal, and the only clue to the existence of these anomalies may come from a history of chest pain or syncope with exercise. Typically, however, these individuals have voiced no complaints prior to their deaths, and autopsy findings are the initial indication of cardiac disease.

Valvar Aortic Stenosis

Obstruction of left-ventricular outflow from restricted aortic valve mobility is probably the most common form of heart disease in children that predisposes to sudden death with exercise (Lambert et al., 1974). In this case, however, the presence of significant valvar obstruction is obvious by physical findings of prominent murmur, ejection click, and systolic thrill (Glew, Varghese, Krovetz, Dorst, & Rowe, 1969). Children with sufficient stenosis to be at risk are typically identified early and restricted from competitive athletics, and they often undergo surgical or balloon dilatation relief of their stenosis.

In summary, the chance of sudden death during exercise from occult cardiac disease in children is exceedingly small. Moreover, only a minority of children with recognized heart disease need to be restricted from physical activities. A careful assessment by the physician of both normal children and those with heart disease is important in ensuring that exercise risks are minimal.

MUSCULOSKELETAL PROBLEMS

The true frequency is unknown, but the number of pubertal and prepubertal athletes involved in serious competitive training in sports such as running, cycling, gymnastics, and swimming appears to be increasing dramatically (Caine & Lindner, 1985). These youngsters are training many hours a day with regimens that once would have been considered rigorous even by adult standards.

Training and Musculoskeletal Growth

Can the stresses imposed on developing bones and joints by this kind of intense exercise impair growth in children? No one knows for certain, but concern has led to recommendations that child and adolescent runners be prohibited from long-distance competitive events (American Academy of Pediatrics, 1982) and limited in training and competitive miles (Micheli, 1981). Most attention has been focused on long-distance running, but all weight-bearing athletic events, including ballet, are suspect (Caine & Lindner, 1985; Kozar & Lord, 1983).

Physical stress is a necessary stimulant to normal bone growth, and in its absence (as in prolonged bed rest) bone atrophy eventually ensues. Within limits, then, exercise can be viewed as an important contributor to normal skeletal development, but beyond a certain threshold—as yet undefined—exercise stress becomes potentially injurious.

Growth of long bones occurs primarily in the cartilage of the epiphyseal plate. These growth centers are vulnerable to traumatic injury, because their strength is estimated to be 2 to 5 times less than that of the surrounding fibrous joint capsule and ligaments (Caine & Lindner, 1984). Major physical blows to epiphyseal plates result in fractures that can eventually impair normal growth of the affected limb. A cross-body block, which might cause a ligament or tendon injury in an adult with closed epiphyses, can therefore result in an epiphyseal fracture of serious consequence in the growing child (Figure 11.1).

This type of *macrotrauma* is not typically encountered in endurance sports such as running or cycling. However, repetitive *microtrauma* from these activities might inflict similar damage. Will the stress effects of 7,500 footstrikes incurred in a 10-mi run, multiplied by 4 or 5 such runs per week, result in damage to leg-bone growth centers? Can such injury cause long-term disturbances in skeletal development and ultimate stature?

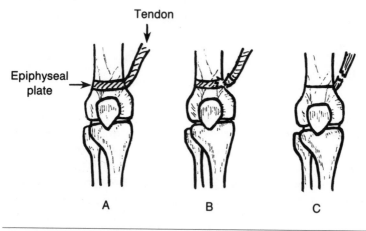

Tendon

Epiphyseal plate

A　　　　　B　　　　　C

Figure 11.1　In a child's knee (A), a blow to the side may cause a fracture of the soft epiphyseal plate (B). In the adult with a closed epiphysis, similar trauma results in tendon/ligament damage (C).

No long-term studies on the effects of exercise training during the growing years have yet been performed to answer these questions. Short-term and cross-sectional studies of high school and college endurance athletes have not demonstrated any abnormalities of skeletal growth (Bailey, Malina, & Rasmussen, 1978; Malina, 1969). These data do not provide any evidence that physical activity even of high intensity or duration will adversely affect normal development of stature (Broekhoff, 1986; Zimmerman, 1987). At large sports medicine clinics, prepubertal athletes present with the same high frequency of overuse musculoskeletal injuries as do adults, but only rarely do these injuries involve epiphyseal growth centers (Cahill, 1977; Godshall, Hansen, & Rising, 1981).

Inflammatory and degenerative changes observed in the distal humerus of Little League baseball pitchers demonstrate, however, that epiphyseal injury can occur from chronic stress. Adams (1976) described separation, fragmentation, and premature closure of the medial epicondylar ephiphysis in these athletes, and although this is not a growth plate, these findings do indicate the potential for epiphyseal damage.

The observation that children have been reported to train for and participate in adult-oriented athletic events (e.g., marathon races) without adverse effects is not altogether reassuring. As Kozar and Lord (1983) emphasized, "The fact that a few genetically exceptional individuals are capable of withstanding strenuous, long-term training loads does not mean that less talented youngsters will not suffer from overuse injuries that may prevent them from continuing in sports" (p. 118).

Overuse Injuries

Because the threshold intensity of exercise that might cause epiphyseal damage is unknown, attention has turned to the significance of overuse injuries in young athletes. These are the "wear-and-tear" problems (e.g., muscle strains, "shin splints," tendinitis, stress fractures) common particularly among endurance competitors; their incidence appears as high in prepubertal as in older athletes (Rowland & Walsh, 1985). These injuries result from repetitive microtrauma, and although they do not typically involve growth plates, they are valuable markers of excessive physical stress that could place the child at risk for epiphyseal damage. Prevention and early management of overuse injuries in young athletes, then, appears to be a rational approach to reducing risks of intensive training in the prepubertal age group.

The importance of identifying specific risk factors that predispose to overuse injuries in children and adolescents has been emphasized (Micheli, 1983). These include the following:

- Training errors, particularly sudden increases in training intensity
- Anatomical malalignment of the legs, such as leg-length discrepancies and abnormal hip rotation
- Improper footwear
- Hard playing surfaces
- Associated disease states of the lower extremity

The growth process itself may predispose the athlete to overuse injuries, as disproportionate growth of muscle–tendon units, bones, and ligaments can result in loss of flexibility during the adolescent growth spurt.

Recommendations

It is important to reemphasize that epiphyseal damage from endurance exercise during childhood generally is possible only in those involved in intense training regimens. The child who wishes to run 1 or 2 miles three times a week can do so without risk of serious musculoskeletal injury. But for children involved in more rigorous training, several guidelines are important:

- Participation should be the child's idea, not a response to the desires of others, including parents.
- Overuse injuries are best prevented and performance is optimized when the serious child athlete is supervised by an individual who is knowledgeable about proper equipment and training techniques. Usually this person is not the athlete's parents. A high school or college coach is often a good candidate.
- Young athletes need to be educated in ways to prevent and treat overuse injuries as well as burnout (see the following discussion).
- Training and competition should not exceed certain limits.

That last item is where the going gets thorny, because exercise thresholds for physical and psychological side effects are not known and presumably differ markedly from one individual to the next. For running, it has been recommended that children not participate in marathon races and that those under 14 years of age not train or compete at distances greater than 10K (American Academy of Pediatrics, 1982; Micheli, 1981). Considering the unknown risks for these activities, such guidelines are prudent at present. Some would argue, though, that there is no clear-cut scientific basis for excluding appropriately trained and supervised prepubertal athletes from these events. It would seem likely, too, that despite official recommendations many children will continue to become involved in intense training regimens. These athletes deserve close medical supervision to assess physical responses to training and competition, hopefully to minimize any adverse effects that may result.

SPORT INJURIES

Physical injury is an inherent risk in sport participation and to a certain extent must be considered an inevitable cost of athletic training and competition. Fortunately, athletic injuries to children and adolescents almost always are minor and carry no long-lasting consequences. Moreover, injuries from sport participation can be minimized through player conditioning, proper equipment, rule enforcement, safe playing fields, and adequate coaching (Mueller & Blyth, 1982). Physicians and parents can help by ensuring that their patients or children are participating in well-organized programs that take care to minimize injuries.

One of the easiest ways to reduce the risks of athletic participation is through the proper selection of sport events. Many researchers have tried to assess the relative risks of different forms of athletics, but their reports suffer from differences in injury definition, lack of consideration of playing time, analysis of select populations, and absence of a uniform means of grading injury. In general, however, these studies verify a predictable analysis of risk: The older and bigger the athlete, the higher the chances for injury, and the more contact involved in the sport, the greater the severity of injury—but only after the onset of puberty. Micheli (1988a) has noted that the risk of injury from contact sports such as football and hockey in the preteen years is low; in fact, such activities may actually be *safer* for this age group than sports characterized by repetitive training (e.g., gymnastics and swimming) because of the latter's high incidence of overuse injuries.

Football

Over a million pre–high school youngsters participate on organized youth football teams despite the reputed injury risks in this sport (Goldberg, Rosenthal, & Nicholas, 1984). In reality, the chances for significant injury from playing football in this age group are small, probably because low levels of muscular strength lessen the force of body impact. Goldberg, Rosenthal, & Nicholas (1984) reported an injury rate of 8.4 percent during a competitive season among 143 football players aged 9 to 12 years (65 to 100 lb), mostly sprains and contusions. Only one major injury occurred in this group (a joint dislocation), and there were no severe or permanent disabilities.

Once these players become older and larger, and hit harder, the risks of injury rise. Goldberg, Rosenthal, & Nicholas (1984) indicated incidence figures of 12.7 and 23.9 percent in weight groups 80 to 115 and 100 to 130 lb, respectively. Injury rates of 50 to 80 percent have been observed at the high school level (Garrick & Requa, 1978), and at this age injuries are typically more crippling.

Soccer

Many parents view their child's participation in soccer as a healthy alternative to the risks of football. Among prepubertal athletes this is probably not true, as their injury incidence from soccer is approximately 7 to 15 percent, again usually sprains, muscle strains, and contusions (Backous, Friedl, Smith, Parr, & Carpine, 1988). As with football, a significant jump in injury frequency is observed after puberty, but at the high school level soccer is clearly safer than playing football; the risk of significant injury in football is 2 to 5 times higher than in soccer, and the severity of injury is also greater (Ward, 1987).

Ice Hockey

Ice hockey is one of the fastest and most violent sports; players can be injured by sticks, skates, and pucks, and they're at risk for musculoskeletal stresses from rapid acceleration and deceleration (Sim & Simonet, 1988). Top hockey players in youth leagues often skate at 20 mph and can propel a 6-oz puck at speeds of 60 to 100 mph. It is not surprising, then, that body collisions, hockey sticks, and pucks account for 75 to 80 percent of all injuries in this sport.

Improvements in protective equipment, particularly helmets and face masks, have lowered the incidence of hockey injuries. In college and professional hockey, the average player still receives 2.5 to 3.0 injuries per year. The incidence of all types of injuries in youth hockey is significantly lower, reportedly 2 per 100 players each year (Sunderland, 1976).

Other Sports

Chandy and Grana (1985) reported the results of a large 3-year study assessing injury rates among high school track, cross-country, swimming, tennis, volleyball, basketball, and baseball players. The overall injury rate was 2.6 percent in the boys and 3.6 percent in the girls, a difference accounted for entirely by a greater number of basketball injuries in the females. This suggests the particular importance of adequate conditioning for girls before basketball participation. The incidence of basketball injuries (5.6 percent in males and 7.8 percent in females) was 5 to 10 times that of the other activities but still significantly lower than previous reports of injury rates in football and other contact sports.

In sports such as wrestling, swimming, running, and gymnastics there are little data identifying risks specifically for prepubertal athletes. At the high school level the incidence of significant wrestling injuries is similar to that in football (Requa & Garrick, 1981). Gymnastics ranks high in injury incidence, particularly for girls, and in one report was fourth in frequency behind football, wrestling, and softball in high school athletes (Shively, Grana, & Ellis, 1981).

Likelihood of Injury

How should parents and physicians view the chances of injury for children involved in organized competitive sport programs? Despite earlier concerns of both educators and physicians, the risk of significant injury appears to be very small. Martens (1980), in fact, contended that

children have less chance of being injured playing baseball than riding their bicycles to the game, less chance of serious injury in wrestling or ice hockey than when skateboarding, and substantially less chance of dying playing tackle football than riding in the school bus or the family car. (p. 384)

PSYCHOLOGICAL RISKS

For most children, participation in sport is an enjoyable, enriching experience. Reacting to the stress of competition builds self-confidence, teaches how to respond to winning and losing, and places a value on self-discipline. But for a small minority the anxiety from competitive sport results in abnormal degrees of stress that can prove psychologically unhealthy. Psychologists have repeatedly emphasized that these children may be guided into more emotionally healthy responses to athletics by a realignment of parental attitudes and coaching approaches. At the other end of the competitive scale, the elite child athlete is perceived to be at risk for psychosocial disturbances from an early and intense commitment to success in sports. An extensive literature has developed surrounding the psychological responses of children to sport participation (Feltz & Ewing, 1987; Martens, 1978; Martens, 1988). The following review briefly summarizes these concerns.

Stress From Competition

Controversy continues to rage on the emotional risks and benefits of competitive sport for prepubertal children. Martens (1988) provides a convincing argument that the problem of excessive anxiety during sport participation has been greatly overemphasized. Most children exhibit transient anxiety during athletics that is no greater than during other life events and has no long-term psychological implications. Certain predisposed youngsters, however, may be vulnerable to the stresses of competition and deserve careful attention.

Characteristics of psychologically at-risk athletes include those who do the following (Martens, 1988; Smilkstein, 1980):

- Perceive that they are not meeting the expectations of their peers, coach, or parents
- View physical abilities as indicators of self-worth
- Feel uncertain about their capacity to face the performance challenge
- Attach a great deal of importance to the outcome of the competition

Many of these features can be prevented or modified by supportive and sensitive coaches and parents. In particular, the emphasis on winning can be particularly detrimental to children. Losing has a powerful influence on perceptions of self-worth in some children; when a child feels high levels of stress from failing to "succeed" by winning, the goals of participation in sports need to be reoriented (Martens, 1980).

Psychological Effects on Young Elite Athletes

A great deal of concern has been expressed by both lay and medical groups over the psychological implications of prepubertal children's participation in world-class athletic competition (Nash, 1987). The pressure to succeed drives these youngsters into intensive training schedules, to the exclusion of normal school and social activities. Families who alter their lifestyles to accommodate these training regimens further intensify the importance of achievement, winning, and gaining competitive goals. Are children emotionally prepared for these stresses? Does early elite-level competition create lasting psychological scars? Can these psychological effects lead to early burnout and discontinued participation in sport activities?

The few psychological studies performed on elite child athletes do not adequately answer these questions (Feltz & Ewing, 1987). Researchers assessing anxiety levels in these young athletes do not, in general, show any differences from those of nonathletes. In fact, some athletes have indicated that nervousness surrounding competition enhances their performance. Early attrition from international levels of competition appears common (Feigley, 1984), but the reasons have not been adequately spelled out.

Elite athletes of all ages are at increased risk for burnout, a poorly-defined complication of intense training that impairs performance and may lead to dropping out of sport participation altogether. Symptoms of lethargy, weight loss, insomnia, anorexia, and depression are common, and disinterest in athletic competition may follow (Feigley, 1984). Whether burnout is a physiological or psychological response to overtraining is unclear (Barron, Noakes, Levy, Smith, & Millar, 1985). Rest is the only therapy, which often needs to be prolonged and may not always be completely effective in restoring the athlete's interest and energy to competitive levels. The most effective preventive measure is to protect against

---

Indicators for Overtraining ("Burnout")

- Rise in morning waking heart rate (> 5 beats/min)
- Post-workout fall in weight
- Decreased sleeping hours
- Later time to bed
- Less fluid intake

burnout by monitoring morning heart rates, postworkout weight, and sleeping hours (Dressendorfer, Wade, & Scaff, 1985; Round Table, 1983) (see box).

Anorexia Nervosa

Physicians need to be aware that some adolescents with anorexia nervosa may develop compulsive exercise habits as a means of losing weight. Smith (1980) noted that excessive weight loss and food aversion in athletes could be separated from true anorexia nervosa by the lack of underlying psychopathology in the former. These athletes need to be counseled that reducing fatness by limiting caloric intake will not improve performance in most sport events.

REPRODUCTIVE DYSFUNCTION

The increasing participation of young females in athletics has raised concern about the effects of physical training on the development of reproductive function. Delayed menarche is observed more commonly among athletes, and there is a higher incidence of menstrual irregularities and amenorrhea in those engaged in intensive training regimens. Are these changes dangerous? What causes them? Are they reasons for limiting exercise intensity in young girls? Will they influence future reproductive function? The answers are not all in, but the available information is reassuring. Such changes deserve medical attention, but there is no evidence that they are deleterious during the growing years or that they influence ultimate reproductive capacity. Several excellent reviews have addressed these issues (Baker, 1981; Frisch, 1987; Malina, 1983; Wells, 1986b; Wells & Plowman, 1988).

Delayed Menarche

Considerable data indicate that menarche is significantly delayed in many young female athletes (Brisson, Dulac, Peronnet, & Ledoux, 1982; Malina, Harper, Avent, & Campbell, 1973). The average age at onset of menses is 12.3 to 12.8 years among healthy American girls, but most studies indicate that those who participate strenuously in sports experience menarche at age 13 to 14 years and sometimes even later (Malina, Spirduso, Tate, & Baylor, 1978; Marker, 1981). This phenomenon has been reported in most sports activities. Swimming has been considered an exception, as an early study indicated that Swedish swimmers experienced menarche *before* nonathletic girls (Åstrand et al., 1963). More recently, however, Stager, Robertshaw, and Miescher (1984) described delayed menarche in swimmers as well.

The age of menarche is apparently related to the number of years of training before onset of menses; on the average, a 0.4-year delay in menarche can be expected for each year of prepubertal training (Frisch et al., 1981).

Two theories have evolved to explain this phenomenon:

- Intense exercise before puberty delays menstrual function by creating energy loss or preventing the achievement of a critical body weight or fat content.
- The physical characteristics associated with delayed puberty (e.g., slender body habitus, long legs) are those more likely to be related to athletic success.

Frisch and Revelle (1971) and Frisch and McArthur (1974) championed the idea that attainment of specific weight (48 kg) and/or percent body fat (17 percent) were necessary to initiate menses. According to this concept, menarche is delayed when the effects of athletic training prevent reaching these anthropometric thresholds. The experimental methodology by which the authors drew these conclusions has been criticized (Scott & Johnston, 1982; Wells & Plowman, 1988), and the concept of a specific threshold weight and fat percentage for onset of menses is not generally accepted. Still, data do support a role for body compositional changes and exercise stress in delaying menarche (Rogol, 1988; Vandenbroucke, van Laar, & Valkenburg, 1983).

Malina (1983) contended that the observed association between delayed menarche and athletic training does not necessarily imply a causal relationship between the two. As an equally plausible explanation, girls with delayed menarche may more often engage in sport activities. Menarche is associated with timing of epiphyseal closure and increase in body fat; those with delayed puberty are characterized by having narrow hips, slender physique, longer legs, and less body fat—all features that would help girls excel in most sports. According to this theory, then, the athletic training–delayed menarche phenomenon is a result of a selective process. Menarche is normally later in some girls, who by their body habitus are more likely to be successful in sports.

Should physicians, parents, and athletes be concerned about retarded pubertal development and late menarche associated with sport participation? The hypoestrogenic state related to delayed menses can result in slowed growth of bone density, but this risk is not significant if menarche occurs by age 18 years. Shangold (1986) suggested estrogen replacement therapy if menses do not occur by that time, because significant impairment of bone mineralization can occur. It has also been recommended that girls who do not display secondary sexual development by the age of 14 years or menarche by 16 undergo a diagnostic evaluation; erroneously ascribing pubertal delay to exercise training may cause pathological conditions such as tumors or hormonal deficiencies to be overlooked.

Exercise-Induced Amenorrhea

Intensive physical training suppresses normal menstrual patterns in many postpubertal females, particularly those involved in endurance sports. Depending on the definitions employed, from 1 to 43 percent of these athletes will experience either irregular menstrual periods or amenorrhea during training (Rogol, 1988). With decreased activities or during rest periods, normal menses resume, and fertility appears unaffected (Eriksson et al., 1978; Warren, 1980). The influence of exercise on menstrual function depends on the intensity of training. In distance running, for instance, amenorrhea might not result from regimens of less than 15 to 20 training miles per week (Feicht, Johnson, Martin, Sparkes, & Wagner, 1978).

The proposed explanations for the cause of exercise-induced amenorrhea are similar to those suggested for delayed menarche (leanness, low body weight, energy drain, physical or emotional stress), but the precise mechanism is unclear (Baker, 1981; Wells, 1986b). Investigation of the hormonal status of amenorrheic athletes has not revealed a uniform picture. Several disturbances of endocrinological function have been described, including a shortened luteal phase and decreased luteinizing hormone pulse frequency (Rogol, 1988; Shangold, Freeman, Thysen, & Gatz, 1979). Some amenorrheic athletes have low estrogen levels, whereas others are anovulatory and euestrogenic.

Secondary amenorrhea in the adolescent from athletic training appears to be benign. Athletes who are anovulatory with normal estrogen levels may have an increased incidence of endometrial hyperplasia and adenocarcinoma, but there is no significant risk for the athlete who has been amenorrheic for less than 5 years or who is under age 20 years (Shangold, 1986). Those who have low estrogen levels need to be concerned about the negative effects on bone density. Again, many years of decreased estrogen are necessary for this effect, and estrogen/progestin replacement therapy is generally not recommended for these women until at least age 18. It is important to remember that secondary amenorrhea in the athlete can have causes other than sports training.

Based on current information, there is no reason to withhold pre- or postpubertal girls from intense athletic training because of concerns over effects on reproductive function (Lutter & Cushman, 1982). These responses are benign (at least through the teenage years), reversible, and in some cases potentially beneficial. Lack of regular menstrual flow may help prevent iron deficiency, and the athlete will not be encumbered by dysmenorrhea or monthly menses. It is important to note that exercise-induced amenorrhea may not protect against pregnancy, and sexually active athletes should utilize an effective means of birth control (Rogol, 1988).

Reproductive Changes in Males

Little is known about the effects of physical training on reproductive function in males. Specifically, there is virtually no information available regarding the influence of athletic participation on pubertal development in boys. Malina (1984) reviewed anthropometric studies on sexual and skeletal maturity of champion swimmers and baseball players aged 9 to 16 years and found these athletes developmentally advanced compared to their nonathletic peers. In this respect, male athletes differ from their female counterparts: In many sports (e.g., football, hockey, wrestling) *early* pubertal development in boys favors successful athletic participation.

Rowland, Morris, Kelleher, Haag, & Reiter (1987) measured serum levels of total and free testosterone in 15 adolescent postpubertal male cross-country runners during the course of a competitive season (Figure 11.2).

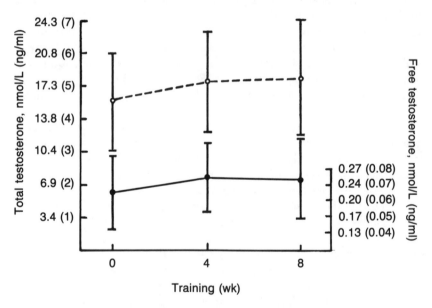

Figure 11.2 Mean ($\pm$ SD) levels of total and free testosterone in male high school cross-country runners during a competitive season. *Note*. From "Serum Testosterone Response to Training in Adolescent Runners" by T.W. Rowland, A.H. Morris, J.F. Kelleher, B.L. Haag, and E.O. Reiter, 1987, *American Journal of Diseases of Children*, **141**, p. 882. Copyright 1987 by the American Medical Association. Reprinted by permission.

No significant changes were observed during the 8-week period, suggesting that running training does not influence the hypothalamic–pituitary–gonadal axis in high school male athletes. However, adult men (mean age 33 years) who ran at least 64 km per week have been reported to have lower serum testosterone and prolactin levels (Wheeler, Wall, Belcastro, & Cumming, 1984).

CONVULSIVE DISORDERS

Concerns about exercise in children with seizure disorders has centered around the possibility that physical activity might predispose to convulsions through fatigue, hyperventilation, or head trauma, and the risks that might be incurred by the child or spectators if a seizure should occur during certain types of activities (e.g., swimming, archery). Such occurrences have been thought to be very infrequent, but their incidence is not known for certain. Other than anecdotal information no epidemiological data are available on the relationship of convulsions to exercise. Seizures can occur during physical activity, and rare cases have been reported of exercise specifically triggering convulsions (Ogunyemi,

---

Exercise Prescription Guidelines for Children With Seizure Disorders

- The decision whether a patient with a seizure disorder should participate in sport depends on the degree of seizure control, type of activity, and history of prior seizure experience with exercise. Such a decision should be shared by the parents, child, and physician.
- In general, physical activity should be promoted as much as possible.
- There is no contraindication for participation in exhaustive activities or collision sports (except boxing).
- Activities such as swimming, mountain climbing, horseback riding, or bicycling are permitted when the child is supervised but only by patients whose seizures are well controlled by medication. Likewise, sports in which the child's participation might pose a danger to spectators (e.g., discus throwing, archery) should not be allowed for uncontrolled epileptic patients.
- Patients should not engage in forms of exercise known to precipitate seizures.

Gomez, & Klass, 1988). But the experience of large clinics is that, in general, there is little connection between sport participation and epilepsy (Livingston, 1971).

There is a general impression among practitioners that seizures are actually more likely to occur during times of inactivity (Cowart, 1986). Seizure discharges on electroencephalograms may, in fact, be decreased by physical activity (Gotze, Kubicki, Hunter, & Teichmann, 1967). There is no evidence that any particular form of athletics—including contact sports—is more likely than others to precipitate seizures.

For these reasons there has been a trend to encourage patients with epilepsy to become involved in physical activities as much as possible (Livingston & Berman, 1973). Most children's epilepsy is well-controlled with medication, and the adverse psychological effects of being unable to play in sports are usually far greater than the small risk of seizures during athletic participation. Accordingly, guidelines have been recommended by the American Academy of Pediatrics (1983a) and Bar-Or (1983), and can be found in the box on the preceding page.

IMPAIRED THERMOREGULATION

Children do not respond as well physiologically to heat stress as do adults. Bar-Or (1980, 1984) has reviewed the anatomical and physiological liabilities and has reported that the following characteristics place children at higher risk for hyperthermia during exercise in warm, humid climates:

• **Ratio of body surface area to mass.** Children have a greater ratio of body surface area to mass than adults. This means that when environmental temperatures approach body temperature the child has a more difficult time losing body heat through convection and radiation.

• **Ratio of heat to body mass**. Prepubertal subjects generate more heat per kilogram of body mass during exercise. This occurs at both a given work load as well as at maximum exercise.

• **Cardiac output.** At a given oxygen uptake, children demonstrate lower cardiac output than adults, which may interfere with skin perfusion and limit convection and radiation heat loss.

• **Sweat production.** Children produce less sweat per unit of skin surface area (Figure 11.3). In hot environments this may amount to no more than 60 to 70 percent of adult sweating capacity. The difference is due to maturity-related sweating rates, because the number of sweat glands in adults and children are equal.

• **Heat acclimatization.** When confronted with a new, warm environment the body adjusts by reducing heart rate and core temperature while increasing sweating rate. Children demonstrate a slower rate of this heat acclimatization than do adults.

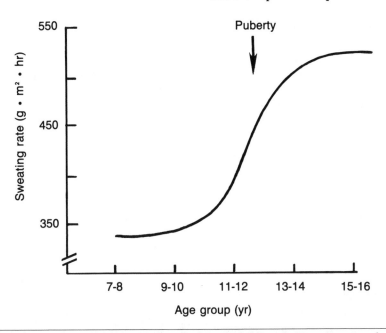

Figure 11.3 Increasing sweating rates during childhood. *Note.* Reprinted from *Sports Medicine: Health Care for Young Athletes,* copyright © 1983 by the American Academy of Pediatrics. Reprinted by permission.

Do these findings have real implications for children exercising in the heat? Adequate heat dissipation is important for maximizing performance, and children are more impaired than adults in their ability to exercise in a hot environment (Drinkwater, Kupprat, Denton, Crist, & Horvath, 1977). The actual risk of clinical hyperthermia with exercise in children is not known, but based on the considerations described, particular attention to preventing heat injuries is important in athletic events that involve prepubertal competitors (Rowland & Hoontis, 1985). These should take place in cool weather or early in the morning if warm days cannot be avoided. Events for children should be postponed when either temperature or humidity are high, because these factors create additive risk for heat-stress injury. Adequate fluids should be available before, during, and after sport competitions.

SUMMARY

The anatomical, physiological, and psychological immaturity of children may place them at greater risk during athletic training and competition. Potential hazards are greatly minimized when the athlete and his or her physician, coach, and parents are aware of these issues.

- It is extremely infrequent that cardiac disease in children presents a risk for sudden death with exercise. Moreover, high-risk abnormalities are often detectable by routine history and clinical examination.
- Whether extensive endurance training can damage growth centers in the bones of growing children is uncertain. There is no direct evidence that even intensive exercise regimens can be expected to produce microtraumatic injury. Still, caution is advised until further research clarifies this question.
- Traumatic injury during sport participation must be viewed as an integral risk of athletics. Injury risks can be lessened, however, by ensuring optimal playing conditions and equipment, proper training techniques, and maturity-matching of competitors.
- Emotional reactions to sport participation are positive for most children. Some children may respond adversely to the stresses of competition, however, particularly if coaches and parents inappropriately stress performance and winning.
- Menarche occurs earlier and oligoamenorrhea more frequently in competitive athletes, but there appear to be no long-term effects on reproductive capabilities.
- With a few common-sense constraints, children with controlled seizure disorders should be encouraged to participate in physical activities.
- Children are at higher risk for heat-stress injury during exercise and deserve particular attention to fluid replacement and environmental conditions in athletic events.

PART III

Strategies for Improving Exercise Habits of Children

Every body continues in its state of rest . . . unless it is compelled to change that state by forces impressed upon it.

Newton (1686)

When Newton formulated his laws of motion he probably did not have the inertia of sedentary human beings in mind. But in this principle lies the greatest problem faced by medical professionals who encourage exercise for healthy living. It is easier to sit than to run, more convenient to watch television than to swim, more tempting to ride elevators than to climb stairs. More recently Bar-Or (1983) has described a contemporary corollary to Newton's laws: Hypoactive children are at great risk of becoming increasingly sedentary. An inactive life depresses the level of physical fitness, which in turn causes the child to avoid exercise even more. The result is a self-perpetuating cycle that results in a poorly fit, overweight youngster with the desire to do little more than watch television and consume snack foods.

Who is responsible for identifying these children who are "turned off" to exercise? What kinds of physical activity programs are available to get them back on track? Traditionally, this has been the role of school physical education classes, but it is apparent that gym class has not been successful in stimulating hypoactive children to enjoy physical activities. The shortcomings of these programs have been appreciated and remedies proposed. But even in the best of physical education curricula there is insufficient time to establish and encourage individual lifestyle changes for increasing physical activity. Schoolteachers cannot be expected to singlehandedly alter the exercise habits of their students. The responsibility needs to be shared.

The family has a major influence on child behavior and needs to be reminded of its vital role in shaping the attitudes and actions of its members. Social forces, however, work against the family. Priorities of job, financial security, marital stress, and self-interest frequently supersede responsibilities to other family members, and the family's ability to favorably influence the activities of its children may be eroded. Sport coaches, older athletes, scout leaders, government officials, and those who control the presentation of sport in the media may also shape attitudes toward physical activity.

The physician needs to be part of this team. Regular physical activity is a powerful effector of good health and deserves the attention of the medical community. Physicians need to promote health-related behaviors in children, and adopting a physically active lifestyle is certainly an important one.

Sheehan (1983) writes of a current epidemic of "exercise deficiency," which he terms "undoubtedly the most prevalent cause of ill health in America" (p. 53). The importance of lifelong exercise to good health dictates that physicians should view this deficiency with the same serious attention they would give a child who is failing to thrive because of caloric deprivation or a patient who is low in body iron. The deficiency needs to be diagnosed, treatment instituted, and progress assessed.

Little has been done to determine whether and how physicians caring for children can alter the exercise habits of their patients and whether successful results can be sustained. In a survey questionnaire of 779 primary care pediatricians, over half considered it important to counsel children over age 6 regarding exercise (Nader, Taras, Sallis, & Patterson, 1987). Interestingly, however, only a fourth felt that pediatricians were likely to be effective in changing the exercise habits of their patients.

This section is aimed at improving both of these proportions. By understanding factors that motivate children to exercise, physicians can offer realistic goals and specific exercise recommendations to habitually inactive children. Equally important, counseling of parents regarding physical activity during the child's early years may pay dividends in preventing the later development of sedentary habits.

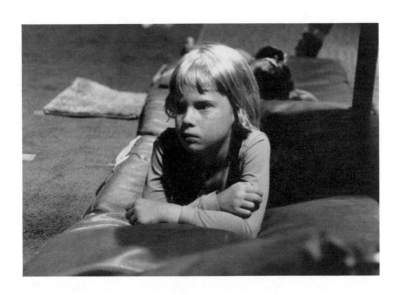

CHAPTER 12

Clinical Approaches to the Sedentary Child

Question: Which of the following do you judge to be the most appropriate goal for the primary care physician in promoting exercise for children and adolescents?

   a. Improve physical fitness.
   b. Make the child an athlete.
   c. Create habits for lifelong exercise.
   d. Increase habitual activity.
   e. All of the above.

Answer: You probably selected answer (e), but that gets you only partial credit. The best answer is actually (b)—turn the child into an athlete. "Athlete," that is, as the word was originally defined—an individual who fulfills to the maximum his or her given physical capabilities. The ancient Greeks firmly believed in this goal. They embodied "being an athlete" into the basic definition of health: soundness of mind, body, and spirit. Becoming a true athlete, then, is within the abilities of all children and is the core issue in improving exercise habits as a means to good health.

This is fine philosophy, but how about in the reality of the physician's office? What is the goal of the physician facing the indolent teenager? What is he or she really trying to accomplish? To improve strength, flexibility, and cardiovascular fitness? To introduce activities like running or swimming as a start to lifetime habits? To educate the patient on the role of exercise in attaining good health?

It is important that realistic, specific goals be defined, because getting that sedentary adolescent off the sofa is not going to be easy. Sallis (quoted in Monahan, 1986b) will receive little argument with his contention that "exercise is the most difficult health habit to alter" (p. 205); it's a truism that gives all the more impetus to early physician intervention with distinct exercise objectives. Unfortunately, effecting changes in children's exercise habits from the physician's office is a new concept, and appropriate goals and methods have not become part of common practice. Certainly these will vary depending on the patient's previous exercise levels, family characteristics, geographical and social setting, body composition, sex, and age. The following discussion, however, is an attempt to formulate a rational approach based on the current understanding of how exercise behaviors affect health.

The information presented in Part II of this book, which reviewed the scientific grounds for viewing exercise as beneficial to health, makes it apparent that health-related outcomes of exercise do not often relate to how *well* physical activities can be performed. Reduction in coronary risk factors, relief of anxiety, prevention and treatment of obesity—all appear to be more a function of *amount* of exercise, the number of calories expended, than of quality of skill. Based on current knowledge about the exercise–health connection, then, promotion of physical activity rather than physical fitness seems to be a logical approach for physicians.

Health officials have used the results of mass fitness testing in children as a marker of the risk for diseases brought on by sedentary lifestyle for the pediatric population as a whole. In counseling individual patients, however, the physician cannot conclude that those who run slower or perform fewer chin-ups than national norms are truly at a health risk, because of the large genetic influence on physical skills.

It follows, then, that *the best working goal for physicians is to first identify sedentary children and then get them moving.* The credo: Every child should be participating regularly in some form of physical activity. It doesn't really matter what children do, or even how much. Getting the overweight boy who is driven to school and who does nothing but work his computer and play video games to go bowling one night a week is a major success (Bar-Or, 1983).

Making exercise an enjoyable experience—one that will become perpetuated through intrinsic motivation—is a requisite objective for getting children into regular exercise habits. It would be nice if all children would participate in aerobic sports 3 to 4 times per week on an ongoing basis, but the obese child and clumsy adolescent won't do it. They view those activities as unpleasant, and there is little chance that their negative attitudes toward exercise will be erased. The point: Limiting exercise interventions to those viewed as beneficial to health will impede success. The more immediate goal of increasing *any* physical activity through finding exercise that is enjoyable to the individual patient is more realistic.

THE DIAGNOSIS OF EXERCISE DEFICIENCY

In most clinical situations, deficiency states can be detected through laboratory testing (e.g., serum ferritin levels for iron depletion) and typical physical findings (e.g., tetany with hypocalcemia). Replacement therapy is based on a knowledge of threshold values for good health and a recognition that overly zealous treatment not only is unnecessary but can produce toxic side effects. Not so with exercise deficiency. Identification of children who need more exercise is currently based on subjective information, and, lacking a dose–effect curve for exercise and health outcomes, the prescription is empirical. As noted in Part I of this book, questions such as "Is this child getting sufficient exercise?" and "How much is enough (or too much)?" can't yet be answered with scientific confidence. But certain guidelines are useful.

Children at greater risk for exercise deficiency are often easily identified. Those with chronic illness (e.g., diabetes or congenital heart disease), obesity, or sedentary parents are unlikely to be participating in physical activities to their full potential. So are children who don't like gym class, who have a strong interest in sedentary hobbies, or who cringe when asked about their involvement in sport.

History taking is the most convenient diagnostic tool. In some future time physicians will provide each of their young patients with a small portable device that accurately records their physical activities over a week's time. After reviewing the results, a quantitative diagnosis of exercise deficiency can be made and a specific prescription provided for needed improvement. Unfortunately, despite significant improvements in their design, such devices currently are not ready for such wide-scale use (Freedson, in press). In the meantime, patients (or their parents) can be asked to keep a log of all activities over a period of days, much the same way a dietary diary is recorded for nutritional analysis, or a questionnaire can be provided to the patient and parent to complete while they are in the waiting room. Questionnaires for this purpose can be extensive, like the "Sample Activity Questionnaire" adapted from Bar-Or (1983), or simple, limited to 2 or 3 questions regarding level of habitual activity and involvement on sports teams (Rowland, 1986). Logs and questionnaires often lack sufficient accuracy as research tools but should give adequate information to determine whether recommendations for improving exercise are indicated.

Sample Activity Questionnaire

1. During the past 3 months, what would best describe your child's usual level of physical activity? (circle letter)

   A. Inactive. Watches television, reads, or does homework after school; has ride to school; no extracurricular sports.
   B. Occasionally active. Prefers sedentary activities but sometimes plays outside.
   C. Moderately active. Takes opportunities to become involved in physical activity when available and enjoys it.
   D. Active. Takes initiative to participate in physical exercise and prefers this to sedentary activities. At least three times a week involved in vigorous exercise.
   E. Very active. Participates regularly in extracurricular sports. Great deal of energy. Dislikes sedentary activities.

2. How would you compare the physical activity of your child with that of her/his friends?

   Equally active
   More active
   Less active

3. During the last 6 months was your child involved in an organized sport or exercise program (such as YMCA, basketball league, gymnastics, dancing classes) outside of regular school physical education?

   Yes   Describe
   No

(Cont.)

Sample Activity Questionnaire (Continued)

4. During the last 6 months was he/she involved in regular athletic training (running, bicycling, swimming, etc.)?

   Yes   Describe

   No

5. In your opinion, is your child as physically active as she/he should be?

   Yes

   Too active

   Not active enough

6. If you feel your child is not sufficiently active, what do you feel is the reason?

   Not interested

   Doesn't feel talented in sports

   Too busy

   Illness

   Exercise is uncomfortable

   Friends aren't interested

   Other reason

Adapted from Bar-Or (1983).

Directly questioning the child or parent will usually, however, provide sufficient information about exercise habits. "What are you [is he/she] doing for exercise?" and "Do you think you are [he/she is] getting enough physical activity?" are two opening questions that most parents and children will respond to honestly and accurately (watch for the cringe!). Follow-up queries concerning use of leisure time, involvement with school or community sports teams, performance in physical education class, and ability to keep up with peers during play will provide a more complete picture.

The definition of exercise deficiency may vary from one patient to the next. What kinds of parameters should the physician use to decide whether a child needs more exercise? It's a difficult question to answer, because what's appropriate physical activity will vary from child to child. The adolescent who was previously a star swimmer and runner but who now only bicycles 1/2 hr twice a week is obviously a physical underachiever. On the other hand, for the obese child who has engaged in little physical activity, to muster enough self-discipline to perform that same amount of exercise might be a minor miracle.

Certainly exercise interventions should be strongly considered in the following situations:

- If the child is not involved in some out-of-school exercise 2 or 3 times a week
- If the child does not exercise on a *regular* basis
- If a negative response is received from the child (or parent) to the question "Do you think you get [he/she gets] enough exercise?"
- If the child is overweight or suffers from chronic physical or emotional illness

It is useful to investigate the family's interest and involvement in physical activities. The exercise prescription for the inactive child deserves to be a family project, and the physician's understanding of the activity habits of all household members is important. This gives clues to the child's genetic-based capabilities for exercise performance as well as to the support she or he is likely to receive for improving exercise habits. Hereditary fitness potential is difficult to assess, but asking about the parents' previous participation in school athletics might provide a reasonable estimate.

Physical fitness testing is of questionable value. Comments have already been made (p. 260) regarding the inappropriateness of improving the physical fitness of pediatric patients as a primary goal for physicians. Tests of fitness (muscle strength, power, and endurance; flexibility; cardiovascular endurance; body composition) can be performed or at least organized from the physician's office, or scores can be made available from testing in the schools. But the value of relating these findings in a given patient to both need for exercise and health outcomes must be seriously questioned. Not all medical authorities share such a negative viewpoint; however, this author cautions against reliance on physical fitness test scores as indicators of need for exercise intervention, for the following reasons:

- An individual's physical fitness does not always correlate well with level of physical activity, which appears more related to health outcomes. There is no information available relating percentile performance on fitness testing with present or future health. Dennison, Straus, Mellits, and Charney (1988) did show, however, that children who scored below the 20th percentile on the 600-yd run in school were less likely to exercise regularly as adults.
- The strong genetic influence on fitness, the variability in biological development at a given chronological age, and the vagaries of sub-

ject motivation make interpretation of results difficult. If a 10-year-old girl scores at the 25th percentile for her age in the mile run, is she "out of shape"? Or genetically less endowed than the average? Overweight or undermotivated? A late maturer compared to the average 10-year-old? At greater risk for coronary artery disease? All are possible, confusing the implications for intervention. Indeed, if this girl is performing at her maximum capability she needs less physician help than the genetically well-endowed child who is underachieving with scores at the 60th percentile.

• Following patients with serial fitness tests to assess progress in exercise programs has been suggested as a motivating "carrot." But here, too, caution is suggested. How does one interpret a 9:10 finish for a mile at the beginning of a running program compared with an 8:48 time at its completion 6 months later? Did the training improve fitness? Or would the time have fallen as a result of growth alone? If the child had been tested the *day* after the first test would the biological variability in performance be enough to get an 8:48 result?

EARLY EXERCISE INTERVENTIONS

The cornerstone of preventive medicine in the practice of pediatrics is the concept that positive health-related habits initiated early in life provide the basis for lifelong well-being. This idea has never been adequately tested experimentally. Observational evidence is strong, however, that how the child eats, exercises, relates to other people, and responds to stress are largely established early in life, strongly influenced by family behavior, and perpetuated into adulthood. Moreover, experience indicates that as these behaviors become established during the developing years they are increasingly difficult to change. This all means that physicians caring for children have both a responsibility and a unique opportunity to make a major impact on the future health of their patients.

How about exercise? Will being raised in a family of physically active individuals who involve the child from an early age help ensure a lifetime of regular exercise habits? No one knows for certain, but a physician who has attempted in vain to get a sedentary 14-year-old into regular activities will find great appeal in the idea of getting them started early. Not that young children aren't physically active. In normal preschoolers the drive for motor activities is intense. But making exercise a regular, family-oriented habit—beginning even in early infancy—may establish exercise patterns that carry over to later years when spontaneous activity wanes.

To this end physicians should encourage parents to plan out regular daily exercise periods with their infant, toddler, or older preschooler.

Some excellent books provide imaginative activities for parents and children in this age group:

Exercise Books for Preschool Children

Diem, L. (1974). *Children learn physical skills. Vol. 1.* Washington, D.C.: American Alliance for Health, Physical Education, Recreation and Dance.

Grasselli, R.N. & Hegner, P.A. (1981). *Playful parenting.* New York: Richard Marek.

Levy, J. (1975). *The baby exercise book.* New York: Random House.

Parents need to understand that the goal of these sessions is neither to make the infant or toddler more fit nor to accelerate motor development. The objective, from a preventive medicine standpoint, is to make exercise an expected, habitual activity that is both enjoyable and stimulating.

Physical exercise for infants and their parents obviously has much broader ramifications. Motor activity is the means by which infants and toddlers get to know their environments (Diem, 1974). Exercise is an essential component of the child's cognitive development and a means for achieving physical closeness and communication with parents. For the mother and father this is an opportunity for making parenting an imaginative and rewarding experience (Grasselli & Hegner, 1981).

MOTIVATIONAL FACTORS

Young children don't need to be motivated to exercise. To the contrary, the preschool youngster appears to be tanked up with an inexhaustible energy supply: "They like to move, play, run, climb, jump, and spin—they *pursue* vertigo" (Round Table, 1987, p. 121). Researchers have long tried to figure out why (Ellis & Scholtz, 1978). Perhaps these youngsters are burning off surplus energy, or maybe, as Freud suggested, there is direct pleasure gained from muscular activity. Some contemporary scientists view children's play as a form of stimulation or arousal-seeking behavior, generated to escape monotony. Others contend that the prevalence of play activity in young children suggests that it is an intrinsic drive, independent of other biological drives. Information discussed earlier in this book suggesting the existence of an activity center in the brain supports this idea, as does the fact that activity levels parallel basal metabolic rate during the growing years. But how can such a drive be explained? What would be its biological value?

Whyever it exists, the high spontaneous activity level of children begins to wane as they age, a decline representing—to a certain extent—a normal concomitant of biological development. The "metabolic fires" of older children, adolescents, and adults do not burn as fiercely as in the preschool child. Whatever factors stimulate young children to boundless physical activity fade as they grow. One can suppose, but not prove, that both social and personal factors can be implicated in speeding this decline in many youngsters—the increasing prevalence of obesity, the tempting passivity of television, the ease of "energy-saving" technology, the failure to succeed in organized sports.

To counter these influences many older children and adolescents must be actively motivated to exercise. The game plan:

- Introduce the inactive child to physical activity.
- Create a "positive" experience.
- Stimulate motivation from the intrinsic enjoyment of the activity.
- Set the stage for regular exercise habits that will be continued throughout life.

The approach is rational, but what are the chances for success without careful attention to those factors (shown in the box that follows) that turn a child "on" or "off" to exercise? Slim—at best. If one could reawaken the exercise drives (for want of a better term) of early childhood, or at least understand their basis, the task would be easier. Certainly some of the factors remain in later years: There is joy in physical exercise, there is a stimulation—even exhilaration—that replaces boredom. But other personal and social factors are important to consider when formulating strategies for getting the older sedentary child moving.

Motivational Keys to Exercise

"Turn-ons"	*"Turnoffs"*
• Fun	• Discomfort
• Success	• Failure
• Peer support	• Embarrassment
• Family participation	• Competition
• Variety	• Boredom
• Enthusiastic leaders	• Injuries
• Freedom	• Regimentation

The exercise must be fun. Exercise programs for children have little hope for success unless they are enjoyable. What is fun for one child, of course, may not be fun for another. But for most inactive children, a session of sweating, panting, and straining will prompt a rapid return to the television set and a bag of corn chips.

How to make it fun? First, aerobic-training regimens are inappropriate. Improving cardiovascular fitness in children—if it can be achieved at all—calls for at least three 1/2-hr sessions per week of sustained endurance exercise at an intensity that raises the heart rate to approximately 170 bpm (Rowland, 1985; Rowland & Green, 1989). That degree of physical activity may improve aerobic capacity and reduce coronary risk factors, but it will probably also destroy any desire of the previously sedentary child to continue with regular exercise. This is no place for "no gain without pain." The initial gain here is getting the inactive child into some form of physical activity, not improving cardiovascular fitness. So, having fun means being comfortable, starting slowly, and participating in enjoyable activities (more on this later). If children don't like an activity, they won't do it for long.

Having fun also means not being embarrassed. Any activity that causes a child to fail or look poor in front of peers will be a turnoff (consider, for instance, the embarrassment obese children might feel at having to appear in swimsuits in front of their lean classmates). The element of freedom also appears to be important (Iso-Ahola, 1979). Children, like adults, balk at activities they feel forced to do.

The child needs to be successful. Most children and adolescents who are athletically talented do not need to be motivated to exercise. It's the sedentary child who has failed in organized sport or who feels incapable of "making the team" who needs to be encouraged. These are the youngsters who have become disenchanted with exercise because they cannot throw a football, shoot a basket, or hit a baseball as well as other children. They retire from regular exercise because they are short on the physical skills to make them a "winner." Nothing extinguishes interest like failure. No one likes to do what they don't do well.

Exercise programs for sedentary children therefore need to be designed to create "successes" that are not based on competing with other children. Individual progress is a strong motivating factor, whether it be simply sticking with the program or increasing the distance cycled per week. Fortunately, the child with initial low levels of physical fitness can often make very substantial progress in a relatively short time if regular exercise can be sustained at all. These children are much more likely to continue exercise if progress is visible—and applauded.

The influence of family and peers is important. Many factors have bearing on the child's attitude to exercise, but probably none is more influential than the support and role models of parents and siblings. The family has tremendous power to mold children's life habits at an early age. Even when mothers work, fathers are away on trips, and siblings are insufferable, their attitudes, expectations, and behaviors affect the child

(Dishman et al., 1985; Lewko & Greendorfer, 1982; Monahan, 1986b). Parent support was cited as a major motivating factor in a structured exercise program for children (Rowland, 1986) as well as by a group of prepubertal runners (Rowland & Walsh, 1985). Sallis, Patterson, McKenzie, and Nader (1988) studied correlates of physical activity habits of preschool children and found significant positive relationships with the amount of exercise performed by parents.

Parents should be encouraged to organize regular family activities, such as bike rides and camping trips, that foster positive attitudes toward exercise. The parents' own exercise habits can be expected to be mimicked by their children. Success in improving children's physical activity may depend heavily on whether their parents can be equally persuaded to exercise regularly. As Pate and Blair (1978) noted, "Perhaps the most certain way to ensure that a child develops positive attitudes toward exercise is to place that child in a home in which the parents are physically active" (p. 272).

The assessment of exercise habits of parents and the frequency of activity time they spend with their children, however, is discouraging. The National Children and Youth Fitness Study II found that less than a third of parents of first- through fourth-graders participated in moderate to vigorous exercise three times a week (Ross & Pate, 1987). Moreover, neither parent spent more than one occasion a week exercising with the child. Shephard (1982) pointed out the problems involved in focusing on families for promoting exercise. The disruption of the nuclear family, high divorce rate, and large percentage of families with both parents working outside of the home make a family-based exercise program (much less an evening meal together!) difficult in many homes.

As a child grows older, the influence of peers on physical activity grows (Dishman et al., 1985). It is probably true, too, that by the time of adolescence, youngsters tend to select friends who have a similar outlook on sport and exercise. Social factors may be important in causing children to persist in exercise programs, and the influence of group affiliation can be utilized as a strong motivational tool. It can be expected that most children will stick to an exercise program better if they are participating along with their friends. Others who tend to be loners might do as well in individual activities (such as distance running), but few prepubertal children possess sufficient self-discipline to persist in these types of activities by themselves for long.

The use of extrinsic motivational techniques (e.g., bribes) may sometimes be justified. A survey of exercise programs for children—particularly those for obese youngsters—would uncover a surprising number using material rewards to motivate subjects to persist in physical activities. Unabashedly these children are offered T-shirts, sweatbands, athletic tickets—even money—to stick with the program. Smith, Smith, and Smoll (1983) warned against using such extrinsic motivators, claiming that these rewards can become the focus of a child's desire to participate and replace the joy of exercise for its own sake. The end result will be an early dropout from physical activity.

There is another side to this argument, however. When a child is successful and has fun in physical activities, the desire to exercise is perpetuated. These are intrinsic motivating factors that, once achieved, can become powerful forces for continuing regular exercise. The problem is, how can sedentary children become initiated into exercise long enough to build intrinsic motivation? If these children can be at least temporarily motivated into physical activity by the desire for a T-shirt or pennant, they may discover the enjoyment of exercise and plant the seeds of longer-lasting intrinsic motivators.

Motivational factors in structured programs may differ from those for adults. A great deal of attention has been focused on factors that affect exercise compliance and adherence in adults, particularly as they relate to cardiac rehabilitation programs. Spouse reinforcement, program time and location, perceived health benefits, and personality factors typically rank high as key aspects of maintaining exercise participation (Dishman et al., 1985). Little has been done, however, to examine similar factors in children.

Rowland (1986) reported the results of a motivation questionnaire completed by parents of diabetic children participating in a 12-week YMCA aerobic exercise program. The items that scored highest were enthusiastic leadership with individualized attention, parent support, and giving the child a sense of accomplishment and self-worth. Rewards (T-shirts, certificates), competition between participants, and absence of a program fee were ranked low as motivators. Interestingly, the desire to improve health and diabetic control were cited as strong motivating factors. Others have noted that concern over health is unlikely to influence exercise habits of well children, who do not view themselves as vulnerable to future illness (Mirotznik, Speedling, Stein, & Bronz, 1985). For children who have chronic disease, however, knowledge that exercise may directly benefit their well-being may be a strong inducement to regular physical activity.

Geographical proximity of the exercise site is another practical consideration. Because children often need to be transported by automobile, the availability and motivation of the *parents* can become a critical issue determining attendance at exercise sessions.

EXERCISE RECOMMENDATIONS

To review: The best chance for putting sedentary children into motion is to provide them with activities they will enjoy and that permit success in a noncompetitive atmosphere, provide variety and avoid monotony, and build on social reinforcers by including family or peers. Extrinsic motivators, such as rewards for progress and perseverance, are not to be eschewed. Regimens for improving cardiovascular fitness usually are not appropriate for inactive children and adolescents; instead, the desired goal is to increase physical activity. Getting inactive children moving with any form of exercise on a regular basis is the initial objective.

Programs

What form of exercise to recommend? Many options are available, but the best choice is an activity that the particular child finds enjoyable. Asking the child is the simplest way of finding this out. Most children, even those who are sedentary, will say that they like *some* form of exercise (particularly swimming, riding a bicycle, or jumping rope). If there is no positive response, suggest something they might not have considered, like dancing, bowling, Ping-Pong, or walking through shopping malls, zoos, or museums. The simple judgment, "You need to get more exercise," is not going to work. The physician's encouragement hopefully will be a strong motivator to improve exercise habits, but recommendations will probably have little effect unless specific proposals for the inactive patient are provided, and close follow-up is planned. Several "prescription" options are available:

Strategy #1: Increasing Daily Activity. This is the technique described for obese children earlier in this book. "Increasing animation" is the way Lindner (1980) described this approach, something valuable for *all* patients but particularly for those whose lifestyles have been very inactive. Children are taught ways to increase their caloric output during daily activities, particularly standing more, using the body instead of machines, adding movement during idle time, and increasing activity levels during routine movements. Doing more household chores (mowing the lawn, raking leaves) can be an important part of this approach. The boxed quiz on page 156, which is modified from Lindner (1980), can allow children to score their increased daily activities, and rewards can be offered when a particular total is reached.

This lifestyle counseling can be extended to problems of time management for children. For instance, Strong (1987) recommended that children should not be allowed to do homework after school (an immediately attractive idea to many patients!). "The child has already logged a long, often tedious day in an activity-restricted atmosphere. After school, children need a break to enhance their physical abilities, to 'let off steam.' They do not need to do homework or watch television before supper. They can do their homework in the evening following supper and after chores, when it is becoming dark. If they still have time after homework, they can watch a special television program" (p. 488).

Strategy #2: Organized Community or School Activities. Many children are more likely to exercise as part of a social experience they can enjoy with their friends. Likewise, group activities are often more fun and variable; they almost always involve a director or coach who has the opportunity to provide enthusiastic leadership and role modeling. On the negative side, group activities may not be positive experiences if the child feels he or she is failing in front of peers. Also, many organized activities require that the child be transported by the parents.

Community athletic teams in sports such as soccer and baseball, or gymnastics or karate classes are excellent ways to get children who are not highly athletic into sport activities. So are swimming or outdoors programs offered by organizations such as the YMCA. Many offer aerobic exercise programs specifically designed for children.

Physicians have the responsibility to know what exercise programs are available for children in their communities. Brochures and other printed material can be given to children and their families in the doctor's office when the exercise "prescription" is made. Directors or coaches of these programs will be happy to provide such materials, but communication lines must be opened so that these leaders are aware of the physician's interest.

Strategy #3: Individual Sport Activities. Individual sports such as running, cycling, and walking are enjoyable, but most children in unsupervised programs are not likely to persist in these activities unless particularly motivated by peers or family. Still, these sports are ideal for starting lifelong exercise habits, and some children may find enjoyment, success, or even hidden talent in these activities that will serve as strong motivating factors. Specific guidelines and information for patients are provided in the next chapter. One way to help children stick with these aerobic activities is to rotate activities at regular intervals (e.g., running in the summer, soccer in the fall, swimming in the winter, and cycling in the spring). Again, ensuring family or peer involvement might be the best key to success.

Follow-Up

Having provided the child with specific instructions for improving activity, the physician must create an effective way to assess progress and to motivate the child to further exercise. A quick 5- to 10-min check in the office at regular intervals may be sufficient. This situation is also a good opportunity for the physician to call on the help of parent and coach or director. Creating a "team" to support and monitor exercise habits will strengthen the effectiveness of the physician's recommendations.

PHYSICIANS CAN DO MORE

There are a number of things physicians can do to encourage their patients to begin and maintain a habitual physical fitness program. The following suggestions are just a few.

Become an advocate for exercise programs for children. The credibility of physicians as spokespersons for child health carries substantial weight for those who organize athletic programs for youngsters. School administrators, directors of community recreation departments, sports editors, the town electorate—they all need to hear the word from the medical profession that sport is more than play, that exercise programs for *all* children are an important aspect of good health. Community resources need to be provided to give youngsters with a broad range of athletic talent the opportunity to participate in physical activities.

Maintain personal physical fitness. Physicians can influence exercise behaviors not only by what they say but also by how they act. Participation in regular exercise demonstrates a commitment to physical activity that goes far beyond simply preaching advice to patients.

Make educational materials about exercise available to patients and their families. Excellent books have been written to help parents help their children improve exercise habits as well as participate in specific sport activities. A few of these are listed here. In addition, notices about local exercise programs and sport opportunities for children should be posted in the doctor's office.

Books for Parents

Fish, H.T., Fish, R.B. & Golding, L.A. (1989). *Starting out well: A parents' approach to physical activity & nutrition.* Champaign, IL: Leisure Press.

Lorin, M.I. (1978). *The parents' book of physical fitness for children.* New York: Atheneum.

Rotella, R.J., & Bunker, L.K. (1987). *Parenting your superstar.* Champaign, IL: Leisure Press.

Smith, N.J., Smith, R.E., & Smoll, F.L. (1983). *Kidsports. A survival guide for parents.* Reading, MA: Addison-Wesley.

Help organize a road race, swim meet, bicycle tour, or other event for children. The participation of physicians in these projects reinforces for children and their families the importance the doctor places on exercise in their lives. Contact local sports clubs to get started.

Keep informed about new knowledge regarding exercise and health. The present understanding of how exercise influences health is far from complete but growing at a rapid pace. Joining the American College of Sports Medicine, subscribing to exercise-related journals (such as *Pediatric Exercise Science* or *The Physician and Sportsmedicine*), and attending workshops and symposia are good ways to keep current.

Make exercise just a part of the promotion of wellness. Physical activity should not be isolated as a panacea to good health. Exercise is but one ingredient of a positive lifestyle that includes the prevention of obesity, proper diet, and avoidance of smoking and drug abuse. As "lifestyle counselors," physicians have the opportunity to promote in children behavior that will pay lifelong dividends of good health.

SUMMARY

Improving exercise habits is a difficult task once "exercise deficiency" is long-standing. This chapter provided some strategies for physicians to use to help the sedentary patient become more active.

- The chronically sedentary child will not quickly abandon his or her usual lifestyle for what is viewed as an uncomfortable, odius activity.
- Most sedentary children have been given no encouragement or guidance in how to become more physically active, and the positive support offered by the physician may be critical for interrupting the hypoactivity–low fitness–hypoactivity cycle.
- The key to success lies in preventing the child from getting into that situation to start with: Beginning exercise-promotion interventions early in life, making the entire family part of the treatment plan, providing incentives and strong support, and creating a multifactorial approach that includes diet, behavior modification, and alterations in daily exercise patterns.

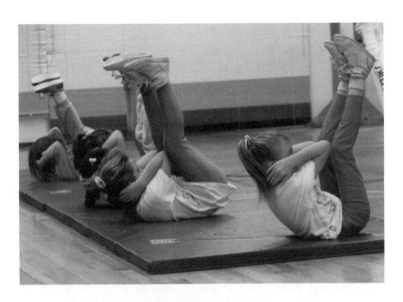

CHAPTER 13

Exercise Activities for Children

As noted previously, structured exercise training programs are not likely to be attractive to most sedentary children and adolescents. Yet certain youngsters and their friends or families wish to participate in sport activities that call for a designed schedule of exercise workouts. These patients often approach their physicians for guidance in prudent training regimens. This chapter is designed to help practitioners offer this advice.

The chapter begins with a section on warming up and cooling down, an important start and finish to all the forms of exercise in the sections that follow. The remainder of the chapter provides an overview of different exercise activities, and is appended with special sections, designed specifically for the child, that the physician can use as handouts.

WARMING UP AND COOLING DOWN

Warming up is generally considered important before all forms of exercise, although there is little scientific documentation that preliminary calisthenics and stretching actually improve performance or prevent injuries. Warming up increases blood flow to muscles, raising their temperature and improving oxygen delivery at the onset of exercise (Inbar and Bar-Or, 1975). The muscles become more compliant with warm-up, and speed of contraction and force-generating capacity may be improved. Myocardial ischemia at the start of exercise may be averted by preliminary increases in coronary blood flow (although this may not be relevant for children). Injuries may be prevented by gradually increasing stresses on the musculoskeletal system during warming up, particularly in sudden, high-burst activities such as sprinting.

Warming up consists of these three phases:

1. Mild activities increase blood supply to the muscle and raise core temperature. This is best accomplished by a short period of walking, slow running, or gentle calisthenics such as swinging arms, body twists, or jumping jacks.
2. Follow this with a brief series of stretching exercises designed to improve the pliability of major muscle groups.
3. Finally, the specific exercise about to be performed should be conducted slowly or with low intensity.

At the end of the exercise session the warm-up should be repeated in reverse order to cool down. The guidelines on pages 284-287 in the appendix can be duplicated and provided to children involved in any exercise program.

STRENGTH TRAINING

As reviewed in chapter 5, a growing number of studies support the importance of resistance training both for prepubertal athletes and as a component of overall fitness programs for children. These reports indicate that strength gains from weight training can be achieved in both boys and girls before puberty, safely and without loss of body flexibility.

Improvements in strength may enhance athletic performance, reduce risk of injury, speed rehabilitation if injuries occur, relieve emotional stress, and help prevent long-term musculoskeletal disease such as back strain and osteoporosis.

In the best of situations, the prepubertal or adolescent athlete has access to formal weight-training facilities with a wide variety of equipment and expert supervision as provided by schools or community organizations such as the YMCA. In these settings weight training can be conducted according to guidelines for children set forth by the National Strength and Conditioning Association (1985) and several authors (American Academy of Pediatrics, 1983b; Fleck & Kraemer, 1987; Leard, 1984). These include the recommendation that children should not weight train without proper supervision or "spotting" and that coaching should emphasize proper technique and form. Examples of specific resistance exercises for children in these supervised programs have been outlined (Fleck & Kraemer, 1987; Rooks & Micheli, 1988).

However, these programs are not available to many children who wish to begin weight training. Suppose a 10-year-old boy has received a set of barbells from his grandparents as a birthday gift and is determined to "pump iron" to improve his physical appearance, and that a prepubertal girl who is trying out for a recreational soccer team wants to lift weights to increase her strength and muscle endurance. Their parents, wary about the advisability of children "lifting weights," seek advice from their physician: Is it safe to weight train at home? If so, what training regimen should be used?

Strength training can be performed by children safely in the home setting provided the child adheres to certain guidelines, which can be overseen by parents. These recommendations are set forth on pages 288-292 in the appendix in a form that can be duplicated and supplied to the prospective weight-training patient. Parents should become familiar with this program to ensure compliance by the child. Included are strength exercises that involve either no weights or use of weights that do not pose a serious risk even for the unsupervised child. In most cases this means that weights are not lifted above or over the head or trunk. Still, the child should be made conscious of the fact that lifting weights is serious business, in which proper technique is important and "horseplay" may increase risk of injury.

Central to all recommendations is the principle that children should lift weights with a high number of repetitions (minimum 7 to 10). No maximal lifts (powerlifting, weight lifting) should be attempted during training or competition until approximately 16 years of age (depending on pubertal development). Children should not compete with each other; specifically, "seeing who can lift the heaviest weight" is forbidden.

WALKING

Walking is an activity particularly well suited to young children or older youngsters with little previous physical activity, and it has many positive features for subjects of all ages. Walking is a lifetime activity, one that can be performed by most everybody over the age of 1 year without special skill or training. Being less intense than sports such as running and cycling, walking can be enjoyed without the risks and discomfort of musculoskeletal stress. This is particularly important for keeping the previously sedentary subject motivated to continue exercising. A couple of bad side-stitches and blisters from running will rapidly make exercise a turnoff for these children.

Another attractive aspect of walking is that during this activity one can socialize, refresh oneself mentally, and get in touch with the environment. Walking can therefore provide pleasures that reinforce regular exercise habits. Insufficient skill, failure as an "athlete," and discomfort from exercise—all strong negative factors—are avoided.

Sweetgall and Neeves have written extensively on walking programs for children and the promotion of walking in school curricula. In their book *Walking for Little Children* (1987) they describe their philosophy of programs for young walkers:

> Competition . . . is great for those kids who make the starting team, but what about the other 99% who become sideline spectators and TV-loving lounge lizards? Walking de-emphasizes competition. Walking lets everyone win. Today we are so busy testing kids for fitness and ranking them on how fast they can run a mile. These tests are painful and distasteful to many children. They teach youngsters to dislike exercise. By failing physical fitness tests, our kids are losing self-esteem. Walking gives every child a sense of accomplishment. (p. 2)

Family walks can, of course, begin when children are very young. Walking programs for children should start simply, and trips to stores, zoos, museums, and farms can serve to increase the pleasure of this activity. Hikes in parks and nature preserves are particularly enjoyable. Here is a chance for parents to stay in communication with their children and an opportunity for youngsters to foster relationships with other children as they walk. Walking becomes an activity not just for improving physical fitness but for stimulating social, emotional, and intellectual growth. Few other forms of exercise can offer these advantages.

As discussed in chapter 7, walking is an excellent adjunct to a weight loss program for obese children. Dietary restriction needs to be included, because weight loss by walking is slow. At a moderate walking pace a 50-kg child burns about 30 to 35 cal every 10 min, or 70 cal/mi (Bar-Or,

1983). Walking 30 min a day (1-1/2 mi), 5 days a week, adds up to a yearly caloric expenditure equivalent of just over 7 lb.

Children's cardiovascular responses to walking training have not been well studied. Sedentary and obese children may show benefit, but active, slender youngsters are unlikely to demonstrate increases in $\dot{V}O_2$max after walking training (Rowland, 1989). This is a reflection of subtarget heart rates, which are usually not greater than 150 bpm, during walking at this age. Long-term cardiovascular benefits may be eventually achieved by these children if they carry regular walking habits into adulthood (Porcari et al., 1987). The guidelines on pages 293-294 in the appendix can be duplicated and given to children who want to begin a walking program.

RUNNING

Running offers several advantages as a way for those of all ages to enjoy regular exercise and improve physical fitness. This is an inexpensive sport that is safe, requires no special skill, and does not require transportation to an exercise facility (translated, no car pooling). It can be practiced at any age, with or without company. Progress can be easily measured, and one can be as competitive as one desires (Lorin, 1978). In terms of caloric expenditure condensed into a short time, running ranks high. A 35-kg child expends 60 cal every 10 min running at 5 mph (a comfortable jog) but only 23 cal during a slow walk over the same period of time (Bar-Or, 1983). This is a very aerobic sport that is useful for building endurance; as a lifetime activity running therefore is particularly valuable for its preventive health effects of controlling weight and maintaining cardiovascular fitness.

All young children like to run, but before the preteen years most do not have the discipline, attention span, and motivation required for formal running training. During these years, jogging along with parents or older siblings as the latter begin or end a running session may be enough to stimulate interest in more regular running later on. In older childhood running at least 1/2 hr for a minimum of three times a week is an appropriate goal. Many children, particularly those who have previously been sedentary, will need to start slowly and progress gradually to this level of exercise. The training regimen outlined on pages 295-296 in the appendix can be adapted for individual prescription, depending on initial fitness and speed of progress. An even more gradual schedule for entering a running program has been provided by Strong and Alpert (1982). This was devised for children who have recently had cardiac surgery but would also be useful for subjects who have particularly low physical capacities.

Children and young adolescents who wish to train and run competitively deserve special attention. They are best referred to an individual who has expertise in proper training regimens and injury prevention (probably a high school or college cross-country coach). Treacy and Cunningham (1986) have outlined training schedules for high school cross-country runners that can be adapted for younger competitors.

SWIMMING

The National Children and Youth Fitness Study II, which evaluated exercise factors in 4,678 6- to 9-year-old children, found that swimming ranked first for both boys and girls as the physical activity most frequently performed in community organizations (Ross & Pate, 1987). This sport is popular at all ages and provides excellent cardiovascular conditioning without many of the musculoskeletal stresses experienced in weight-bearing activities. Swimming is therefore a particularly suitable form of exercise for obese children, and the high heat and humidity in many swimming settings make this sport a good choice for those with asthma. On the negative side, swimming with sufficent intensity to improve fitness or expend calories requires a certain amount of skill, and lack of easy accessibility to swimming facilities may be another barrier to participation.

Encouraging children to become comfortable in the water from an early age is important from a safety standpoint and as a starting point for a lifetime of aquatic activity. The physician can most effectively introduce swimming to an older child as a means of increasing physical activity by referral to a structured, supervised school or community program. This setting is more likely to produce health-related benefits, because learning proper stroke techniques is particularly important for enhancing performance and enjoyment, and expenditure of calories requires disciplined, repetitive laps, which may not be as dutifully performed in non-supervised surroundings. "Playing around" in the water is fun but does little to improve health. Effective fitness training, on the other hand, probably requires at least 30 min of steady swimming several times per week. The crawl stroke is the most calorically demanding, followed by the breast and back strokes (Bar-Or, 1983).

For children who wish to swim independently, Maglischo (1982) offered daily training guidelines for beginners. These guidelines are found on page 297 in the appendix and can be duplicated and given to patients.

BICYCLING

Riding a bicycle is a favorite activity of children, and even the sedentary, TV-addicted youngster will claim to getting on a bike once in a while. Children say they like to cycle because it is not as boring as walking or as arduous as running (although neither is necessarily true). Bicycling can be exhilarating, and, with the efficiency of modern-day 10-speed bikes, can be performed without a great deal of effort. Recommending cycling as a means of getting sedentary children into regular exercise habits is therefore a good way to start. Hopefully, the child will get "hooked" by the fun of cycling to either persist in more intense cycling or extend sport participation to other activities.

It is difficult to create specific guidelines for cycle exercise, because bicycle riding can range from a very leisurely to a very physically demanding sport, depending on terrain, weather, gear selection, and pedaling frequency. A child cycling slowly at 6 mph expends one third the calories of a subject jogging comfortably at 5 mph. A 35-kg child burns up about 200 cal/hr when cycling at 10 mph (Bar-Or, 1983). Starting out at 20 to 30 min per day, three or four times per week, would be reasonable for most children, aiming at a goal of 1-hr sessions. Youngsters who wish to become more involved in cycle training can contact local cycling clubs for more guidance.

Once some cycling endurance is gained, opportunities abound. Cross-country touring trips, competitive racing, family expeditions, and off-road cycling offer variety and enjoyment that can reinforce the value of regular cycling exercise. For some children the joys of learning how to repair and maintain their bicycles is an added incentive.

Safety, of course, is a particularly important concern with cycling. Any child who takes to the roads on a bicycle should be well informed, through instruction or reading, on cycling safety and etiquette. Helmets are mandatory. Several excellent books are available (Allen, 1981; Howard, 1984).

The guidelines on pages 298-299 in the appendix are geared to the preteenager or early adolescent who has limited previous cycling experience. They can be duplicated and given to interested patients.

SUMMARY

The material in this chapter provides a starting point for helping youngsters become involved in specific activities.

- Children (and their parents) who are interested in specific sports activities are often eager for direction from physicians regarding safe training regimens.
- The particularly talented child athlete can be referred to a high school or college coach for further guidance in proper training schedules.
- Physician supervision is equally important for these children as they face the physical and psychological stresses of intensive training and competition.

APPENDIX
Patient Guidelines
for Specific Activities

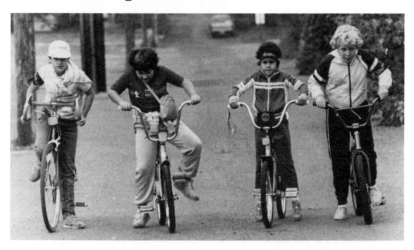

- Getting Ready for Exercise
- Tips for Getting Stronger Safely
- Walking: Getting in Shape the Easy Way
- A Running Schedule for Children: Getting Started
- Getting Fit by Swimming
- Getting Started Cycling

GETTING READY FOR EXERCISE

You should warm up before and after each time you exercise. Warming up gets your body ready for physical activity. Muscles become more flexible, and that helps prevent injury. The heart rate and blood flow to the muscles increase, too. That means that when you warm up, more energy is immediately available when the exercise starts. Exercise can actually make some muscles stiffer, and that's one reason why it's important to "cool down" after exercise with the same exercises you used to warm up. Both warming up and cooling down should take you about 10 minutes.

Begin your warm-up with some gentle exercises to get the blood going to your muscles. Walking or slow running for 1 to 3 minutes is best, or do some mild calisthenics such as swinging your arms, body twists, or jumping jacks. Then you are ready for stretching exercises, which are designed to loosen up all the major muscles. Some of these are described below. When you do these exercises it's important to hold the position for 10 to 15 seconds without "bouncing." Do each stretch at least twice. After you finish the stretches, do the exercise you are about to perform at a slower rate (runners jog, rowers take a moderate cadence, swimmers stroke leisurely). When you cool down after the exercise, do the warmups in reverse order.

Stretching Exercises

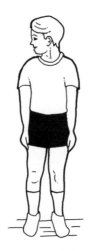

Neck Flexibility. Lower your chin slowly toward your chest, then raise it until you are looking at the ceiling. Turn your head slowly to the left, until you are looking over your left shoulder, then repeat on the right. Each stretch should be held for 15 seconds.

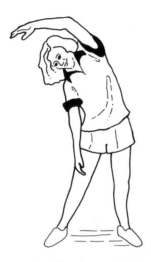

Side Stretch. Stand straight with your legs spread apart and slightly bent. Stretch one arm up as high as it will go while bending your body at the waist to the opposite side. Hold for 15 seconds, and repeat with the other side.

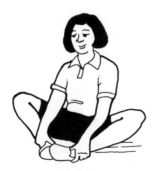

Groin Muscles. Sit on the floor with your legs bent and the soles of your feet together. Lower your knees toward the floor (using your arms) until the muscles on the inside of your legs become tense. Hold for 15 seconds.

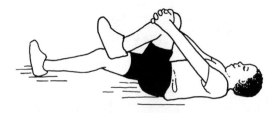

Hip Flexors. While lying on the floor on your back, pull one leg up tight to the chest, using your arms, while the other leg stays straight. Hold for 15 seconds, and then use the other leg.

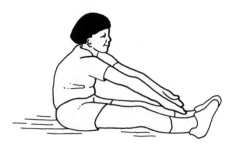

Hamstrings. Sit on the floor. With your legs straight, bend forward and extend your arms down to touch your toes. Hold for 15 seconds.

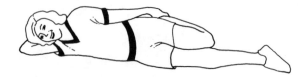

Quadriceps. Lie on your left side. Grab your right foot with your right hand and pull back until the thigh muscles are tight. Hold for 15 seconds. Then lie on your right side and repeat with the other leg.

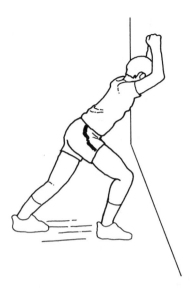

Wall Calf and Achilles Stretch.   Hold yourself against a wall or post with outstretched arms and your feet together. Slide one foot backward about two feet, keeping both heels flat on the floor or ground. Bend the forward leg and lean forward until stretch is felt in the calf of the back leg, which should be kept straight. Hold for 15 seconds, and then repeat with the other leg. Now repeat this stretch with *both* legs straight.

TIPS FOR GETTING STRONGER SAFELY

If you regularly perform the exercises described here you will increase the strength of your muscles. This should allow you to perform better in sports, particularly in those that require strength (such as football or wrestling), and will help prevent your being injured. Remember that strength will only improve in those muscles that are exercised. That's why it's important to perform exercises that stress all the major muscle groups of the arms, trunk, and legs. You should also realize that although boys and girls of all ages can benefit from these exercises, increasing muscle *size* is likely only if you are over 13 or 14 years old.

Exercises should be performed three times a week, always with a day of rest in between. Each session should begin with a 5- to 10-minute warm-up of stretches and calisthenics. This increases the blood flow to the muscles and helps reduce the chance of muscle strain. And at the end, repeat these exercises to "cool down" for a similar period of time.

Muscle strength is gained by repeatedly working the muscle through the use of weights or exercises. As you progress, you will gain in strength, and the amount of weight you can lift or exercise you can perform will increase. To begin, use very light weights (or few exercises) until the form and proper technique are learned. Then experiment to find the weight that you can just lift for 10 times, or repetitions ("reps"). This is the weight you should use until you become strong enough that it can be lifted 15 times. When this happens, increase the amount of weight so that, again, you can only lift it 10 times (this will probably be an increase of 2-1/2 to 5 pounds). Keep repeating this change in weight as strength increases.

Performing a lift through 10 to 15 reps is called a *set*. Do one set for each of the exercises listed below, then repeat the entire series two more times during each training session. Lift the weights and perform the exercises smoothly, under control, and in a steady manner while avoiding jerking motions. Move the weights through the entire range of motion of the joint involved. Work hard, but do not strain, keeping proper form at all times. It is important not to hold your breath during strength training, because this puts stress on your heart. Many lifters pattern their breathing during exercise, breathing out as the weight is lifted and back in when it is returned to the starting position.

Do not lift any weight that you cannot lift at least 10 times. Maximum lifts (a single lift to see how much you can raise) are dangerous and should not be performed. Do not lift weights above your head or body (e.g., bench press or military press). These types of lifts are only safe when a trained "spotter" is in attendance.

You may experience mild muscle soreness on the day after your training session. This is to be expected and is a signal that the muscles have worked hard. The soreness should disappear in a day or two. Training can continue if the discomfort is mild. Otherwise, postpone training for a short period until the pain is gone, and then begin again with a slightly decreased exercise frequency or weight load.

Make a chart to keep track of your progress. Good luck!

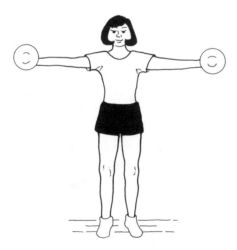

Lateral Raises (Shoulder and Back). Hold a dumbbell in each hand, with the palms facing in toward your body. Keeping your arms straight, raise the weights up until they are as high as your shoulders, then slowly lower.

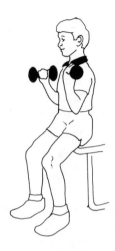

Arms Curls (Biceps). Sit on a bench or chair with a dumbbell in one or both hands. Keeping your back straight, bend your arm and bring the weight up as far as it will go. Then return it to the starting position.

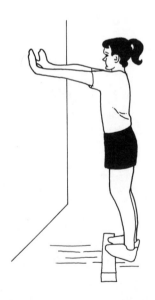

Heel Raises (Calf Muscles). Place a piece of wood (such as a 2-by-4) on the floor, and place the forward parts of your feet on it to raise the toes above the heels. Hold on to a wall or other support if necessary to keep your balance. Raise your heels up as far as possible, hold for 1 to 2 seconds, and then lower them to the starting position. If you can do 15 of these, make it harder by holding a dumbbell in your hands.

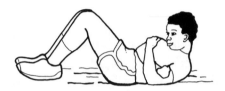

Bent-Knee Sit-Ups (Abdominal Muscles). Lie on your back with your knees bent and feet on the floor. Cross your hands over your chest, and curl up about half way, until you feel your abdominal ("stomach") muscles tighten. Hold for 1 to 3 seconds, and then slowly return to the starting position. This exercise can be made more difficult by holding the arms to the front of your chest with a weight.

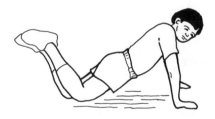

Push-Ups (Shoulder and Upper Arm). Do these sometimes with your hands at shoulder width (straight down) and other times with them out a bit wider (this exercises different muscles). If you can't do more than a few push-ups, start by performing them with your knees touching the ground.

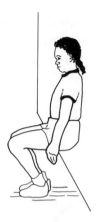

Wall Sits (Thigh).   Stand about 6 inches away from a wall, facing away, and place your back on it. Slowly slide down until your thighs are parallel to the floor. Hold for 3 seconds, then slowly slide back up.

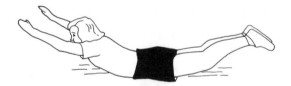

Superhero Exercise (Back Muscles).   Lie on your stomach with your arms extended forward. Raise your outstretched arms, shoulders, hips, and legs off the floor as far as they will go. Hold this position for 10 seconds.

WALKING: GETTING IN SHAPE THE EASY WAY

You will like walking. This is an exercise that improves your body's fitness at the same time as you enjoy the outdoors, the company of others, and interesting sights along the way. Walking is good for your muscles, bones, and heart, and it will help you control your weight. It will make you feel better about yourself, too. Best of all, walking is a sport that can provide these benefits without leaving you uncomfortable from exhaustion. This activity gives you "gains without pain."

Most anyone can walk, but how far, where, and how often are important considerations. Some experts think that you should try to walk (weather permitting) every day, 7 days a week. Others recommend three or four times a week. Do whichever is most comfortable for you. The idea is that it is important to make walking a regular habit, just like brushing your teeth or eating dinner. Make a schedule and stick to it. Even if you "don't feel like it," go out for at least 5 or 10 minutes. You may find that starting out walking actually makes you feel better with *more* energy. Walking isn't like running and other high-intensity sports that require days of rest to prevent injury.

Start gradually, trying to work up to a mile a day. If you walk rapidly you will be going about 3-1/2 to 4 miles per hour, but if you go slower your pace will be 2-1/2 to 3 miles per hour. So your initial target is to walk at a medium speed for about 15 to 20 minutes. If this is too much to start, begin walking 10 minutes every other day and then increase distance and time as you feel stronger. Walk continuously, without stopping. With increasing experience you will be able to walk farther. A good long-range goal is 15 to 25 miles per week. Keep a chart to mark your progress, making a few notes about how you felt, the weather, or what you saw.

Walking is much more fun when you do it with someone else. It's a good chance to get "caught up" with friends or enjoy the company of your family. Walking interesting places makes it exciting, too. Try walking at a zoo, around a shopping mall, or at a farm. Hikes in parks are a natural. Or pick some destination (bank, movie, post office). Do different kinds of walks—fast, slow, flat, with hills, in the city, in the country. If one day's walk leaves you tired, do just a short one the next day. The amount of walking can be flexible, but stick to your regular schedule.

Proper walking technique is important. Stand straight up, without slouching. Relax your shoulders and let your arms swing back and forth. This helps give you momentum and keeps your walking rhythm. Walk heel-to-toe, landing first on your heel and then pushing off with your toes. If you land on your toes first it hurts your back and feet—not to mention your shoes! You will walk most efficiently if you walk with your body as straight as possible.

Before you start, it's important to get your muscles warmed up. Begin by walking slowly for a short distance, then stop and do some stretching exercises. This loosens up the muscles and gets the heart and lungs ready for more vigorous exercise. Repeat these exercises at the end of your daily walk to "cool down."

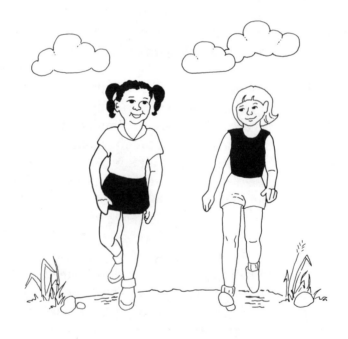

From *Exercise and Children's Health* by T.W. Rowland, 1990, Champaign, IL: Human Kinetics. Copyright 1990 by Thomas W. Rowland.

A RUNNING SCHEDULE FOR CHILDREN: GETTING STARTED

The running schedule described in the table that follows is designed so that you can gradually increase distance and time over a 6-month period. It isn't important, though, that you move through the stages in the time period described. Instead, progress only as rapidly as feels comfortable for you. The idea is to start slowly and gradually, putting an emphasis on the distance you can run rather than how fast you can do it. Keep a chart at home to record your progress.

The first stage is devoted to sessions of alternating run and walk. Stage 2 increases running distance. Completing stages 3 through 6 requires increasing speed and distance.

Running on a track is a good way to measure distance, because each lap is usually 1/4 mile. For variety, though, it is often more fun to run on sidewalks or fields (such as around a golf course). Have your parents measure off distances of 1/8, 1/4, 1/2, and 1 mile using their automobile odometer, if they have a car. Do not run in the street. Timed distances (stages 3 through 6) might be best done at the track with a parent using a stopwatch.

Spend 5 minutes before each session warming up with stretching exercises, and at the completion of your run, walk briefly and repeat the stretches to "cool down." Avoid running in very hot or humid weather, and on warm days try to run early in the morning. Don't forget to drink plenty of water, too.

Well-constructed "sneakers" are fine to use as you get started in your running program. As you get more involved with longer periods of running, it would be a good idea to buy a good pair of running shoes. These provide well-padded soles, flexibility, and a stable heel, and they are lightweight. Several brands are available in children's sizes.

Some leg-muscle soreness is expected following running, particularly early in the program. With a day's rest between sessions this should disappear without problems. If you have persistent or severe pain, particularly in your joints, you should be more concerned, and you should consult your doctor.

A Running Program for Children

Stage	Week	Monday	Wednesday	Friday	Week total
I	1	Run 1/8 mile Walk 1/8 mile Run 1/8 mile Walk 1/8 mile	Same	Same	1-1/2
	2	Run 1/4 mile Walk 1/4 mile Run 1/4 mile Walk 1/4 mile	Same	Same	3
	3	Run 1/2 mile Walk 1/4 mile Run 1/2 mile Walk 1/4 mile	Same	Same	4-1/2
	4	Run 3/4 mile Walk 1/4 mile Run 3/4 mile Walk 1/4 mile	Same	Same	6
II	1	Run 1 mile	Same	Same	3
	2	Run 1-1/2 miles			4-1/2
	3	Run 2 miles			6
	4	Run 2-1/2 miles			7-1/2
III	1-4	Run 3 miles	Same	Run 3 miles under 30 min	9
IV	1-4	Run 3-4 miles	Same	Run 3 miles under 27 min	9-11
V	1-4	Run 3-5 miles	Same	Run 3 miles under 24 min	9-13
VI	1-4	Run 3-5 miles	Same	Run 3 miles under 21 min	9-13

GETTING FIT BY SWIMMING

Swimming is a fun activity and it is good exercise, especially when it is hot outdoors. Swimming strengthens your heart and muscles if you do it regularly.

The best way to start a regular swimming program is to join a community center that has a swimming pool. If you don't know how to swim yet, make sure you learn from a qualified instructor. Most of the time community centers have classes that teach all ability levels. Practice hard so that you can learn proper swimming strokes. Learning the crawl stroke, breast stroke, and back stroke is necessary before you can get the full benefits of a swimming program.

After you know how to swim, you can begin your exercise program. If you swim for 30 minutes three or four times each week, you will be working hard enough to become physically fit. It is fun to just play in the water, but you have to swim steadily if you want to get fit. The crawl stroke will give you the most fitness benefits, followed by the breast stroke, then the back stroke.

If you are swimming in a community center program, your instructor can help you figure out how long and how far you should swim to get the most out of your swimming program. If you are swimming on your own, though, the following guidelines will help you know how far to swim each time you work out.

Suggested Beginning Distances for Physical Fitness Through Swimming

Age (years)	Distance (yards)
Under 8	400
8 to 10	600 to 1200
11 to 12	1000 to 2000
13 to 14	2000 to 4000

From *Swimming Faster* by E.W. Maglischo, 1982. Mountain View, CA: Mayfield.

As your skill and endurance increase, increase the suggested distances by two or three times.

From *Exercise and Children's Health* by T.W. Rowland, 1990, Champaign, IL: Human Kinetics. Copyright 1990 by Thomas W. Rowland.

GETTING STARTED CYCLING

If you know how to ride a bike, getting into cycling is easy. If you don't, get someone to teach you! Biking does good things for your muscles, heart, and lungs while it helps burn off extra body fat. To do this, however, you need to bike *regularly*, and you need to cycle over a sustained period of time without stopping (more on this later). BMX, or "dirt bikes," are great fun, but stunts on this equipment don't help your health very much. For distance cycling you will find a standard 1-speed, 3-speed, or 10-speed bike more appropriate.

Before you start cycling there are 3 things you must do:

1. First, make sure your bike is working properly. Have it checked at a local bike shop if you have any questions.
2. You must next become acquainted with the rules of the road. When you are cycling on streets, you are competing with some pretty dangerous traffic. You need to know how to avoid accidents and keep you and your bike safe. There may be a short course in bicycle safety you can take in your town, or get a cycling book from the library or bookstore.
3. Finally, buy a helmet, and always wear it when you ride.

Begin your cycling program gradually. Bike slowly for 15 to 20 minutes on easy rides every other day for a few weeks. Cycle with a constant, even cadence. Don't start out too fast; if you don't pace yourself you will become exhausted halfway through your ride. You will find that your endurance will improve quickly, and as you get stronger you will be able to cycle longer. Aim eventually to get up to 45 to 60 minutes, four times a week. Then you can try different kinds of rides—some hard, up hills, others easy and short. Try to avoid heavy traffic routes and busy times of day as much as possible. Keep a chart to follow your progress.

Before and after each cycling session be sure that you warm up and cool down with calisthenics and stretches. Then when you start cycling, pedal with a slow cadence for 5 to 10 minutes to get your legs limbered up.

Dress appropriately. Remember that in cooler weather you will feel even colder when you are riding because of the wind factor. On long rides drink plenty of water, particularly on warm, humid days.

Learn how to take care of your bike. You will find your riding is more enjoyable if the equipment is in top shape and if you know how to make repairs (such as fixing a flat tire).

If you feel you want to do more with cycling, such as training for competition, the best route is through the guidance of a local cycling club. Get more information from a cycling shop.

Have fun!

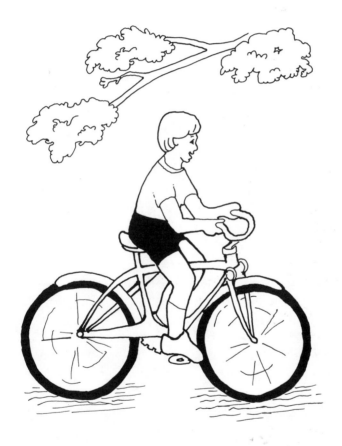

References

Abraham, S., & Nordsieck, M. (1960). Relationship of excess weight in children and adults. *Public Health Reports, 75,* 263-273.

Adams, J.E. (1976). The Little League survey. *The American Journal of Sports Medicine, 4,* 207-209.

Adams, W.C. (1967). Influence of age, sex, and body weight on energy expenditures of bicycle riding. *Journal of Applied Physiology, 22,* 539-545.

Allen, J.S. (1981). *The complete book of bicycle commuting.* Emmaus, PA: Rodale Press.

Allison, M.T. (1982). Sportsmanship: Variations based on sex and degree of competitive experience. In A.O. Dunleavy, A.W. Miracle, & C.R. Rees (Eds.), *Studies in the sociology of sport* (pp. 153-165). Fort Worth, TX: Texas Christian University Press.

Allon, N. (1980). Sociological aspects of overweight youth. In P.J. Collipp (Ed.), *Childhood obesity.* (3rd ed., pp. 139-156). Littleton, MA: PSG Publishing.

Alpert, B.S., Bloom, K.R., Gilday, D., & Olley, P.M. (1979). The comparison between non-invasive and invasive methods of stroke volume determination in children. *American Heart Journal, 98,* 763-766.

American Academy of Pediatrics (1976). Fitness in the preschool child. *Pediatrics, 58,* 88-89.

American Academy of Pediatrics (1982). Risks of long-distance running for children. *The Physician and Sportsmedicine, 10,* 82-86.

American Academy of Pediatrics (1983a). Sports and the child with epilepsy. *Pediatrics, 72,* 884-885.

American Academy of Pediatrics (1983b). Weight training and weight lifting: Information for the pediatrician. *The Physician and Sportsmedicine, 11,* 157-161.

American Academy of Pediatrics (1987). Physical fitness and the schools. *Pediatrics, 80,* 449-450.

American Alliance for Health, Physical Education, Recreation and Dance (1980). *Youth fitness test manual.* Washington, DC: Author.

American College of Sports Medicine (1978). Position statement on the recommended quantity and quality of exercise for developing and maintaining fitness in healthy adults. *Medicine and Science in Sports and Exercise, 10,* vii-x.

Anand, B.K. (1961). Nervous regulation of food intake. *Physiologic Reviews, 41,* 677-708.

Andersen, K.L., Seliger, V., Rutenfranz, J., & Messel, S. (1974). Physical performance capacity of children in Norway. *European Journal of Applied Physiology*, **33**, 265-274.

Anderson, B. (1980). Activity and diabetic vitreous hemorrhages. *Ophthalmology*, **87**, 173-175.

Anderson, S.D., & Godfrey, S. (1971). Cardiorespiratory response to treadmill exercise in normal children. *Clinical Science*, **40**, 433-442.

Anderson, S.D., Silverman, M., Konig, P. & Godfrey, S. (1975). Exercise-induced asthma. *British Journal of Diseases of the Chest*, **69**, 1-39.

Andreasson, B., Jonson, B., Kornfaldt, R., Nordmark, E., & Sandstrom, S. (1987). Long-term effects of physical exercise on working capacity and pulmonary function in cystic fibrosis. *Acta Paediatrica Scandinavica*, **76**, 70-75.

Aristimuno, G.G., Foster, T.A., Voors, A.W., Srinivasan, S.R., & Berenson, G.S. (1984). Influence of persistent obesity in children on cardiovascular risk factors: The Bogalusa Heart Study. *Circulation*, **69**, 895-904.

Arnold, P.J. (1986). Moral aspects of an education in movement. In G.A. Stull & H.M. Eckert (Eds.), *Effects of physical activity on children* (pp. 14-21). Champaign, IL: Human Kinetics.

Asano, K., & Hirakoba, K. (1984). Respiratory and circulatory adaptation during prolonged exercise in 10-12 year old children and adults. In J. Ilmarinen & I. Valimaki (Eds.), *Children and sport* (pp. 119-128). Berlin: Springer.

Ashton, N.J. (1983). Relationship of chronic physical activity levels to physiologic and anthropometric variables in 9-10 year old girls (abstract). *Medicine and Science in Sports and Exercise*, **15**, 143.

Asmussen, E., & Heeboll-Nielsen, K. (1955). Physical performance and growth in children. Influence of sex, age, and intelligence. *Journal of Applied Physiology*, **8**, 371-380.

Åstrand, I. (1960). Aerobic work capacity in men and women with special reference to age. *Acta Physiologica Scandinavica*, **49**(Suppl. 169), 1-57.

Åstrand, P.O. (1952). *Experimental studies of physical working capacity in relationship to sex and age.* Copenhagen: Munksgaard.

Åstrand, P.O., Engstrom, I., Eriksson, B.O., Karlberg, P., Nylander, I., Saltin, B., & Thoren, C. (1963). Girl swimmers, with special reference to respiratory and circulatory adaptation and gynaecological and psychiatric aspects. *Acta Paediatrica Scandinavica*, **147**(Suppl.), 1-75.

Åstrand, P.O., & Rodahl, K. (1977). *Textbook of work physiology. Physiologic basis of exercise* (2nd ed.). New York: McGraw-Hill.

Åstrand, P.O., & Rodahl, K. (1986). *Textbook of work physiology. Physiologic basis of exercise* (3rd ed.). New York: McGraw-Hill.

Atomi, Y., Iwaoka, K., Hatta, H., Miyashita, M., & Yamamoto, Y. (1986). Daily physical activity levels in preadolescent boys related to $\dot{V}O_2$max and lactate threshold. *European Journal of Applied Physiology*, **55**, 156-161.

Atomi, Y., Kuroda, Y., Asami, T., & Kawahara, T. (1986). HDL$_2$-cholesterol of children (10 to 12 years of age) related to $\dot{V}O_2$max, body fat, and sex. In J. Rutenfranz, R. Mocellin, & F. Klimt (Eds.), *Children and exercise XII* (pp. 167-172). Champaign, IL: Human Kinetics.

Backous, D.D., Friedl, K.E., Smith, N.J., Parr, T.J., & Carpine, W.D. (1988). Soccer injuries and their relation to physical maturity. *American Journal of Diseases of Children*, **142**, 839-842.

Baevre, H., Sovik, O., Wisnes, A., & Heiervang, E. (1985). Metabolic responses to physical training in young insulin-dependent diabetics. *Scandinavian Journal of Clinical Laboratory Investigation*, **45**, 109-114.

Bailey, D.A. (1973). Exercise, fitness, and physical education for the growing child—a concern. *Canadian Journal of Public Health*, **64**, 421-430.

Bailey, D.A., Malina, R.M., & Rasmussen, R.L. (1978). The influence of exercise, physical activity, and athletic performance on the dynamics of human growth. In F. Falkner & J.M. Tanner (Eds.), *Human growth* (pp. 475-505). New York: Plenum Press.

Bailey, D.A., Ross, W.D., Mirwald, R.L., & Weese, D. (1978). Size dissociation of maximal aerobic power during growth in boys. *Medicine and Sport*, **11**, 140-151.

Baker, E.R. (1981). Menstrual dysfunction and hormonal status in athletic women: A review. *Fertility and Sterility*, **36**, 691-696.

Balfour, I., Drimmer, A., & Nouri, S. (1986). Pediatric cardiac rehabilitation: Exercise training and prescription. *Journal of the Medical Association of Georgia*, **5**, 676-678.

Bar-Or, O. (1980). Climate and the exercising child—a review. *International Journal of Sports Medicine*, **1**, 53-65.

Bar-Or, O. (1983). *Pediatric sports medicine for the practitioner. From physiologic principles to clinical applications*. New York: Springer.

Bar-Or, O. (1984a). Children and physical performance in warm and cold environments. In R.A. Boileau (Ed.), *Advances in pediatric sport sciences* (pp. 117-129). Champaign, IL: Human Kinetics.

Bar-Or, O. (1984b). The growth and development of children's physiologic and perceptional responses to exercise. In J. Ilmarinen & I. Valimaki (Eds.), *Children and sport* (pp. 3-17). Berlin: Springer.

Bar-Or, O. (1986). Pathophysiological factors which limit the exercise capacity of the sick child. *Medicine and Science in Sports and Exercise*, **18**, 276-282.

Barron, B.L., Noakes, T.D., Levy, W., Smith, C., & Millar, R.P. (1985). Hypothalamic dysfunction in overtrained athletes. *Journal of Endocrinology and Metabolism*, **60**, 803-806.

Baum, V.C., Levitsky, L.L., & Englander, R.M. (1987). Abnormal cardiac function after exercise in insulin-dependent diabetic children and adolescents. *Diabetes Care*, **10**, 319-323.

Becker, D.M., & Vaccaro, P. (1983). Anaerobic threshold alterations caused by endurance training in young children. *Journal of Sports Medicine*, **23**, 445-449.

Becque, M.D., Katch, V.L., Rocchini, A.P., Marks, C.R., & Moorehead, C. (1988). Coronary risk incidence of obese adolescents: Reduction by exercise plus diet intervention. *Pediatrics*, **81**, 605-612.

Bell, R.D., MacDougall, J.D., Billeter, R., & Howald, H. (1980). Muscle fiber types and morphometric analysis of skeletal muscle in six-year-old children. *Medicine and Science in Sports and Exercise*, **12**, 28-31.

Ben-Dov, I., Bar-Yishay, E., & Godfrey, S. (1982). Refractory period after exercise-induced asthma, unexplained by respiratory heat loss. *American Review of Respiratory Diseases*, **125**, 530-534.

Bennett, P.H. (1981). Diabetes and heart disease—the magnitude of the problem. In R.C. Scott (Ed.), *Clinical cardiology and diabetes* (Vol. I, pp. 3-12). Mount Kisco, NY: Futura.

Ben Schachar, G., Fuhrman, B.P., Wang, Y., Lucas, R.V., & Lock, J.E. (1982). Rest and exercise hemodynamics after the Fontan procedure. *Circulation*, **65**, 1043-1048.

Bentgsson, E. (1956). The working capacity in normal children, evaluated by submaximal exercise on the bicycle ergometer and compared with adults. *Acta Medica Scandinavica*, **154**, 91-109.

Berenson, G.S. (1986). Evolution of cardiovascular risk factors in early life: Perspectives on causation. In G.S. Berenson (Ed.), *Causation of cardiovascular risk factors in children* (pp. 1-26). New York: Raven.

Berryman, J.W. (1982). The rise of highly organized sports for preadolescent boys. In R.A. Magill, M.J. Ash, & F.L. Smoll (Eds.), *Children in sport* (pp. 2-15). Champaign, IL: Human Kinetics.

Bevegard, S., Eriksson, B.O., Graff-Lonnevig, V., Kraepelien, S., & Saltin, B. (1976). Respiratory function, cardiovascular dimensions, and work capacity in boys with bronchial asthma. *Acta Paediatrica Scandinavica*, **65**, 289-296.

Bhasin, S.S., Khullar, S.C., & Weissler, A.M. (1980). Value of blood pressure response to exercise in the recognition of latent or early borderline hypertension (abstract). *American Journal of Cardiology*, **45**, 489.

Bierman, C.W., Kawabori, I., & Pierson, W.E. (1975). Incidence of exercise-induced asthma in children. *Pediatrics*, **56** (Suppl.), 847-850.

Biersner, R.J., Gunderson, E.K.E., & Rahe, R.H. (1972). Relationships of sports interests and smoking to physical fitness. *Journal of Sports Medicine and Physical Fitness*, **12**, 124-127.

Björntorp, P. (1978). Physical training in the treatment of obesity. *International Journal of Obesity*, **2**, 149-156.

Blair, S.N. (1985). Physical activity leads to fitness and pays off. *The Physician and Sportsmedicine*, **13**, 153-157.

Blair, S.N., Goodyear, N.N., Gibbons, L.W., & Cooper, K.H. (1984). Physical fitness and incidence of hypertension in healthy normotensive men and women. *Journal of the American Medical Association, 252,* 487-490.

Bombeck, E. (1971). *"Just wait till you have children of your own!"* Garden City, NY: Doubleday.

Bonanno, J.A., & Lies, J.E. (1974). Effects of physical training on coronary risk factors. *American Journal of Cardiology, 33,* 760-764.

Bouchard, C. (1986). Genetics of aerobic power and capacity. In R.M. Malina & C. Bouchard (Eds.), *Sport and human genetics* (pp. 59-88). Champaign, IL: Human Kinetics.

Bradfield, R.B., & Jourdan, M.H. (1973). Relative importance of specific dynamic action in weight reduction diets. *The Lancet, 22,* 640-643.

Bradley, L.M., Galioto, F.M., Vaccaro, P., Hansen, D.A., & Vaccaro, J. (1985). Effect of intense aerobic training on exercise performance in children after surgical repair of tetralogy of Fallot or complete transposition of the great arteries. *American Journal of Cardiology, 56,* 816-818.

Bray, G.A. (1983). The energetics of obesity. *Medicine and Science in Sports and Exercise, 15,* 32-40.

Brisson, G.R., Dulac, S., Peronnet, F., & Ledoux, M. (1982). The onset of menarche: A late event in pubertal progression to be affected by physical training. *Canadian Journal of Applied Sports Science, 7,* 61-67.

Broekhoff, J. (1986). The effect of physical activity on physical growth and development. In G.A. Stull & H.M. Eckert (Eds.), *The effects of physical activity on children* (pp. 75-87). Champaign, IL: Human Kinetics.

Brown, B.J. (1977). The effect of an isometric strength program on the intellectual and social development of trainable retarded males. *American Corrective Therapy Journal, 31,* 44-48.

Brown, E.W., & Kimball, R.G. (1983). Medical history associated with adolescent powerlifting. *Pediatrics, 72,* 636-644.

Brown, J.D., & Lawton, M. (1986). Stress and well-being in adolescence: The moderating role of physical exercise. *Journal of Human Stress, 12,* 125-131.

Brown, M., Klish, W., Hollander, J., Campbell, M., & Forbes, G. (1983). A high protein, low calorie liquid diet in the treatment of very obese adolescents: Long term effects on lean body mass. *American Journal of Clinical Nutrition, 38,* 20-31.

Brown, R.S. (1982). Exercise and mental health in the pediatric population. *Clinics in Sports Medicine, 1,* 515-527.

Brownell, K.D., Bachorik, P.S., & Ayerle, R.S. (1982). Changes in plasma lipid and lipoprotein levels in men and women after a program of moderate exercise. *Circulation, 65,* 477-484.

Brownell, K.D., & Kaye, F.S. (1982). A school-based behavior modification, nutrition education, and physical activity program for obese children. *The American Journal of Clinical Nutrition, 35,* 277-283.

Bruce, R.A., Kusumi, F., & Hosmer, D. (1973). Maximal oxygen intake and nomographic assessment of functional aerobic impairment in cardiovascular disease. *American Heart Journal, 85,* 546-562.

Bryant, J.G., Garett, H.L., & Dean, M.S. (1984). Coronary heart disease. The beneficial effects of exercise to children. *Journal of the Louisiana State Medical Society*, **136**, 15-17.

Bullen, B.A., Reed, R.B., & Mayer, J. (1964). Physical activity of obese and non-obese adolescent girls, appraised by motion picture sampling. *American Journal of Clinical Nutrition*, **14**, 211-223.

Bureau, M.A., Lupien, L., & Begin, R. (1981). Neural drive and ventilatory strategy of breathing in normal children and in patients with cystic fibrosis and asthma. *Pediatrics*, **68**, 187-194.

Burke, E.J. (1975). Validity of selected laboratory and field tests of physical working capacity. *Research Quarterly*, **47**, 95-104.

Burmeister, W. (1966). Body cell mass as the basis of allometric growth function. *Annales Paediatrici*, **204**, 65-72.

Burr, M.L., Eldridge, B.A., & Borysiewicz, L.K. (1974). Peak expiratory flow rates before and after exercise in school children. *Archives of Disease of Childhood*, **49**, 923-926.

Cahill, B.R. (1977). Stress fracture of the proximal tibial epiphysis: A case report. *The American Journal of Sports Medicine*, **5**, 186-187.

Caine, D.J., & Lindner, K.J. (1984). Growth plate injury: A threat to young distance runners? *The Physician and Sportsmedicine*, **12**, 118-124.

Caine, D.J., & Lindner, K.J. (1985). Overuse injuries of growing bones: The young female gymnast at risk? *The Physician and Sportsmedicine*, **13**, 51-62.

Campaigne, B.N., Gilliam, T.B., Spencer, M.L., Lampman, R., & Schork, B. (1984). Effects of a physical activity program on metabolic control and cardiovascular fitness in children with insulin-dependent diabetes mellitus. *Diabetes Care*, **7**, 57-63.

Campaigne, B.N., Landt, K.W., Mellies, M.J., James, F.W., Glueck, C.J., & Sperling, M.A. (1985). The effects of physical training on blood lipid profiles in adolescents with insulin-dependent diabetes mellitus. *The Physician and Sportsmedicine*, **13**, 83-89.

Canny, G.J., & Levison, H. (1987). Exercise response and rehabilitation in cystic fibrosis. *Sports Medicine*, **4**, 143-152.

Cantu, R.C. (1982). *Diabetes and exercise*. New York: E.P. Dutton.

Cantwell, J.D. (1986). Marfan's syndrome: Detection and management. *The Physician and Sportsmedicine*, **14**, 51-55.

Carruthers, M., Taggart, P., Somerville, W. (1970). Plasma catecholamine estimations. *Lancet*, **2**, 421.

Caspersen, C.J., Powell, K.E. & Christenson, G.M. (1985). Physical activity, exercise, and physical fitness: Definitions and distinctions for health-related research. *Public Health Reports*, **100**, 126-131.

Cavagna, G.A., Franzetti, P., & Fuchimoto, T. (1983). The mechanics of walking in children. *Journal of Physiology*, **343**, 323-339.

Cavanagh, P.R., & Kram, R. (1985). Mechanical and muscular factors affecting the efficiency of human movement. *Medicine and Science in Sports and Exercise*, **17**, 326-331.

Cerny, F.J., Pullano, T.P., & Cropp, G.J.A. (1982). Cardiorespiratory adaptations to exercise in cystic fibrosis. *American Review of Respiratory Disease*, **126**, 217-220.

Chandler, L.A. (1985). *Children under stress* (2nd ed.). Springfield, IL: Charles C Thomas.

Chandy, T.A., & Grana, W.A. (1985). Secondary school athletic injury in boys and girls: A three year comparison. *The Physician and Sportsmedicine*, **13**, 106-111.

Charney, E., Goodman, H.C., McBride, M., Lyon, B., & Pratt, R. (1976). Childhood antecedents of adult obesity. Do chubby infants become obese adults? *New England Journal of Medicine*, **295**, 6-9.

Chasey, W.C., Swartz, J.D., & Chasey, C.G. (1974). Effect of motor development on body image scores for institutionally mentally retarded children. *American Journal of Mental Deficiency*, **78**, 440-445.

Chasey, W.C., & Wyrick, W. (1970). Effect of a gross motor development program on form perception skills of educable mentally retarded children. *Research Quarterly*, **41**, 345-352.

Christie, J., Sheldahl, L.M., Tristani, F.E., Sagar, K.B., Ptacin, M.J., & Wann, S. (1987). Determination of stroke volume and cardiac output during exercise: Comparison of two-dimensional and Doppler echocardiography, Fick oximetry, and thermodilution. *Circulation*, **76**, 539-547.

Clarke, D.H. (1986). Children and the research process. In G.A. Stull & H.M. Eckert (Eds.), *Effects of physical activity on children* (pp. 9-13). Champaign, IL: Human Kinetics.

Clarke, H.H. (1973). National adult physical fitness survey. *President's Council on Physical Fitness and Sports Newsletter*. Washington, D.C.

Coates, A.L., Boyce, P., Muller, D., Mearns, M., & Godfrey, S. (1980). The role of nutritional status, airway obstruction, hypoxia, and abnormalities in serum lipid composition in limiting exercise tolerance in children with cystic fibrosis. *Acta Paediatrica Scandinavica*, **69**, 353-358.

Coates, T.J., & Thoresen, C.E. (1978). Treating obesity in children and adolescents: A review. *American Journal of Public Health*, **68**, 143-151.

Collipp, P.J. (1980a). Obesity programs in public schools. In P. Collipp (Ed.), *Childhood obesity* (pp. 297-308). Littleton, MA: PSG Publishing.

Collipp, P.J. (1980b). *Childhood obesity*. Littleton, MA: PSG Publishing.

Committee on Nutrition (1968). Measurement of skinfold thickness in children. *Pediatrics*, **42**, 538-543.

Committee on Nutrition of the Mother and Preschool Child, Food and Nutrition Board (1978). Fetal and infant nutrition and susceptibility to obesity. *The American Journal of Clinical Nutrition*, **31**, 2026-2030.

Cook, D.L. (1962). The Hawthorne Effect in educational research. *Phi Delta Kappan,* **44,** 116-122.

Cooper, D.M., Kaplan, M.R., Baumgarten, L., Weiler-Ravell, D., Whipp, B.J., & Wasserman, K. (1987). Coupling of ventilation and CO_2 production during exercise in children. *Pediatric Research,* **21,** 568-572.

Cooper, K.H., Pollock, M.L., Martin, R.P., White, S.R., Linnerud, A.C., & Jackson, A. (1976). Physical fitness levels vs. selected coronary risk factors. *Journal of the American Medical Association,* **236,** 166-169.

Cooper, R.S. (1984). Juvenile diabetes and the heart. *Pediatric Clinics of North America,* **31,** 653-663.

Corbin, C.B. (1987). Youth fitness, exercise, and health: There is much to be done. *Research Quarterly for Exercise and Sport,* **58,** 308-314.

Corbin, C.B., & Pletcher, P. (1968). Diet and physical activity patterns of obese and nonobese elementary school children. *Research Quarterly,* **39,** 922-928.

Corder, W.W. (1966). Effects of physical education on the intellectual and social development of educable mentally retarded boys. *Exceptional Children,* **32,** 357-364.

Costill, D.L., Cleary, P., & Fink, W.J. (1979). Training adaptations in skeletal muscle of juvenile diabetes. *Diabetes,* **28,** 818-822.

Cotes, J.E. (1979). *Lung function. Assessment and application in medicine.* Oxford: Blackwell Scientific Publications.

Cowart, V.S. (1986). Should epileptics exercise? *The Physician and Sportsmedicine,* **14,** 183-191.

Cowart, V.S. (1987). How does heredity affect athletic performance? *The Physician and Sportsmedicine,* **15,** 134-140.

Cresanta, J.L., Srinivasan, S.R., Webber, L.S., & Berenson, G.S. (1984). Serum lipid and lipoprotein cholesterol grids for cardiovascular risk screening of children. *American Journal of Diseases of Children,* **138,** 379-387.

Crews, D.J., & Landers, D.M. (1987). A meta-analytic review of aerobic fitness and reactivity to psychosocial stressors. *Medicine and Science in Sports and Exercise,* **19**(Suppl.), S114-S120.

Crews, D.J., Landers, D.M., O'Connor, J.S., & Clark, J.S. (1988). Psychosocial stress response following training (abstract). *Medicine and Science in Sports and Exercise,* **20**(Suppl.), S85.

Cropp, G.J., Pullano, T.P., Cerny, F.J., & Nathanson, I.T. (1982). Exercise tolerance and cardiorespiratory adjustments at peak work capacity in cystic fibrosis. *American Review of Respiratory Disease,* **126,** 211-216.

Cropp, G.J.A. & Tanakawa, N. (1977). Cardiorespiratory adaptations of normal and asthmatic children to exercise. In J.A. Dempsey & C.E. Reed (Eds.), *Muscular exercise and the lung* (pp. 265-278). Madison, WI: University of Wisconsin Press.

Cumming, G.R. (1977). Hemodynamics of supine bicycle exercise in "normal" children. *American Heart Journal,* **93,** 617-622.

Cumming, G.R., Everatt, D., & Hastman, L. (1978). Bruce treadmill test in children: Normal values in a clinic population. *American Journal of Cardiology*, **41**, 69-75.

Cumming, G.R., Garand, T., & Borysyk, L. (1972). Correlation of performance in track and field events with bone age. *Journal of Pediatrics*, **80**, 970-973.

Cumming, G.R., & Hnatiuk, A. (1980). Establishment of normal values for exercise capacity in a hospital clinic. In K. Berg & B.O. Eriksson (Eds.), *Children and exercise IX* (pp. 79-92). Baltimore: University Park Press.

Cumming, G.R., & Langford, S. (1985). Comparison of nine exercise tests used in pediatric cardiology. In R.A. Binkhorst, H.C.G. Kemper, & W.H.M. Saris (Eds.). *Children and exercise XI* (pp. 58-68). Champaign, IL: Human Kinetics.

Cunningham, D.A., Paterson, D.H., & Blimkie, C.J.R. (1984). The development of the cardiorespiratory system with growth and physical activity. In R.A. Boileau (Ed.), *Advances in pediatric sport sciences* (pp. 85-116). Champaign, IL: Human Kinetics.

Cunningham, D.A., Paterson, D.H., Blimkie, C.J.R., & Donner, A.P. (1984). Development of cardiorespiratory function in circumpubertal boys: A longitudinal study. *Journal of Applied Physiology*, **56**, 302-307.

Cunningham, D.A., Stapleton, J.J., MacDonald, I.C., & Paterson, D.H. (1981). Daily energy expenditure of young boys as related to maximal aerobic power. *Canadian Journal of Applied Sports Science*, **6**, 207-211.

Cureton, K.J. (1987). Commentary on "Children and fitness: A public health perspective." *Research Quarterly for Exercise and Sport*, **58**, 315-320.

Dahl-Jorgenson, K., Meen, H.D., Hanssen, K.F., & Aagenaes, O. (1980). The effect of exercise on diabetic control and hemoglobin A1 (HbA1) in children. *Acta Paediatrica Scandinavica*, Suppl. 283, 53-56.

Dahlkoetter, J., Callahan, E.J., & Lindton, J. (1979). Obesity and the unbalanced energy equation: Exercise versus eating habit change. *Journal of Consulting and Clinical Psychology*, **47**, 898-905.

Daniels, J.T. (1985). The physiologist's view of running economy. *Medicine and Science in Sports and Exercise*, **17**, 332-338.

Davies, C.T.M. (1980). Metabolic cost of exercise and physical performance in children with some observations on external loading. *European Journal of Applied Physiology*, **45**, 95-102.

Davies, C.T.M., Barnes, C., & Godfrey, S. (1972). Body composition and maximal exercise performance in children. *Human Biology*, **44**, 195-214.

Davies, C.T.M., & Thompson, M.W. (1979). Aerobic performance of female marathon and male ultramarathon athletes. *European Journal of Applied Physiology*, **41**, 233-245.

Dawber, T.R., Kannel, W.B., & Kagan, A. (1967). Environmental factors in hypertension. In J. Stamler, R. Stamler, & T.N. Pullman (Eds.), *The epidemiology of hypertension* (p. 255). New York: Grune & Stratton.

Dawson, T.J., & Taylor, C.R. (1973). Energetic cost of locomotion in kangaroos. *Nature*, **246**, 313-314.

Day, L. (1981). The testing, prediction, and significance of maximal aerobic power in children. *Australian Journal of Sport Sciences*, **1**, 18-22.

The DCCT Research Group (1988). Are continuous studies of metabolic control and microvascular complications in insulin-dependent diabetes mellitus justified? *New England Journal of Medicine*, **318**, 246-249.

Deal, E.C., McFadden, G.R., Ingram, R.H., Breslin, F.J., & Jaeger, J.J. (1980). Airway responsiveness to cold air and hyperpnea in normal subjects and those with hay fever and asthma. *American Review of Respiratory Diseases*, **121**, 621-628.

Deal, E.C., McFadden, E.R., Ingram, R.H., & Jaeger, J.J. (1979). Esophageal temperature during exercise in asthmatic and non-asthmatic subjects. *Journal of Applied Physiology*, **46**, 484-490.

DeBenedette, V. (1988). Getting fit for life: Can exercise reduce stress? *The Physician and Sportsmedicine*, **16**, 185-200.

DeLorme, T.L., Ferris, B.G., & Gallagher, J.R. (1952). Effect of progressive exercise on muscular contraction time. *Archives of Physical Medicine*, **33**, 86-97.

Dennison, B.A., Straus, J.H., Mellits, N., & Charney, E. (1988). Childhood physical fitness tests: Predictor of adult physical activity levels? *Pediatrics*, **82**, 324-330.

deVries, H.A., & Gray, D.E. (1963). After effects of exercise upon resting metabolism rate. *Research Quarterly*, **34**, 314-321.

Diem, L. (1974). *Children learn physical skills. Vol. 1.* Washington DC: American Alliance for Health, Physical Education, and Recreation.

Dietz, W.H. (1983). Childhood obesity: Susceptibility, cause, and management. *Journal of Pediatrics*, **103**, 676-686.

diPrampero, P.E., & Cerretelli, P. (1969). Maximum muscular power (aerobic and anaerobic) in African natives. *Ergonomics*, **12**, 51-59.

Dishman, R.K. (1986). Mental health. In V.S. Seefeldt (Ed.), *Physical activity and well-being* (pp. 303-341). Reston, VA: American Alliance for Health, Physical Education, Recreation and Dance.

Dishman, R.K., Sallis, J.F., & Orenstein, D.R. (1985). The determinants of physical activity and exercise. *Public Health Reports*, **100**, 158-171.

Ditzel, J., Kawahava, R., & Mourits-Andersen, T. (1981). Changes in blood glucose, glycosylated hemoglobin, and hemoglobin-oxygen affinity following meals in diabetic children. *European Journal of Pediatrics*, **137**, 171-174.

Dlin, R. (1986). Blood pressure response to dynamic exercise in healthy and hypertensive youths. *Pediatrician*, **13**, 34-43.

Docherty, D., Wenger, H.A., & Collis, M.L. (1987). The effects of resistance training on aerobic and anaerobic power of young boys. *Medicine and Science in Sports and Exercise*, **19**, 389-392.

Dressendorfer, R.H., Wade, C.E., & Scaff, J.H. (1985). Increased morning heart rate in runners: A valid sign of overtraining? *The Physician and Sportsmedicine,* **13,** 77-86.

Drinkwater, B.L., Kupprat, I.C., Denton, J.E., Crist, J.L., & Horvath, S.M. (1977). Response of prepubertal girls and college women to work in the heat. *Journal of Applied Physiology,* **43,** 1046-1053.

Driscoll, D.J., Feldt, R.H., Mottram, C.D., Puga, F.J., Schaff, H.V., & Danielson, G.K. (1987). Cardiorespiratory response to exercise after definitive repair of univentricular atrioventricular connection. *International Journal of Cardiology,* **17,** 73-81.

Duda, M. (1986). Prepubescent strength training gains support. *The Physician and Sportsmedicine,* **14,** 157-161.

Dudley, G.A., & Fleck, S.J. (1987). Strength and endurance training. Are they mutually exclusive? *Sports Medicine,* **4,** 79-85.

Dufaux, B., Assmann, G., & Hollman, W. (1982). Plasma lipoproteins and physical activity: A review. *International Journal of Sports Medicine,* **3,** 123-136.

Duncan, J.J., Hagan, R.D., Upton, J., Farr, J.E., & Oglesby, M.E. (1983). The effects of an aerobic exercise program on sympathetic neural activity and blood pressure in mild hypertension (abstract). *Circulation,* Suppl. 68, III-285.

DuRant, R.H., Linder, C.W., Harkess, J.W., & Gray, R.G. (1983). The relationship between physical activity and serum lipids and lipoproteins in black children and adolescents. *Journal of Adolescent Health Care,* **4,** 55-60.

DuRant, R.H., Linder, C.W., & Mahoney, O.M. (1983). Relationship between habitual physical activity and serum lipoprotein levels in white male adolescents. *Journal of Adolescent Health Care,* **4,** 235-240.

Durnin, J.V.G.A., Lonergan, M.E., Good, J., & Ewan, A. (1974). A cross-sectional nutritional and anthropometric study, with an interval of 7 years, on 611 young adolescent school children. *British Journal of Nutrition,* **32,** 169-179.

Durnin, J.V.G.A., & Passmore, R. (1967). *Energy, work, and leisure.* London: Heinemann Educational Books.

Dustan, H.P. (1980). Obesity and hypertension. In R.M. Lauer & R.B. Shekelle (Eds.), *Childhood prevention of atherosclerosis and hypertension* (pp. 305-312). New York: Raven.

Dwyer, J., & Bybee, R. (1983). Heart rate indices of the anaerobic threshold. *Medicine and Science in Sports and Exercise,* **15,** 72-76.

Dwyer, T., Coonan, W.E., Leitch, D.R., Hetzel, B.S., & Baghurst, R.A. (1983). An investigation of the effects of daily physical activity on the health of primary school students in South Australia. *International Journal of Epidemiology,* **12,** 308-313.

Earls, F.J. (1983). An epidemiologic approach to the study of behavior problems in very young children. In S.B. Guze, F.J. Earls, & J.E. Barret

(Eds.) *Childhood psychopathology and development* (pp. 1-15). New York: Raven.

Eaton, W.O., & Enns, L.R. (1986). Sex differences in human motor activity level. *Psychological Bulletin*, **100**, 19-28.

Edholm, O.G., Fletcher, J.G., Widdowson, E.M., & McCane, R.A. (1955). The energy expenditure and food intake of individual men. *British Journal of Nutrition*, **9**, 286-300.

Edlund, L.D., French, R.W., Herbst, J.S., Ruttenberg, H.D., & Ruhling, R.D. (1986). Effects of a swimming program on children with cystic fibrosis. *American Journal of Diseases of Children*, **140**, 80-88.

Edmunds, A.T., Tooley, M., & Godfrey, S. (1978). The refractory period after exercise-induced asthma, its duration and relation to the severity of exercise. *American Review of Respiratory Diseases*, **177**, 247-254.

Eggleston, P.A. (1975). The cycloergometer as a system for studying exercise-induced asthma. *Pediatrics*, **56**(Suppl.), 899-903.

Eidsmoe, R.M. (1951). The facts about the academic performance of high school athletes. *Journal of Health, Physical Education and Recreation*, **32**, 20.

Eisenman, P. (1986). Physical activity and body composition. In V. Seefeldt (Ed.), *Physical activity & well-being* (pp. 163-182). Reston, VA: American Alliance for Health, Physical Education, Recreation and Dance.

Ekelund, L.G., Haskell, W.L., Johnson, J.L., Whaley, F.S., Criqui, M.H., & Sheps, D.S. (1988). Physical fitness as a predictor of cardiovascular mortality in asymptomatic North American men. *New England Journal of Medicine*, **319**, 1379-1384.

Ellis, M.J., & Scholtz, J.L. (1978). *Activity and play of children*. Englewood Cliffs, NJ: Prentice Hall.

Elsom, S.D. (1981). Self-management of hyperactivity: Children's use of jogging. *Dissertation Abstracts International*, **41**, 3176-B.

Engerbretson, D.L. (1965). The effects of exercise on diabetic control. *Journal of the Association for Physical Medicine and Rehabilitation*, **19**, 74-78.

Enos, W.F., Beyer, J.C., & Holmes, R.H. (1955). Pathogenesis of coronary disease in American soldiers killed in Korea. *Journal of the American Medical Association*, **158**, 912-914.

Epstein, L.H., Koeske, R., Zidansek, J., & Wing, R.R. (1983). Effects of weight loss on fitness in obese children. *American Journal of Diseases of Children*, **137**, 654-657.

Epstein, L.H., & Wing, R.R. (1980). Aerobic exercise and weight. *Addictive Behaviors*, **5**, 371-388.

Epstein, L.H., Wing, R.R., Koeske, R., Ossip, D., & Beck, S. (1982). A comparison of lifestyle change and programmed aerobic exercise on weight and fitness changes in obese children. *Behavior Therapy*, **13**, 651-665.

Epstein, S.E., & Maron, B.J. (1986). Sudden death and the competitive athlete, perspectives on preparticipation screening studies. *Journal of the American College of Cardiology, 7, 220-230.

Eriksson, B.O. (1972). Physical training, oxygen supply, and muscle metabolism in 11-13 year old boys. *Acta Physiologica Scandinavica,* Suppl. 384, 1-48.

Eriksson, B.O. (1980). Muscle metabolism in children—a review. *Acta Paediatrica Scandinavica,* Suppl. 283, 20-27.

Eriksson, B.O., Engstrom, L., Karlberg, P., Lundin, A., Saltin, B., & Thoren, C. (1978). Long-term effect of previous swim training in girls: A 10-year followup on the "girl swimmers." *Acta Paediatrica Scandinavica, 67,* 285-291.

Eriksson, B.O., Gollnick, P.D., & Saltin, B. (1973). Muscle metabolism and enzyme activities after training in boys 11-13 years old. *Acta Physiologica Scandinavica, 87,* 485-497.

Eriksson, B.O., Karlsson, J., & Saltin, B. (1971). Muscle metabolites during exercise in pubertal boys. *Acta Paediatrica Scandinavica, 217*(Suppl.), 154-157.

Eriksson, B.O., & Koch, G. (1973). Effect of physical training on hemodynamic response during maximal and submaximal exercise. *Acta Physiologica Scandinavica, 87,* 27-39.

Eriksson, B.O., & Saltin, B. (1974). Muscle metabolism during exercise in boys aged 11 to 16 years compared to adults. *Acta Paediatrica Belgium, 28*(Suppl.), 257-261.

Farrell, P.A., & Barbariak, J. (1980). The time course of alterations in plasma lipid and lipoprotein concentrations during eight weeks of endurance training. *Atherosclerosis, 37,* 231-238.

Farrell, P.A., Maksud, M.G., Pollock, M.L., Foster, C., Anholm, J., Hare, J., & Leon, A.S. (1982). A comparison of plasma cholesterol, triglycerides, and high density lipoprotein-cholesterol in speed skaters, weight-lifters, and non-athletes. *European Journal of Applied Physiology, 48,* 77-82.

Feicht, C.B., Johnson, T.S., Martin, B.J., Sparkes, K.E., & Wagner, W.W. (1978). Secondary amenorrhoea in athletes. *The Lancet, 2,* 1145-1146.

Feigley, D.A. (1984). Psychological burnout in high-level athletes. *The Physician and Sportsmedicine, 12,* 109-119.

Fein, F.S., & Sonnenblick, E.H. (1985). Diabetic cardiomyopathy. *Progress in Cardiovascular Diseases, 27,* 255-270.

Feinleib, M., Garrison, R.J., & Havlik, R.J. (1980). Environmental and genetic factors affecting the distribution of blood pressure in children. In R.M. Lauer & R.B. Shekelle (Eds.), *Childhood prevention of atherosclerosis and hypertension* (pp. 271-279). New York: Raven.

Feltz, D.L., & Ewing, M.E. (1987). Psychologic characteristics of elite young athletes. *Medicine and Science in Sports and Exercise, 19*(Suppl.), S98-S105.

Fiddler, G.I., Tajik, A.J., Weidman, W.H., McGoon, D.C., Ritter, D.G., & Giuliani, E.R. (1978). Idiopathic hypertrophic subaortic stenosis in the young. *The American Journal of Cardiology*, **42**, 793-799.

Fielding, J.E. (1985). Smoking: Health effects and control. *New England Journal of Medicine*, **313**, 491-498.

Fish, H.T., Fish, R.B., & Golding, L.A. (1989). *Starting out well: A parents' approach to physical activity & nutrition*. Champaign, IL: Leisure Press.

Fisher, A.G., & Brown, M. (1982). The effects of diet and exercise on selected coronary risk factors in children (abstract). *Medicine and Science in Sports and Exercise*, **14**, 171.

Fitch, K.D. (1975a). Comparative aspects of available exercise systems. *Pediatrics*, **56**(Suppl.), 904-907.

Fitch, K.D. (1975b). Exercise-induced asthma and competitive athletics. *Pediatrics*, **56**(Suppl.), 942-943.

Fitch, K.D. (1986). The use of anti-asthmatic drugs. Do they affect sports performance? *Sports Medicine*, **3**, 136-150.

Fitch, K.D., Blivitch, J.D., & Morton, A.R. (1986). The effect of running training on exercise-induced asthma. *Annals of Allergy*, **57**, 90-94.

Fitch, K.D., Morton, A.R., & Blanksby, S. (1976). Effects of swimming training on children with asthma. *Archives of Disease in Childhood*, **51**, 190-194.

Fixler, D.E. (1978). Epidemiology of childhood hypertension. In W.B. Strong (Ed.), *Atherosclerosis: Its pediatric aspects* (pp. 177-192). New York: Grune & Stratton.

Fixler, D.E., Baron, A., Laird, W.P., Fayers, P., Shinebourne, E.A., & de Swiet, M. (1984). Tracking of blood pressure during childhood. In J.M.H. Loggie, M.J. Horan, A.B. Gruskin, A.R. Hohn, J.B. Dunbar, & R.J. Havlik (Eds.), *NHLBI workshop on juvenile hypertension* (pp. 37-49). New York: Biomedical Information Corporation.

Fixler, D.E., Laird, W.P., & Dana, K. (1985). Usefulness of exercise stress testing for prediction of blood pressure trends. *Pediatrics*, **75**, 1071-1075.

Fleck, S.J., & Kraemer, W.J. (1987). *Designing resistance training programs*. Champaign, IL: Human Kinetics.

Folkins, C.H., Lynch, S., & Gardner, M.M. (1972). Psychological fitness as a function of physical fitness. *Archives of Physical Medicine and Rehabilitation*, **53**, 503-510.

Fontaine, E., Savard, R., Tremblay, A., Despres, J.P., Poehlman, E., & Bouchard, C. (1985). Resting metabolic rate in monozygotic and dizygotic twins. *Acta Geneticae Medicae et Gemellologiae*, **34**, 41-47.

Fortney, V.L. (1983). The kinematics and kinetics of the running pattern of two-, four-, and six-year-old children. *Research Quarterly for Exercise and Sport*, **54**, 126-135.

Foss, M.L., Lampman, R.M., & Schteingart, D.E. (1980). Extremely obese patients: Improvements in exercise tolerance with physical training and weight loss. *Archives of Physical Medicine and Rehabilitation, 61,* 119-124.

Fox, E.L. (1984). *Sports physiology* (2nd ed.). Philadelphia: Saunders.

Francis, R.J., & Rarick, G.L. (1959). Motor characteristics of the mentally retarded. *American Journal of Mental Deficiency, 63,* 792-811.

Fraser, G.E. (1986). *Preventive cardiology.* New York: Oxford University Press.

Fraser, G.E., Phillips, R.L., & Harris, R. (1983). Physical fitness and blood pressure in school children. *Circulation, 67,* 405-412.

Freedson, P. (in press). Field monitoring of physical activity in children. *Pediatric Exercise Science.*

Freedson, P.S., Katch, V.L., Gilliam, T.B., & MacConnie, S. (1981). Energy expenditure in prepubescent children: Influence of sex and age. *The American Journal of Clinical Nutrition, 34,* 1827-1830.

Freis, E.D. (1982). Should mild hypertension be treated? *New England Journal of Medicine, 307,* 306-309.

Friedman, N.E., Levitsky, L.L., & Edidin, D.V. (1982). Echocardiographic evidence for impaired myocardial performance in children with type I diabetes mellitus. *American Journal of Medicine, 73,* 846-850.

Fripp, R.R., & Hodgson, J.L. (1987). Effect of resistive training on plasma lipid and lipoprotein levels in male adolescents. *Journal of Pediatrics, 111,* 926-931.

Frisch, R.E. (1987). Body fat, menarche, fitness, and fertility. *Human Reproduction, 2,* 521-533.

Frisch, R.E., & McArthur, J.W. (1974). Menstrual cycles: Fatness as a determinant of minimum weight for height necessary for their maintenance or onset. *Science, 185,* 949-951.

Frisch, R.E., & Revelle, R. (1971). Height and weight at menarche and a hypothesis of menarche. *Archives of Diseases of Childhood, 46,* 695-701.

Froelicher, V.F. (1983). *Exercise testing & training.* New York: LeJacq.

Gabriele, A.J., & Marble, A. (1949). Experiences with 116 juvenile campers in a new summer camp for diabetic boys. *American Journal of Medical Science, 218,* 161-165.

Gadhoke, S., & Jones, N.L. (1969). The responses to exercise in boys aged 9-15 years. *Clinical Science, 37,* 789-801.

Garrick, J.C., & Requa, R.K. (1978). Injuries in high school sports. *Pediatrics, 61,* 465-469.

Garrow, J.S. (1986). The effect of exercise on obesity. *Acta Medica Scandinavica,* Suppl. 711, 67-73.

Gettman, L.R., & Pollock, M.L. (1981). Circuit weight training: A critical review of its physiological benefits. *The Physician and Sportsmedicine, 9,* 44-60.

Geva, T., Hegesh, J., & Frand, M. (1987). The clinical course and echo-cardiographic features of Marfan's syndrome in childhood. *American Journal of Diseases of Children*, **141**, 1179-1182.

Ghory, J.E. (1975). Exercise, the school, and the allergic child. *Pediatrics*, **56**(Suppl.), 948-949.

Gilliam, T.B., & Burke, M.B. (1978). Effects of exercise on serum lipids and lipoproteins in girls, ages 8 to 10 years. *Artery*, **4**, 203-213.

Gilliam, T.B., & Freedson, P.S. (1980). Effects of a 12-week school physical fitness program on peak $\dot{V}O_2$, body composition, and blood lipids in 7 to 9 year old children. *International Journal of Sports Medicine*, **1**, 73-78.

Gilliam, T.B., Freedson, P.S., Geenan, D.L., & Shahraray, B. (1981). Physical activity patterns determined by heart rate monitoring in 6-7 year old children. *Medicine and Science in Sports and Exercise*, **13**, 65-67.

Gilliam, T.B., Katch, V.L., Thorland, W., & Weltman, A.L. (1977). Prevalence of coronary heart disease risk factors in active children, 7 to 12 years of age. *Medicine and Science in Sports*, **9**, 21-25.

Gilliam, T.B., Sady, S., Thorland, W.G., & Weltman, A.L. (1977). Comparison of peak performance measures in children ages 6 to 8, 9 to 10, and 11 to 13 years. *Research Quarterly*, **48**, 695-702.

Girandola, R.N., Wiswell, R.A., Frisch, F., & Wood, K. (1981). Metabolic differences during exercise in pre- and post-adolescent girls (abstract). *Medicine and Science in Sports and Exercise*, **13**, 110.

Glass, D.C., Krakoff, L.R., & Contrada, R. (1980). Effect of harrassment and competition upon cardiovascular and plasma catecholamine responses in type A and type B individuals. *Psychophysiology*, **17**, 453-460.

Glew, R.H., Varghese, P.J., Krovetz, L.J., Dorst, J.P., & Rowe, R.D. (1969). Sudden death in congenital aortic stenosis. *American Heart Journal*, **78**, 615-625.

Godfrey, S. (1974). *Exercise testing in children*. London: W.B. Saunders.

Godfrey, S., Davies, C.T.M., Wozniak, E., & Barnes, C.A. (1971). Cardiorespiratory response to exercise in normal children. *Clinical Science*, **40**, 419-431.

Godfrey, S., & Konig, P. (1975). Suppression of exercise-induced asthma by salbutamol, theophylline, atropine, cromolyn, and placebo in a group of asthmatic children. *Pediatrics*, **56**(Suppl.), 930-934.

Godfrey, S., & Mearns, M. (1971). Pulmonary function and response to exercise in cystic fibrosis. *Archives of Disease in Childhood*, **46**, 144-151.

Godfrey, S., Silverman, M., & Anderson, S.D. (1975). The use of the treadmill for assessing exercise-induced asthma and the effect of varying the severity and duration of exercise. *Pediatrics*, **56**(Suppl.), 893-898.

Godshall, R.W., Hansen, C.A., & Rising, D.C. (1981). Stress fractures through the distal femoral epiphysis in athletes. *The American Journal of Sports Medicine, 9,* 114-116.

Goforth, D., & James, F.W. (1985). Exercise training in noncoronary heart disease. *Cardiovascular Clinics, 15,* 243-260.

Goldberg, B., Fripp, R.R., Lister, G., Loke, J., Nicholas, J.A., & Talner, N.S. (1981). Effect of physical training on exercise performance of children following surgical repair of congenital heart disease. *Pediatrics, 68,* 691-699.

Goldberg, B., Rosenthal, P.P., & Nicholas, J.A. (1984). Injuries in youth football. *The Physician and Sportsmedicine, 12,* 122-132.

Goldberg, B., Veras, G., & Nicholas, J.A. (1978). Sports medicine. Pediatric perspective. *New York Journal of Medicine, 78,* 1406-1409.

Goldberg, L., & Elliot, D.L. (1985). The effect of physical activity on lipid and lipoprotein levels. *Medical Clinics of North America, 69,* 41-55.

Goldberg, L., Elliot, D.L., Schutz, R.W., & Kloster, F.E. (1984). Changes in lipid and lipoprotein levels after weight training. *Journal of the American Medical Association, 252,* 504-506.

Golebiowska, M., & Bujnowski, T. (1986). Effects of an 8-month reducing program on the physical fitness of obese children. In J. Rutenfranz, R. Mocellin, & F. Klimt (Eds.), *Children and exercise XII* (pp. 195-200). Champaign, IL: Human Kinetics.

Gonzalez, E.R. (1979). Exercise therapy "rediscovered" for diabetes, but what does it do? *Journal of the American Medical Association, 242,* 1591-1592.

Gordon, T., Castelli, W.P., Hjortland, M.J., Kannel, W.B., & Dawber, T.R. (1977). HDL as a protective factor against CHD. The Framingham study. *American Journal of Medicine, 62,* 707-714.

Gotze, W., Kubicki, S., Hunter, M., & Teichmann, J. (1967). Effect of physical exercise on seizure threshold. *Diseases of the Nervous System, 28,* 664-667.

Graff-Lonnevig, V., Bevegard, S., Eriksson, B.O., Kraepelien, S., & Saltin, B. (1980). Two years' follow-up of asthmatic boys participating in a physical activity programme. *Acta Paediatrica Scandinavica, 69,* 347-352.

Graham, T.P. (1983). Ventricular performance in adults after operation for congenital heart disease. In M.A. Engle & J.K. Perloff (Eds.), *Congenital heart disease after surgery* (pp. 322-343). New York: Yorke Medical Books.

Grasselli, R.N., & Hegner, P.A. (1981). *Playful parenting.* New York: Richard Marek.

Green, D.E. (1980). Beliefs of teenagers about smoking and health. In R.M. Lauer & R.B. Shekelle (Eds.), *Childhood prevention of atherosclerosis and hypertension* (pp. 223-228). New York: Raven.

Griffiths, M., & Payne, P.R. (1976). Energy expenditure in small children of obese and nonobese parents. *Nature, 260,* 698-700.

Groom, D. (1971). Cardiovascular observations on Tarahumara Indian runners—the modern Spartans. *American Heart Journal*, **81**, 304-314.

Gruber, J.J. (1986). Physical activity and self-esteem development in children: A meta-analysis. In G.A. Stull & H.M. Eckert (Eds.), *Effects of physical activity on children* (pp. 30-48). Champaign, IL: Human Kinetics.

Guyton, A.C. (1966). *Textbook of medical physiology* (3rd ed.). Philadelphia: W.B. Saunders.

Hagan, R.D. (1988). Benefits of aerobic conditioning and diet for overweight adults. *Sports Medicine*, **5**, 144-155.

Hagan, R.D., Marks, J.F., & Warren, P.A. (1979). Physiologic responses of juvenile-onset diabetic boys to muscular work. *Diabetes*, **28**, 1114-1119.

Hagberg, J.M., Ehsani, A.A., Goldring, O., Hernandez, A., Sinacore, D.R., & Holloszy, J.O. (1984). Effects of weight training on blood pressure and hemodynamics in hypertensive adolescents. *Journal of Pediatrics*, **104**, 147-151.

Hagberg, J.M., Goldring, D., Ehsani, A.A., Heath, G.W., Hernandez, A., Schechtman, K., & Holloszy, J.O. (1983). Effect of exercise training on the blood pressure and hemodynamic features of hypertensive adolescents. *American Journal of Cardiology*, **52**, 763-768.

Hage, P. (1983). Primary care physicians: First stop for exercise advice? *The Physician and Sportsmedicine*, **11**, 149-152.

Hamel, P., Simoneau, J., Lortie, G., Boulay, M.R., & Bouchard, C. (1986). Heredity and muscle adaptation to endurance training. *Medicine and Science in Sports and Exercise*, **18**, 690-696.

Hames, C.G., Heyden, S., Prineas, R., Heiss, G., Comberg, H.U., & Sneiderman, J. (1978). The natural history of hypertension in Evans County, Georgia. In W.B. Strong (Ed.), *Atherosclerosis: Its pediatric aspects* (pp. 171-175). New York: Grune & Stratton.

Hamilton, P., & Andrew, G.M. (1976). Influence of growth and athletic training on heart and lung functions. *European Journal of Applied Physiology*, **36**, 27-38.

Hammar, S.L. (1980). Obesity: Early identification and treatment. In P.J. Collipp (Ed.), *Childhood obesity* (2nd ed., pp. 281-295). Littleton, MA: PSG Publishing.

Hampton, M.C., Huenemann, R.L., Shapiro, L.R., Mitchell, B.W., & Behnke, A.R. (1966). A longitudinal study of gross body composition and body conformation and their association with food and activity in a teen-age population. *American Journal of Clinical Nutrition*, **19**, 422-435.

Haskell, W.L. (1985). Physical activity and health: Need to define the required stimulus. *American Journal of Cardiology*, **55**, 4D-9D.

Haskell, W.L., Montoye, H.J., & Orenstein, D. (1985). Physical activity and exercise to achieve health-related fitness components. *Public Health Reports*, **100**, 202-212.

Hauser, W.J., & Lueptow, L.B. (1978). Participation in athletics and academic achievement: A replication and extension. *Sociological Quarterly*, **19**, 304-309.

Hayashi, T., Fujino, M., Shindo, M., Hiroki, T., & Arakawa, K. (1987). Echocardiographic and electrocardiographic measures in obese children after an exercise program. *International Journal of Obesity*, **11**, 465-472.

Heald, F.P. (1972). The natural history of obesity. *Advances in Psychosomatic Medicine*, **7**, 102-115.

Heald, F.P., & Hunt, S. (1965). Caloric dependency in obese adolescents as affected by degree of maturation. *Journal of Pediatrics*, **66**, 1035-1041.

Hebbelinck, M. (1978). Methods of biological maturity assessment. *Medicine and Sport*, **11**, 108-117.

Hellenbrand, W.E., Laks, H., Kleinman, C.S., & Talner, N.S. (1981). Hemodynamic evaluation of the Fontan procedure at rest and with exercise (abstract). *American Journal of Cardiology*, **47**, 432.

Henriksen, J.M., & Nielson, T.T. (1983). Effect of physical training on exercise-induced bronchoconstriction. *Acta Paediatrica Scandinavica*, **72**, 31-36.

Hill, A.V. (1939). The mechanical efficiency of frog's muscle. *Proceedings of the Royal Society of London*, **127**, 434-451.

Hoerr, S.L. (1984). Exercise: An alternative to fad diets for adolescent girls. *The Physician and Sportsmedicine*, **12**, 76-83.

Hofman, A., Walter, H.J., Connelly, P.A., & Vaughan, R.D. (1987). Blood pressure and physical fitness in children. *Hypertension*, **9**, 188-191.

Hogberg, P. (1952). How do stride length and stride frequency influence the energy output during running? *Arbeitsphysiologie*, **14**, 437-442.

Holman, R.L., McGill, H.C., Strong, J.P., & Geer, J.C. (1958). The natural history of atherosclerosis: The early aortic lesions as seen in New Orleans in the middle of the 20th century. *American Journal of Pathology*, **34**, 209-235.

Horton, E.S. (1988). Role and management of exercise in diabetes mellitus. *Diabetes Care*, **11**, 201-211.

Houlsby, W.T. (1986). Functional aerobic capacity and body size. *Archives of Disease in Childhood*, **61**, 388-393.

Howard, J. (1984). *The cyclist's companion*. New York: S. Green Press.

Huenemann, R., Hampton, M., Behnke, A., Shapiro, L., & Mitchell, B. (1974). *Teenage nutrition and physique*. Springfield, IL: Charles C Thomas.

Hunsicker, P., & Reiff, G.G. (1976). *AAPHERD youth test manual*. Reston, VA: American Alliance for Health, Physical Education, Recreation and Dance.

Hurley, B.F., & Kokkinos, P.F. (1987). Effects of weight training on risk factors for coronary artery disease. *Sports Medicine, 4,* 231, 238.

Hurley, B.F., Seals, D.R., Hagberg, J.M., Goldberg, A.C., Ostrove, S.M., Holloszy, J.O., Weist, W.G., & Goldberg, A.P. (1984). High-density lipoprotein cholesterol in body builders and power lifters. *Journal of the American Medical Association, 252,* 507-513.

Inbar, O., & Bar-Or, O. (1975). The effects of intermittent warm-up on 7- to 9-year old boys. *European Journal of Applied Physiology, 34,* 81-89.

Inbar, O., & Bar-Or, O. (1986). Anaerobic characteristics in male children and adolescents. *Medicine and Science in Sports and Exercise, 18,* 264-269.

Ismail, A.H. (1967). The effect of an organized physical education program on intellectual performance. *Research in Physical Education, 1,* 31-38.

Ismail, A.H., & Gruber, J.J. (1967). *Motor aptitude and intellectual performance.* Columbus, OH: Charles E. Merrill.

Iso-Ahola, S. (1976). Evaluation of self and team performance and feelings of satisfaction after success and failure. *International Review of Sport Sociology, 11,* 33-44.

Iso-Ahola, S. (1979). Some social psychological determinants of perceptions of leisure. *Leisure Science, 2,* 305-314.

Iverson, D.C., Fielding, J.E., Crow, R.S., & Christenson, G.M. (1985). The promotion of physical activity in the United States population: The status of programs in medical, worksite, community, and school settings. *Public Health Reports, 100,* 212-224.

James, L., Faciane, J., & Sly, R.M. (1976). Effects of treadmill exercise on asthmatic children. *Journal of Allergy and Clinical Immunology, 57,* 408-416.

James, S.W. (1978). Smoking and atherosclerosis: Epidemiology and means of intervention. In W.B. Strong (Ed.), *Atherosclerosis: Its pediatric aspects* (pp. 193-204). New York: Grune & Stratton.

Janos, M., Janos, M., Tamas, S., & Ivan, S. (1985). Assessment of biological development by anthropometric variables. In R.B. Binkhorst, H.C.G. Kemper, & W.H.M. Saris (Eds.), *Children and exercise XI* (pp. 341-345). Champaign, IL: Human Kinetics.

Jarrett, R.J., Keen, H., & Chakrabarti, R. (1982). Diabetes, hyperglycemia, and arterial disease. In H. Keen & R.J. Jarrett (Eds.), *Complications of diabetes* (pp. 179-204). London: Edward Arnold.

Johnson, C.C., Stone, M.H., Lopez, S.A., Hebert, J.A., Kilgore, L.T., & Byrd, R.J. (1982). Diet and exercise in middle-aged men. *Journal of the American Dietetic Association, 81,* 695-701.

Johnson, M.L., Burke, B.S., & Mayer, J. (1956). Relative importance of inactivity and overeating in the energy balance of obese high school girls. *American Journal of Clinical Nutrition, 4,* 37-44.

Johnson, S.B., & Rosenbloom, A.L. (1982). Behavioral aspects of diabetes mellitus in childhood and adolescence. *Pediatric Clinics of North America, 5,* 357-369.

Jokl, E. (1978). Introduction. In J. Borms & M. Hebbelink (Eds.), *Medicine and Sport* (pp. 1-28). Basel: Karger.

Joslin, E.P. (1959). The treatment of diabetes mellitus. In E.P. Joslin, H.F. Root, P. White, & A. Marble (Eds.), *Treatment of diabetes mellitus* (pp. 243-300). Philadelphia: Lea & Febiger.

Kannel, W.B., & Sorlie, P. (1979). Some health benefits of physical activity. The Framingham study. *Archives of Internal Medicine, 139,* 857-861.

Kannel, W.B., & Thom, T.J. (1984). Declining cardiovascular mortality. *Circulation, 70,* 331-336.

Kanstrup, I., & Ekblom, B. (1984). Blood volume and hemoglobin concentration as determinants of maximal aerobic power. *Medicine and Science in Sports and Exercise, 16,* 256-262.

Kaplan, N.M. (1986). *Clinical hypertension* (4th ed.). Baltimore: Williams & Wilkins.

Karpman, V.L. (1987). *Cardiovascular system and physical exercise.* Boca Raton, FL: CRC Press.

Katch, F.I., & McArdle, W.D. (1983). *Nutrition, weight control, and exercise* (2nd ed.). Philadelphia: Lea & Febiger.

Katch, F.I., Pechar, G.S., McArdle, W.D., & Weltman, A.L. (1973). Relationship between individual differences in a steady pace endurance running performance and maximal oxygen intake. *Research Quarterly, 44,* 206-215.

Katch, V.L. (1983). Physical conditioning of children. *Journal of Adolescent Health Care, 3,* 241-246.

Katch, V.L., & Katch, F.I. (1972). Reliability, individual differences and intra-variation of endurance performance on the bicycle ergometer. *Research Quarterly, 43,* 31-38.

Katch, V.L., Marks, C., & Rocchini, A. (1983). Basal, resting, and maximum exercise metabolic rate of obese adolescents: Influence of body composition (abstract). *Medicine and Science in Sports and Exercise, 15,* 138.

Katsura, T. (1986). Influence of age and sex on cardiac output during submaximal exercise. *Annals of Physiological Anthropology, 5,* 39-57.

Katz, J.F. (1982). Effects of aerobic versus nonaerobic play on selected behaviors of autistic children. Presented at the Midwest Symposium on Exercise and Mental Health, Lake Forest College, Lake Forest, IL. April.

Katz, R.M. (1986). Prevention with and without the use of medications for exercise-induced asthma. *Medicine and Science in Sports and Exercise, 18,* 331-333.

Kay, R.S., Felker, D.W., & Varoz, R.O. (1972). Sports interests and abilities as contributors to self-concept in junior high school boys. *Research Quarterly*, **43**, 208-215.

Keens, T.G. (1979). Exercise training programs for pediatric patients with chronic lung disease. *Pediatric Clinics of North America*, **26**, 517-524.

Keens, T.G., Krastins, I.R.B., Wannamaker, E.M., Levison, H., Crozier, D.N., & Bryan, A.C. (1977). Ventilatory muscle endurance training in normal subjects and patients with cystic fibrosis. *American Review of Respiratory Disease*, **116**, 853-860.

Keesey, R.E. (1980). Neurophysiologic control of body fatness. In R.M. Lauer & R.B. Shekelle (Eds.), *Childhood prevention of atherosclerosis and hypertension* (pp. 167-186). New York: Raven.

Kelly, F.J., & Baer, D.J. (1969). Jenness Inventory and self-concept measures for delinquents before and after participation in Outward Bound. *Psychologic Reports*, **25**, 719-724.

Kemmer, F.W., & Berger, M. (1983). Exercise and diabetes mellitus: Physical activity as a part of daily life and its role in the treatment of diabetic patients. *International Journal of Sports Medicine*, **4**, 77-88.

Kemper, H.C.G., & Verschuur, R. (1985). Maximal aerobic power. In H.C.G. Kemper (Ed.), *Growth, health, and fitness of teenagers* (pp. 107-126). Basel: Karger.

Kidd, T.R., & Woodman, W.F. (1975). Sex orientations toward winning in sport. *Research Quarterly*, **46**, 476-483.

Kinsell, L.W. (1955). Prevention of vascular disease in the diabetic. *Diabetes*, **4**, 298-303.

Kirkendall, D.R. (1986). Effects of physical activity on intellectual development and academic performance. In G.A. Stull & H.M. Eckert (Eds.) *Effects of physical activity on children* (pp. 49-63). Champaign, IL: Human Kinetics.

Kistler, H.W. (1957). Attitudes expressed about behavior demonstrated in certain specific situations. *Proceedings of the College Physical Education Association*, **60**, 55-58.

Klausen, K., Rasmussen, B., Glensgaard, L.K., & Jensen, O.V. (1985). Work efficiency during submaximal bicycle exercise. In R.A. Binkhorst, H.C.G. Kemper, & W.H.M. Saris (Eds.), *Children and exercise XI* (pp. 210-217). Champaign, IL: Human Kinetics.

Klausen, K., Rasmussen, B., & Schibye, B. (1986). Evaluation of the physical activity of school children during a physical education lesson. In J. Rutenfranz, R. Mocellin, & F. Klimt (Eds.), *Children and exercise XII* (pp. 93-102). Champaign, IL: Human Kinetics.

Kleiber, D.A., & Roberts, G.C. (1981). The effects of sport experience in the development of social character: An exploratory investigation. *Journal of Sport Psychology*, **3**, 114-122.

Kleiber, M. (1961). *The fire of life. An introduction to animal energetics*. New York: John Wiley.

Klesges, L.K., & Klesges, R.C. (1987). The assessment of children's physical activity: A comparison of methods. *Medicine and Science in Sports and Exercise*, **19**, 511-517.

Klissouras, V. (1971). Heritability of adaptive variation. *Journal of Applied Physiology*, **31**, 338-344.

Knittle, J.L. (1972). Obesity in childhood: A problem in adipose tissue cellular development. *Journal of Pediatrics*, **81**, 1048-1059.

Knittle, J.L., & Ginsberg-Fellner, F. (1980). Can obesity be prevented? In P.J. Collipp (Ed.), *Childhood obesity* (2nd ed., pp. 63-78). Littleton, MA: PSG Publishing.

Knittle, J.L., & Hirsch, J. (1968). Effect of early nutrition on the development of rat epididymal fat pads: Cellularity and metabolism. *Journal of Clinical Investigation*, **47**, 2091-2098.

Knoebel, L.K. (1963). Energy metabolism. In E.E. Selkurt (Ed.), *Physiology* (pp. 564-579). Boston: Little, Brown.

Kobayashi, K., Kitamura, K., Miura, M., Sodeyama, H., Murase, Y., Miyashita, M., & Matsui, H. (1978). Aerobic power as related to body growth and training in Japanese boys: A longitudinal study. *Journal of Applied Physiology*, **44**, 666-672.

Koch, G. (1974). Muscle blood flow after ischemic work and during bicycle ergometer work in boys aged 12 years. *Acta Paediatrica Belgica*, **28**(Suppl.), 29-39.

Koch, G. (1978). Muscle blood flow in prepubertal boys. Effect of growth combined with intensive physical training. In J. Borms & M. Hebbelink (Eds.), *Medicine and sport, Vol. 11* (pp. 34-46). Basel: Karger.

Koch, G. (1980). Aerobic power, lung dimensions, ventilatory capacity, and muscle blood flow in 12-16 year old boys with high physical activity. In K. Berg & B.O. Eriksson (Eds.), *Children and exercise IX* (pp. 99-108). Baltimore: University Park Press.

Koch, G., & Rocker, L., (1980). Total amount of hemoglobin, plasma and blood volume, and intravascular protein masses in trained boys. In K. Berg & B.O. Eriksson (Eds.), *Children and exercise I* (pp. 109-115). Baltimore: University Park Press.

Koivisto, V.A., & Felig, P. (1978). Effects of leg exercise on insulin absorption in diabetic patients. *New England Journal of Medicine*, **298**, 79-83.

Kozar, B., & Lord, R.M. (1983). Overuse injury in the young athlete: Reasons for concern. *The Physician and Sportsmedicine*, **11**, 116-122.

Krahenbuhl, G.S., Pangrazi, R.P., & Chomokos, E.A. (1979). Aerobic responses of young boys to submaximal running. *Research Quarterly*, **50**, 413-421.

Krahenbuhl, G.S., Pangrazi, R.P., Petersen, G.W., Burkett, L.N., & Schneider, M.J. (1978). Field testing of cardiorespiratory fitness in primary school children. *Medicine and Science in Sports*, **10**, 208-213.

Krahenbuhl, G.S., Skinner, J.S., & Kohrt, W.M. (1985). Developmental aspects of maximal aerobic power in children. *Exercise and Sport Sciences Reviews*, **13**, 503-538.

Kramsch, D.M., Aspen, A.J., Abramowitz, B.M., Kreimendahl, T., & Hood, W.B. (1981). Reduction of coronary atherosclerosis by moderate conditioning exercise in monkeys on an atherogenic diet. *New England Journal of Medicine*, **305**, 1483-1489.

Krebs, H.A. (1950). Body size and tissue respiration. *Biochimica et Biophysica Acta*, **4**, 249-269.

Kucera, M. (1986). A method for assessing the movement activity of normal children and children with cardiovascular diseases. In J. Rutenfranz, R. Mocellin, & F. Klimt (Eds.), *Children and exercise XII* (pp. 111-119). Champaign, IL: Human Kinetics.

Laakso, L., Rimpela, M., & Telema, R. (1979). Relationship between physical activity and some health habits among Finnish youth. *Schriftenreihe des Bundestintitus für Sportwissenschaft*, **36**, 76-81.

Lababidi, Z.A., & Goldstein, D.E. (1983). High prevalence of echocardiographic abnormalities in diabetic youths. *Diabetes Care*, **6**, 18-22.

Laird, W.P., Fixler, D.E., & Huffines, F.D. (1979). Cardiovascular response to isometric exercise in normal adolescents. *Circulation*, **59**, 651-654.

Lambert, E.C., Menon, V.A., Wagner, H.R., & Vlad, P. (1974). Sudden unexpected death from cardiovascular disease in children. *The American Journal of Cardiology*, **34**, 89-96.

LaPorte, R.E., Dearwater, S., Cauley, J.A., Slemenda, C., & Cook, T. (1985). Cardiovascular fitness: Is it really necessary? *The Physician and Sportsmedicine*, **13**, 145-150.

LaPorte, R.E., Dorman, J.S., Tajima, N., Cruickshanks, K.J., Orchard, T.J., Cavender, D.E., & Drash, A.L. (1986). Pittsburgh insulin-dependent diabetes mellitus morbidity and mortality study: Physical activity and diabetic complications. *Pediatrics*, **78**, 1027-1033.

LaPorte, R.E., Montoye, H.J., & Caspersen, C.J. (1985). Assessment of physical activity in epidemiologic research: Problems and prospects. *Public Health Reports*, **100**, 131-146.

Larsson, Y. (1980). Physical exercise and juvenile diabetes—summary and conclusions. *Acta Paediatrica Scandinavica*, Suppl. 283, 120-122.

Larsson, Y. (1984). Physical performance and the young diabetic. In R.A. Boileau (Ed.), *Advances in pediatric sports sciences* (pp. 131-156). Champaign, IL: Human Kinetics.

Larsson, Y., Persson, B., & Sterky, G. (1964). Functional adaptation to vigorous training and exercise in diabetic and non-diabetic adolescents. *Journal of Applied Physiology*, **19**, 629-635.

Larsson, Y., Persson, B., Sterky, G., & Thoren, C. (1964). Effect of exercise on blood lipids in juvenile diabetes. *The Lancet*, **1**, 350-355.

Larsson, Y., Sterky, G., Ekengren, K., & Moeller, T. (1962). Physical fitness and the influence of training in diabetic adolescent girls. *Diabetes*, **11**, 109-117.

Lauer, R.M., & Clarke, W.R. (1980). Immediate and long term prognostic significance of childhood blood pressure levels. In R.M. Lauer & R.B. Shekelle (Eds.), *Childhood prevention of atherosclerosis and hypertension* (pp. 281-290). New York: Raven.

Lauer, R.M., Connor, W.E., Leaverton, P.E., Reiter, M.A., & Clarke, W.R. (1975). Coronary heart disease risk factors in school children: The Muscatine study. *Journal of Pediatrics*, **86**, 697-706.

Lauer, R.M., & Shekelle, R.B. (1980). *Childhood prevention of atherosclerosis and hypertension*. New York: Raven.

Lawrence, R.D. (1926). The effect of exercise on insulin action in diabetes. *British Medical Journal*, **1**, 648-652.

Leard, J.S. (1984). Flexibility and conditioning in the young athlete. In L.J. Micheli (Ed.), *Pediatric and adolescent medicine* (pp. 194-210). Boston: Little, Brown.

Legwold, G. (1982). Does lifting weights harm a prepubescent athlete? *The Physician and Sportsmedicine*, **10**, 141-144.

Legwold, G. (1985). Are we running from the truth about the risks and benefits of exercise? *The Physician and Sportsmedicine*, **13**, 136-148.

Leon, A.S. (1984). Exercise and risk of coronary heart disease. In H.M. Eckert & H.J. Montoye (Eds.), *Exercise and health* (pp. 14-31). Champaign, IL: Human Kinetics.

Leon, A.S. (1985). Physical activity levels and coronary heart disease. *Medical Clinics of North America*, **69**, 3-19.

Letcher, R.L., Pickering, T.G., Chien, S., & Laragh, J.H. (1978). Effects of physical training on plasma viscosity, plasma proteins, and systemic hemodynamics in normal subjects. *Circulation*, **57**, 11.

Levy, J. (1975). *The baby exercise book*. New York: Random House.

Lewko, J.H. & Greendorfer, S.L. (1982). Family influence and sex differences in children's socialization into sport: A review. In R.A. Magill, M.J. Ash, & F.L. Smoll (Eds.), *Children in sport* (pp. 279-293). Champaign, IL: Human Kinetics.

Lieberman, E. (1986). Hypertension in childhood and adolescence. In N.M. Kaplan, *Clinical hypertension* (4th ed., pp. 447-472). Baltimore: Williams & Wilkins.

Linder, C.W., & DuRant, R.H. (1982). Exercise, serum lipids, and cardiovascular disease—risk factors in children. *Pediatric Clinics of North America*, **29**, 1341-1354.

Linder, C.W., DuRant, R.H., Gray, R.G., & Harkess, J.W. (1979). The effects of exercise on serum lipid levels in children (abstract). *Clinical Research*, **27**, 797.

Linder, C.W., DuRant, R.H., & Mahoney, O.M. (1983). The effect of physical conditioning on serum lipids and lipoproteins in white male adolescents. *Medicine and Science in Sports and Exercise*, **15**, 232-236.

Lindner, P. (1980). Techniques of management for the inactive obese child. In P.J. Collipp (Ed.), *Childhood obesity* (pp. 179-205). Littleton, MA: PSG Publishing.

Lipid Research Clinics Program (1984). The lipid research clinics coronary primary prevention trial results. II. The relationship of reduction in incidence of coronary heart disease to cholesterol lowering. *Journal of the American Medical Association*, **251**, 365-374.

Livingston, S. (1971). Should physical activity of the epileptic child be restricted? *Clinical Pediatrics*, **10**, 694-696.

Livingston, S., & Berman, W. (1973). Participation of epileptic patients in sports. *Journal of the American Medical Association*, **224**, 236-239.

Lloyd, J.K., Wolff, O.H., & Whelen, W.S. (1961). Childhood obesity. A long term study of height and weight. *British Medical Journal*, **7**, 142-148.

Lohman, T.G., Boileau, R.A., & Slaughter, M.H. (1984). Body composition in children and youth. In R.A. Boileau (Ed.), *Advances in pediatric sport sciences* (pp. 29-58). Champaign, IL: Human Kinetics.

Longhurst, J.C., Kelly, A.R., Gonyea, W.J., & Mitchell, J.H. (1981). Chronic training with static and dynamic exercise: Cardiovascular adaptation, and response to exercise. *Circulation Research*, **48**(Suppl. 1), I-171-178.

Longmuir, P.E., Turner, J.A.P., Rowe, R.D., & Olley, P.M. (1985). Postoperative exercise rehabilitation benefits children with congenital heart disease. *Clinical and Investigative Medicine*, **8**, 232-238.

Lorin, M.I. (1978). *The parents' book of physical fitness for children*. New York: Atheneum.

Loucks, A.B. (1988). Osteoporosis prevention begins in childhood. In E.W. Brown & C.F. Branta (Eds.), *Competitive sports for children and youth* (pp. 213-223). Champaign, IL: Human Kinetics.

Ludvigsson, J. (1980). Physical exercise in relation to degree of metabolic control in juvenile diabetics. *Acta Paediatrica Scandinavica* **283**(Suppl.), 45-49.

Ludwick, S.K., Jones, J.W., Jones, T.K., Fukuhara, J.T., & Strunk, R.C. (1986). Normalization of cardiopulmonary endurance in severely asthmatic children after bicycle ergometry therapy. *Journal of Pediatrics*, **109**, 446-451.

Lueptow, L.B., & Kayser, B.D. (1973). Athletic involvement, academic achievement, and aspiration. *Sociologic Focus*, **7**, 24-35.

Lutter, J.M., & Cushman, S. (1982). Menstrual patterns in female runners. *The Physician and Sportsmedicine*, **10**, 60-70.

Maccoby, E.E., & Jacklin, C.N. (1974). *The psychology of sex differences*. Stanford, CA: Stanford University Press.

MacDonald, M.J. (1987). Postexercise late-onset hypoglycemia in insulin-dependent diabetic patients. *Diabetes Care*, **10**, 584-588.

MacDougall, J.D., Roche, P.D., Bar-Or, O., & Moroz, J.R. (1979). Oxygen cost of running in children of different ages; maximal aerobic power of Canadian school children. *Canadian Journal of Applied Sports Science*, **4**, 237.

MacDougall, J.D., Tuxen, D., Sale, D.G., Moroz, J.R., & Sutton, J.R. (1985). Arterial blood pressure response to heavy resistance exercise. *Journal of Applied Physiology*, **58**, 785-790.

Máček, M. (1986). Aerobic and anaerobic energy output in children. In J. Rutenfranz, R. Mocellin, & F. Klimt (Eds.), *Children and exercise XII* (pp. 3-9). Champaign, IL: Human Kinetics.

Máček, M., & Vávra, J. (1985). Anaerobic threshold in children. In R.A. Binkhorst, H.C.G. Kemper, & W.H.M. Saris (Eds.), *Children and exercise XI* (pp. 110-118). Champaign, IL: Human Kinetics.

Máček, M., Vávra, J., Benesova, H., & Radvansky, J. (1984). The adjustment of oxygen uptake at the onset of exercise: Relation to age and to work load. In J. Ilmarinen & I. Valimaki (Eds.), *Children and sport* (pp. 129-134). Berlin: Springer.

Máček, M., Vávra, J., & Novosadova, J. (1976). Prolonged exercise in prepubertal boys. I. Cardiovascular and metabolic adjustment. *European Journal of Applied Physiology*, **35**, 291-298.

MacMahon, J.R., & Gross, R.T. (1987). Physical and psychological effects of aerobic exercise in boys with learning disabilities. *Developmental and Behavioral Pediatrics*, **8**, 274-277.

Magill, R.A., Ash, M.J., & Smoll, F.L. (1982). *Children in sport*. Champaign, IL: Human Kinetics.

Maglischo, E.W. (1982). *Swimming faster*. Mountain View, CA: Mayfield.

Malina, R.M. (1969). Exercise as an influence upon growth. *Clinical Pediatrics*, **8**, 16-26.

Malina, R.M. (1983). Menarche in athletes: A synthesis and hypothesis. *Annals of Human Biology*, **10**, 1-24.

Malina, R.M. (1984). Human growth, maturation, and regular physical activity. In R.A. Boileau (Ed.), *Advances in Pediatric Sport Sciences* (pp. 59-83). Champaign, IL: Human Kinetics.

Malina, R.M. (1986). Physical growth and maturation. In V. Seefeldt (Ed.), *Physical activity & well-being* (pp. 3-38). Reston, VA: American Alliance for Health, Physical Education, Recreation and Dance.

Malina, R.M., Harper, A.B., Avent, H.H., & Campbell, D.E. (1973). Age at menarche in athletes and non-athletes. *Medicine and Science in Sports*, **5**, 11-13.

Malina, R.M., Spirduso, W.W., Tate, C., & Baylor, A.M. (1978). Age at menarche and selected menstrual characteristics in athletes at different competitive levels and in different sports. *Medicine and Science in Sports*, **10**, 218-222.

Malone, J.I., Cader, T.C., & Edwards, W.C. (1977). Diabetic vascular changes in children. *Diabetes*, **26**, 673-679.

Maloney, M.P., & Payne, L.F. (1980). Notes on the stability of changes in body image due to sensory-motor training. *American Journal of Mental Deficiency*, **74**, 708.

Maloney, T., & Petrie, B. (1972). Professionalization of attitudes toward play among Canadian school pupils as a function of sex, grade, and athletic participation. *Journal of Leisure Research*, **4**, 184-195.

Mann, G.V., Shaffer, R.D., & Rich, A. (1965). Physical fitness and immunity to heart disease in Masai. *Lancet*, **2**, 1308-1310.

Mantel, R., & Vander Velden, L. (1974). The relationship between the professionalization of attitudes toward play of preadolescent boys and participation in organized sport. In G.H. Sage (Ed.), *Sport in American society* (pp. 172-178). Reading, MA: Addison-Wesley.

Marcotte, J.E., Grisdale, R.K., Levison, H., Coates, A.L., & Canny, G.J. (1986). Multiple factors limit exercise capacity in cystic fibrosis. *Pediatric Pulmonology*, **2**, 274-281.

Marker, K. (1981). Influence of athletic training on the maturity process of girls. *Medicine and Sport*, **15**, 117-126.

Marks, C., Katch, V., Rocchini, A., Becque, M.D., Moorehead, C., & Ballor, D. (1986). Heart rate, blood pressure, and $\dot{V}O_2$ adaptations of obese adolescents after exercise and/or dietary intervention (abstract). *Medicine and Science in Sports and Exercise*, **18**(Suppl.), S51.

Marks, C., Katch, V., Rocchini, A., Beekman, R., & Rosenthal, A. (1985). Validity and reliability of cardiac output by CO_2 rebreathing. *Sports Medicine*, **2**, 432-446.

Maron, B.J., Bonow, R.O., Cannon, R.O., Leon, M.B., & Epstein, S.E. (1987). Hypertrophic cardiomyopathy. *The New England Journal of Medicine*, **316**, 844-852.

Maron, B.J., Epstein, S.E., & Roberts, W.C. (1986). Causes of sudden death in competitive athletes. *Journal of the American College of Cardiology*, **7**, 204-214.

Maron, B.J., Henry, W.L., Clark, C.E., Redwood, D.R., Roberts, W.C., & Epstein, S.E. (1976). Asymmetric septal hypertrophy in childhood. *Circulation*, **53**, 9-19.

Maron, B.J., Roberts, W.C., & Epstein, S.E. (1982). Sudden death in hypertrophic cardiomyopathy: A profile of 78 patients. *Circulation*, **65**, 1388-1394.

Martens, R. (1978). *Joy and sadness in children's sports*. Champaign, IL: Human Kinetics.

Martens, R. (1980). The uniqueness of the young athlete: Psychologic considerations. *The American Journal of Sports Medicine*, **8**, 382-385.

Martens, R. (1988). Competitive anxiety in children's sports. In R.M. Malina (Ed.), *Young athletes. Biological, psychological, and educational perspectives* (pp. 235-244). Champaign, IL: Human Kinetics.

Mason, E. (1970). Obesity in pet dogs. *The Veterinary Record*, **86**, 612-615.

Massey, B.H., & Chaudet, N.L. (1956). Effects of heavy resistance exercise on range of joint movements in young male adults. *Research Quarterly*, **27**, 41-51.

Massicotte, D.R., Gauthier, R., & Markon, P. (1985). Prediction of $\dot{V}O_2$max from the running performance in children aged 10-17 years. *Journal of Sports Medicine*, **25**, 10-17.

Massicotte, D.R., & MacNab, R.B.J. (1974). Cardiorespiratory adaptations to training at specified intensities in children. *Medicine and Science in Sports*, **6**, 242-246.

Master, A.M., & Oppenheimer, E.T. (1929). A simple exercise tolerance test for circulatory efficiency with standard tables for normal individuals. *American Journal of Medical Science*, **177**, 223-243.

Mathews, R.A., Nixon, P.A., Stephenson, R.J., Robertson, R.J., Donovan, E.F., Dean, F., Fricker, F.J., Beerman, L.B., & Fischer, D.R. (1983). An exercise program for pediatric patients with congenital heart disease: Organizational and physiologic aspects. *Journal of Cardiac Rehabilitation*, **3**, 467-475.

Mayer, J. (1980). The best diet is exercise. In P.J. Collipp (Ed.), *Childhood obesity* (2nd ed., pp. 207-222). Littleton, MA: PSG Publishing.

Mayers, N., & Gutin, B. (1979). Physiological characteristics of elite prepubertal cross country runners. *Medicine and Science in Sports and Exercise*, **11**, 172-176.

Mayhew, J.L., & Gifford, D.B. (1975). Prediction of maximal O_2 uptake in pre-adolescent boys from anthropometric parameters. *Research Quarterly*, **46**, 302-311.

McAlister, A.L., Perry, C., & Maccoby, N. (1979). Adolescent smoking: Onset and prevention. *Pediatrics*, **63**, 650-658.

McArdle, W.D., Katch, F.I., & Katch, V.L. (1981). *Exercise physiology. Energy, nutrition, and human performance*. Philadelphia: Lea & Febiger.

McCrory, W.W., Klein, A.A., & Fallo, F. (1984). Predictors of blood pressure: Humoral factors. In J.M.H. Loggie, M.J. Horan, A.B. Gruskin, A.R. Hohn, J.B. Dunbar, & R.J. Havlik (Eds.), *NHLBI Workshop on Juvenile Hypertension* (pp. 181-204). New York: Biomedical Information Corporation.

McGill, H.C. (1980). Morphologic development of the atherosclerotic plaque. In R.M. Lauer & R.B. Shekelle (Eds.), *Childhood prevention of atherosclerosis and hypertension* (pp. 41-49). New York: Raven.

McIntosh, P.C. (1971). An historical view of sport and social control. *International Review of Sport Sociology*, **6**, 5-16.

McMahon, M., & Palmer, R.M. (1985). Exercise and hypertension. *Medical Clinics of North America*, **69**, 57-69.

McMahon, T. (1973). Size and shape in biology. *Science*, **199**, 1202-1204.

McMahon, T.A. (1984). *Muscles, reflexes, and locomotion*. Princeton, NJ: Princeton University Press.

McMillan, D.E. (1975). Deterioration of the microcirculation in diabetes. *Diabetes*, **24**, 944-957.

McMillan, D.E. (1978). Diabetic angiopathy—its lessons in vascular physiology. *American Heart Journal*, **96**, 401-406.

McMillan, D.E. (1979). Exercise and diabetic microangiopathy. *Diabetes*, **28**(Suppl.), 103-106.

McMillan, D.E., Utterback, N.G., & LaPuma, J. (1978). Reduced erythrocyte deformability in diabetes. *Diabetes*, **27**, 895-901.

Micheli, L.J. (1981). Complications of recreational running. *Pediatric Alert*, **6**, 1-2.

Micheli, L.J. (1983). Overuse injuries in children's sports: The growth factor. *Orthopedic Clinics of North America*, **14**, 337-360.

Micheli, L.J. (1988a). The incidence of injuries in children's sports: A medical perspective. In E.W. Brown & C.F. Branta (Eds.), *Competitive sports for children and youth* (pp. 279-284). Champaign, IL: Human Kinetics.

Micheli, L.J. (1988b). Strength training in the young athlete. In E.W. Brown & C.F. Branta (Eds.), *Competitive sports for children and youth* (pp. 99-106). Champaign, IL: Human Kinetics.

Middeke, M., Remien, J., & Holzgrere, H. (1984). The influence of sex, age, blood pressure, and physical stress on beta-2 adrenoceptor density of mononuclear cells. *Journal of Hypertension*, **2**, 261-264.

Miller, H.S. (1985). Supervised versus nonsupervised exercise rehabilitation of coronary patients. *Cardiovascular Clinics*, **5**, 193-200.

Miller, L.G. (1987). Exercise-induced asthma. In R.C. Cantu (Ed.), *The exercising adult* (pp. 213-225). New York: McMillan.

Mirotznik, J., Speedling, E., Stein, R., & Bronz, C. (1985). Cardiovascular fitness program: Factors associated with participation and adherence. *Public Health Reports*, **100**, 13-18.

Mirwald, R.L., & Bailey, D.A. (1981). Longitudinal comparison of aerobic power in active and inactive boys aged 7 to 17 years. *Annals of Human Biology*, **8**, 404-414.

Mirwald, R.L., & Bailey, D.A. (1986). *Maximal aerobic power. A longitudinal analysis*. London, Ontario: Sports Dynamics.

Mirwald, R.L., Bailey, D.A., Cameron, N., & Rasmussen, R.L. (1981). Longitudinal comparison of aerobic power in active and inactive boys aged 7 to 17 years. *Annals of Human Biology*, **8**, 404-414.

Mitchell, S.C. (1973). Introduction. Symposium on prevention of atherosclerosis at the pediatric level. *American Journal of Cardiology*, **31**, 539-541.

Miyamura, M., & Honda, Y. (1973). Maximum cardiac output related to sex and age. *Japanese Journal of Physiology*, **23**, 645-656.

Monahan, T. (1986a). Exercise and depression: Swapping sweat for serenity? *The Physician and Sportsmedicine*, **14**, 193-197.

Monahan, T. (1986b). Family exercise means relative fitness. *The Physician and Sportsmedicine*, **14**, 202-206.

Montoye, H.J. (1986). Physical activity, physical fitness, and heart disease risk factors in children. In G.A. Stull & H.M. Eckert (Eds.), *The effects of physical activity on children* (pp. 127-152). Champaign, IL: Human Kinetics.

Montoye, H.J., Metzner, H.L., Keller, J.B., Johnson, B.C., & Epstein, F.H. (1972). Habitual physical activity and blood pressure. *Medicine and Science in Sports*, **4**, 175-181.

Morgan, W.P. (1981). Psychologic benefits of physical activity. In F.J. Nagle & H.J. Montoye (Eds.), *Exercise in health and disease* (pp. 299-314). Springfield, IL: Charles C Thomas.

Morgan, W.P. (1985). Affective beneficence of vigorous physical activity. *Medicine and Science in Sports and Exercise*, **17**, 94-100.

Morgan, W.P., Roberts, J.A., & Feinerman, A.D. (1971). Psychologic effect of acute physical activity. *Archives of Physical Medicine and Rehabilitation*, **52**, 442-449.

Morganroth, J., Maron, B.J., Henry, W.L., & Epstein, J.E. (1975). Comparative left ventricular dimensions in trained athletes. *Annals of Internal Medicine*, **82**, 521-524.

Morgensen, C.E., & Vittinghaus, E. (1975). Urinary albumin excretion during exercise in juvenile diabetes. *Scandinavian Journal of Clinical and Laboratory Investigation*, **35**, 295-300.

Moritani, T., & deVries, H.A. (1980). Potential for gross hypertrophy in older men. *Journal of Gerontology*, **35**, 672-682.

Morris, J.N., Chave, S.P.W., Adam, C., Sirey, C., Epstein, L., & Sheehan, D.J. (1973). Vigorous exercise in leisure time and the incidence of coronary heart disease. *The Lancet*, **1**, 333-339.

Morris, J.N., Everitt, M.G., Pollard, R., Chave, S.P.W., & Semmence, A.M. (1980). Vigorous exercise in leisure time: Protection against coronary heart disease. *Lancet*, **2**, 1207-1210.

Morse, M., Schultz, F.W., & Cassels, D.E. (1949). Relation of age to physiological responses of the older boy (10 to 17 years) to exercise. *Journal of Applied Physiology*, **1**, 683-709.

Mueller, F., & Blyth, C. (1982). Epidemiology of sports injuries in children. *Clinics in Sports Medicine*, **1**, 343-352.

Mullins, A.G. (1958). The prognosis in juvenile obesity. *Archives of Disease of Childhood*, **33**, 307-314.

Murphy, P. (1986). Youth fitness testing: A matter of health or performance? *The Physician and Sportsmedicine*, **14**, 189-190.

Nader, P.R., Taras, H.L., Sallis, J.F., & Patterson, T.L. (1987). Adult heart disease prevention in children: A national survey of pediatricians' practices and attitudes. *Pediatrics*, **79**, 843-850.

Nash, H.L. (1987). Elite child-athletes: How much does victory cost? *The Physician and Sportsmedicine*, **15**, 129-133.

332 • References

National Strength and Conditioning Association (1985). Position paper on prepubescent strength training. *National Strength and Conditioning Association Journal*, **7**, 27-31.

Neijens, H.J. (1985). Children with lung disease and exercise. In R.A. Binkhorst, H.C.G. Kemper, & W.H.M. Saris (Eds.), *Children and exercise XI* (pp. 81-92). Champaign, IL: Human Kinetics.

Newman, W.P., & Strong, J.P. (1978). Natural history, geographic pathology, and pediatric aspects of atherosclerosis. In W.B. Strong (Ed.), *Atherosclerosis: Its pediatric aspects* (pp. 15-40). New York: Grune & Stratton.

Nickerson, B.G., Bautista, D.B., Namey, M.A., Richards, W., & Keens, T.G. (1983). Distance running improves fitness in asthmatic children without pulmonary complications or changes in exercise-induced bronchospasm. *Pediatrics*, **71**, 147-152.

Nizankowski-Blaz, T., & Abramowicz, T. (1983). Effects of intensive physical training on serum lipids and lipoproteins. *Acta Paediatrica Scandinavica*, **72**, 357-359.

Nudel, D.B., Diamant, S., Brady, T., Jarenwattanon, M., Buckley, B.J., & Gootman, N. (1987). Chest pain, dyspnea on exertion, and exercise induced asthma in children and adolescents. *Clinical Pediatrics*, **26**, 388-392.

Ogilvie, B.C., & Tutko, T.A. (1971, October). Sport: If you want to build character try something else. *Psychology Today*, 61-63.

Ogunyemi, A.O., Gomez, M.R., & Klass, D.W. (1988). Seizures induced by exercise. *Neurology*, **38**, 633-634.

Ojala, C.F. (1987, May). A geography of major interscholastic women's sports in the United States. *The Geographical Bulletin*, 24-43.

Olavi, O., Hirvonen, L., Peltonen, T., & Valimaki, I. (1965). Physical working capacity of normal and diabetic children. *Annale Paediatrica Fenn*, **11**, 25-31.

Oliver, J.N. (1958). The effects of physical conditioning exercises and activities on the mental characteristics of educationally subnormal boys. *British Journal of Educational Psychology*, **28**, 155-165.

Orenstein, D.M., Franklin, B.A., Doershuk, C.F., Hellerstein, H.K., & Germann, K.J. (1981). Exercise conditioning and cardiopulmonary fitness in cystic fibrosis: The effects of a three-month supervised running program. *Chest*, **80**, 392-398.

Orenstein, D.M., Germann, K.J., & Costill, D.L. (1981). Exercise in the heat in cystic fibrosis patients (abstract). *Medicine and Science in Sports and Exercise*, **13**, 91.

Orenstein, D.M., Henke, K.G., & Cerny, F.J. (1983). Exercise and cystic fibrosis. *The Physician and Sportsmedicine*, **11**, 57-63.

Orenstein, D.M., Reed, M.E., Grogan, F.T., & Crawford, L.V. (1985). Exercise conditioning in children with asthma. *Journal of Pediatrics*, **106**, 556-560.

Oscai, L., Babirak, S.P., & Dubach, F.B. (1974). Exercise or food restriction: Effect on adipose tissue cellularity. *American Journal of Physiology*, **227**, 901-904.

Osternig, L.R. (1986). Isokinetic dynamometry: Implications for muscle testing and rehabilitation. *Exercise and Sport Science Reviews*, **14**, 45-80.

Otis, A.B., Fenn, W.O., & Rahn, H. (1950). Mechanics of breathing in man. *Journal of Applied Physiology*, **2**, 592-607.

Paffenbarger, R.S., & Hyde, R.T. (1984). Exercise in the prevention of coronary heart disease. *Preventive Medicine*, **13**, 3-22.

Paffenbarger, R.S., Hyde, R.T., Wing, A.L., & Hsieh, C. (1986). Physical activity, all-cause mortality, and longevity of college alumni. *New England Journal of Medicine*, **314**, 605-613.

Paffenbarger, R.S., Hyde, R.T., Wing, A.L., & Steinmetz, C.H. (1984). A natural history of athleticism and cardiovascular health. *Journal of the American Medical Association*, **252**, 491-495.

Paffenbarger, R.S., Laughlin, M.E., Gina, A.S., & Black, R.A. (1970). Work activity of longshoremen as related to death from coronary heart disease and stroke. *New England Journal of Medicine*, **282**, 1109-1114.

Paffenbarger, R.S., Wing, A.L., Hyde, R.T., & Jung, D.L. (1983). Physical activity and incidence of hypertension in college alumni. *American Journal of Epidemiology*, **117**, 245-257.

Page, L.B. (1980a). Dietary sodium and blood pressure: Evidence from human studies. In R.M. Lauer & R.B. Shekelle (Eds.), *Childhood prevention of atherosclerosis and hypertension* (pp. 291-303). New York: Raven.

Page, L.B. (1980b). Hypertension and atherosclerosis in primitive and acculturating societies. In J.C. Hunt, T. Cooper, E.D. Frohlick, R.W. Gifford, N.M. Kaplan, J.H. Laragh, M.H. Maxwell, & C.G. Strong (Eds.), *Hypertension update: Mechanisms, epidemiology, evaluation, management* (pp. 1-12). Bloomfield, NJ: Health Learning Systems.

Page, L.B., Friedlander, J., & Moellering, R.C. (1977). Culture, human biology, and disease in the Solomon Islands. In G.A. Harrison (Ed.), *Population structure and human variation* (pp. 143-164). Cambridge: Cambridge University Press.

Painter, P.L. (1988). Exercise in end-stage renal disease. *Exercise and Sport Sciences Reviews*, **16**, 305-339.

Panico, S., Celentano, E., Krogh, V., Jossa, F., Farinaro, E., Trevisan, M., & Mancini, M. (1987). Physical activity and its relationship to blood pressure in school children. *Journal of Chronic Diseases*, **40**, 925-930.

Pardy, R.L., Hussain, S.N.A., & MacKlem, P.T. (1984). The ventilatory pump in exercise. *Clinics in Chest Medicine*, **5**, 35-49.

Parizkova, J. (1977). *Body fat and physical fitness*. The Hague: Martinus Nijhoff.

Pate, R.R., & Blair, S.N. (1978). Exercise and the prevention of atherosclerosis: Pediatric implications. In W.B. Strong (Ed.), *Atherosclerosis: Its pediatric aspects* (pp. 251-286). New York: Grune & Stratton.

Paterson, D.H., McLellan, T.M., Stella, R.S., & Cunningham, D.A. (1987). Longitudinal study of ventilation threshold and maximal O_2 uptake in athletic boys. *Journal of Applied Physiology*, 62, 2051-2057.

Pena, M., Barta, L., Regoly-Merei, A., & Tichy, M. (1980). The influence of physical exercise upon the body composition of obese children. *Acta Paediatrica Academiae Scientiarum Hungaricae*, 21, 9-14.

Persson, B., & Thoren, C. (1980). Prolonged exercise in adolescent boys with juvenile diabetes mellitus. *Acta Paediatrica Scandinavica*, Suppl. 283, 62-69.

Pert, C.B., & Bowie, D.L. (1979). Behavioral manipulation of rats causes alterations in opiate receptor occupancy. In E. Usdin, W.E. Bunnery, & N.S. Kline (Eds.), *Endorphins in mental health* (pp. 93-104). New York: Oxford University Press.

Peters, R.K., Cady, L.D., Bischoff, D.P., Bernstein, L., & Pike, M.C. (1983). Physical fitness and subsequent myocardial infarction in healthy workers. *Journal of the American Medical Association*, 249, 3052-3056.

Peterson, C.M., Jones, R.L., Esterly, J.A., Wantz, G.E., & Jackson, R.L. (1980). Changes in basement membrane thickening and pulse volume concomitant with improved glucose control and exercise in patients with insulin-dependent diabetes mellitus. *Diabetes Care*, 3, 586-589.

Petrofsky, J.S., & Phillips, C.A. (1986). The physiology of static exercise. *Exercise and Sport Sciences Reviews*, 14, 1-44.

Pfeiffer, R.D., & Francis, R.S. (1986). Effects of strength training on muscle development in prepubescent, pubescent, and postpubescent males. *The Physician and Sportsmedicine*, 14, 137-143.

Phelan, P., & Hey, E. (1984). Cystic fibrosis mortality in England and Wales and in Victoria, Australia 1976-80. *Archives of Disease in Childhood*, 59, 71-73.

Pierson, W.E., & Bierman, C.W. (1975). Free running test for exercise-induced bronchospasm. *Pediatrics*, 56(Suppl.), 890-892.

Pi-Sunyer, X.F., & Woo, R. (1985). Effect of exercise on food intake in human subjects. *American Journal of Clinical Nutrition*, 42, 983-990.

Pittet, P., Chappius, P., Acheson, K., DeTechtermann, F., & Jequier, E. (1976). Thermic effects of glucose in obese subjects studied by direct and indirect calorimetry. *British Journal of Nutrition*, 35, 281-292.

Poortmans, J.R., Saerens, P., Edelman, R., Vertongen, F., & Dorchy, H. (1986). Influence of the degree of metabolic control on physical fitness in type I diabetic adolescents. *International Journal of Sports Medicine*, 7, 232-235.

Porcari, J., McCarron, R., Kline, G., Freedson, P., Ward, A., Ross, J., & Rippe, J. (1987). Is fast walking an adequate aerobic stimulus for 30- to 69-year old men and women? *The Physician and Sportsmedicine*, 15, 119-129.

Prineas, R.J., Gillum, R.F., & Blackburn, H. (1980). Possibilities for primary prevention of hypertension. In R.M. Lauer & R.B. Shekelle (Eds.), *Childhood prevention of atherosclerosis and hypertension* (pp. 357-366). New York: Raven.

Pyeritz, R.E., & McKusick, V.A. (1979). The Marfan syndrome: Diagnosis and management. *The New England Journal of Medicine, 300,* 772-777.

Raithel, K.S. (1987). Are girls less fit than boys? *The Physician and Sportsmedicine, 15,* 157-163.

Ransford, C.P. (1982). The role for amines in the antidepressant effect of exercise: A review. *Medicine and Science in Sports and Exercise, 14,* 1-10.

Rape, R.N. (1987). Running and depression. *Perceptual and Motor Skills, 64,* 1303-1310.

Rasanen, L., Ahola, M., Kara, R., & Uhari, M. (1985). Atherosclerotic precursors in Finnish children and adolescents. VIII. Food consumption and nutrient intakes. *Acta Paediatrica Scandinavica,* Suppl. 318, 135-153.

Raskin, L.A., Shaywitz, S.E., Shaywitz, B.A., Anderson, G.M., & Cohen, D.J. (1984). Neurochemical correlates of attention deficit disorder. *Pediatric Clinics of North America, 31,* 387-396.

Raskin, P., Marks, J.F., Burns, H., Plumer, M.E., & Siperstein, M.D. (1975). Capillary basement membrane width in diabetic children. *American Journal of Medicine, 58,* 365-371.

Rauh, J.C., Schumsky, D.A., & Witt, M.T. (1967). Heights, weights, and obesity in urban school children. *Child Development, 28,* 515-521.

Ravussin, E., Lillioja, S., Knowler, W.C., Christin, L., Freymond, D., Abbott, W.G.H., Boyce, V., Howard, B.V., & Bogardus, C. (1988). Reduced energy expenditure as a risk factor for body weight gain. *New England Journal of Medicine, 318,* 467-472.

Ready, A.E., & Quinney, H.A. (1982). Alterations in anaerobic threshold as the result of endurance training and detraining. *Medicine and Science in Sports and Exercise, 14,* 292-296.

Reisen, E., Abel, R., Modan, M., Silverberg, D.S., Eliahou, H.E., & Modan, B. (1978). Effect of weight loss without salt restriction on the reduction of blood pressure in overweight hypertensive patients. *New England Journal of Medicine, 298,* 1-5.

Requa, R., & Garrick, J.G. (1981). Injuries in interscholastic wrestling. *The Physician and Sportsmedicine, 9,* 44-51.

Rians, C.B., Weltman, A., Cahill, B.R., Janney, C.A., Tippett, S.R., & Katch, F.I. (1987). Strength training for prepubescent males: Is it safe? *The American Journal of Sports Medicine, 15,* 483-489.

Rice, S.G., Bierman, C.W., Shapiro, G.G., Furukawa, C.T., & Pierson, W.E. (1985). Identification of exercise-induced asthma among intercollegiate athletes. *Annals of Allergy, 55,* 790-793.

Rigotti, N.A., Thomas, G.S., & Leaf, A. (1983). Exercise and coronary heart disease. *Annual Review of Medicine*, **34**, 391-412.

Riley, W.J., & Rosenbloom, A.L. (1980). Exercise and insulin dependent diabetes mellitus. *Journal of the Florida Medical Association*, **67**, 392-394.

Riopel, D.A., Tayler, A.B., & Hohn, A.R. (1979). Blood pressure, heart rate, pressure-rate product, and electrocardiographic changes in healthy children during treadmill exercise. *American Journal of Cardiology*, **44**, 697-703.

Roan, Y., & Galant, S.P. (1981). The ontogeny of neutrophil beta-adrenergic receptors. *Clinical Research*, **29**, 144A.

Roberts, S.B., Savage, J., Coward, W.A., Chew, B., & Lucas, A. (1988). Energy expenditure and intake in infants born to lean and overweight mothers. *New England Journal of Medicine*, **318**, 461-466.

Robinson, S. (1938). Experimental studies of physical fitness in relation to age. *Arbeitsphysiologie*, **10**, 251-323.

Roche, A.F. (1984). Anthropometric methods: New and old, what they tell us. *International Journal of Obesity*, **8**, 509-523.

Rode, A., Bar-Or, O., & Shephard, R.J. (1973). Cardiac output and oxygen conductance. A comparison of Canadian Eskimos and city dwellers. In O. Bar-Or (Ed.), *Pediatric work physiology* (pp. 45-47). Natanya, Israel: Wingate Institute.

Rogol, A.D. (1988). Pubertal development in endurance-trained female athletes. In E.W. Brown & C.F. Branta (Eds.), *Competitive sports for children and youth* (pp. 173-193). Champaign, IL: Human Kinetics.

Rollard-Cachera, M.F., Sempe, M., Guilloud-Bataille, M., Patois, E., Pequignot-Guggenbuhl, F., & Fautrad, V. (1982). Adiposity in children. *American Journal of Clinical Nutrition*, **36**, 178-184.

Romero, T.E., & Friedman, W.F. (1979). Limited left ventricular response to volume overload in the neonatal period: A comparative study with the adult animal. *Pediatric Research*, **13**, 910-915.

Rooks, D.S., & Micheli, L.J. (1988). Musculoskeletal assessment and training: The young athlete. *Clinics in Sports Medicine*, **7**, 641-677.

Rose, H.E., & Mayer, J. (1968). Activity, caloric intake, and the energy balance of infants. *Pediatrics*, **41**, 18-23.

Ross, J.G., Dotson, C., Gilbert, G., & Katz, S. (1985). The National Children and Youth Fitness Study: Maturation and fitness test performance. *Journal of Physical Education, Recreation, and Dance*, **56**, 67-69.

Ross, J.G., & Pate, R.R. (1987). The National Children and Youth Fitness Study II. A summary of findings. *Journal of Physical Education, Recreation, and Dance*, **58**, 51-56.

Rost, R. (1987). *Athletics and the heart*. Chicago: Year Book Medical Publishers.

Rotella, R.J., & Bunker, L.K. (1987). *Parenting your superstar*. Champaign, IL: Leisure Press.

Roth, D.L., & Holmes, D.S. (1985). Influence of physical fitness in determining the impact of stressful life events on physical and psychological health. *Psychosomatic Medicine, 47*, 164-173.

Rotkis, T., Boyden, T.W., Pamenter, R.W., Stanforth, P., & Wilmore, J. (1981). High density lipoprotein cholesterol and body composition of female runners. *Metabolism, 30*, 994-995.

Rotstein, A., Dotan, R., Bar-Or, O., & Tenenbaum, G. (1986). Effect of training on anaerobic threshold, maximal aerobic power, and anaerobic performance of preadolescent boys. *International Journal of Sports Medicine, 7*, 281-286.

Round Table (1983). Overtraining of athletes. *The Physician and Sportsmedicine, 11*, 93-110.

Round Table (1984). Exercise and asthma. *The Physician and Sportsmedicine, 12*, 59-77.

Round Table (1987). The health benefits of exercise. *The Physician and Sportsmedicine, 15*, 115-132.

Routh, D.K., Schroeder, C., & O'Tuama, L. (1974). Development of activity level in children. *Developmental Psychology, 10*, 163-168.

Rowland, T.W. (1981). Physical fitness in children: Implications for the prevention of coronary artery disease. *Current Problems in Pediatrics, 11*, 1-54.

Rowland, T.W. (1985). Aerobic response to endurance training in prepubescent children: A critical analysis. *Medicine and Science in Sports and Exercise, 17*, 493-497.

Rowland, T.W. (1986). Motivational factors in exercise training programs for children. *The Physician and Sportsmedicine, 14*, 122-128.

Rowland, T.W. (1989). [Aerobic responses to walking training in children]. Unpublished raw data.

Rowland, T.W., Auchinachie, J.A., Keenan, T.J., & Green, G.M. (1987). Physiologic responses to treadmill running in adult and prepubertal males. *International Journal of Sports Medicine, 8*, 292-297.

Rowland, T.W., Auchinachie, J.A., Keenan, T.J., & Green, G.M. (1988). Submaximal aerobic running economy and treadmill performance in prepubertal boys. *International Journal of Sports Medicine, 9*, 201-204.

Rowland, T.W., & Green, G.M. (1988). Physiologic responses to treadmill exercise in females: Adult-child differences. *Medicine and Science in Sports and Exercise, 20*, 474-478.

Rowland, T.W., & Green, G.M. (1989). Anaerobic threshold and the determination of target training heart rates in premenarchal girls. *Pediatric Cardiology, 10*, 75-79.

Rowland, T.W., & Hoontis, P.P. (1985). Organizing road races for children: Special concerns. *The Physician and Sportsmedicine, 13*, 126-132.

Rowland, T.W., Morris, A.H., Kelleher, J.F., Haag, B.L., & Reiter, E.O. (1987). Serum testosterone response to training in adolescent runners. *American Journal of Diseases of Children, 141*, 881-883.

Rowland, T.W., Staab, J., Unnithan, V., & Siconolfi, S. (1988). Maximal cardiac responses in prepubertal and adult males (abstract). *Medicine and Science in Sports and Exercise*, **20**(Suppl.), S32.

Rowland, T.W., Swadba, L.A., Biggs, D.E., Burke, E., and Reiter, E.O. (1985). Glycemic control with physical training in insulin-dependent diabetes mellitus. *American Journal of Diseases of Children*, **139**, 307-310.

Rowland, T.W., & Walsh, C.A. (1985). Characteristics of child distance runners. *The Physician and Sportsmedicine*, **13**, 45-53.

Rubler, S., & Arvan, S.B. (1975). Exercise testing in young asymptomatic diabetic patients. *Angiology*, **27**, 539-548.

Rutenfranz, J. (1986). Longitudinal approach to assessing maximal aerobic power during growth: The European experience. *Medicine and Science in Sports and Exercise*, **18**, 270-275.

Ruttenberg, H.D., Adams, T.D., Orsmond, G.S., Conlee, R.K., & Fisher, A.G. (1983). Effects of exercise training on aerobic fitness in children after open heart surgery. *Pediatric Cardiology*, **4**, 19-24.

Ryan, A.J. (1984). Exercise and health: Lessons from the past. In H.M. Eckert & H.J. Montoye (Eds.), *Exercise and health* (pp. 3-13). Champaign, IL: Human Kinetics.

Sady, S.P. (1986). Cardiorespiratory exercise training in children. *Clinics in Sports Medicine*, 493-514.

Sady, S.P., Berg, K., Beal, D., Smith, J.L., Savage, M.P., Thompson, W.H., & Nutter, J. (1984). Aerobic fitness and serum high density lipoprotein cholesterol in young children. *Human Biology*, **56**, 771-781.

Sady, S.P., & Katch, V.L. (1981). Relative endurance and physiological responses: A study of individual differences in prepubescent boys and adult men. *Research Quarterly for Exercise and Sport*, **52**, 246-255.

Safrit, M.J. (1986). Health-related fitness levels of American youth. In G.A. Stull & H.M. Eckert (Eds.), *Effects of physical activity on children* (pp. 153-166). Champaign, IL: Human Kinetics.

Sage, G.H. (1986a). The effects of physical activity on the social development of children. In G.A. Stull & H.M. Eckert (Eds.), *Effects of physical activity on children* (pp. 22-29). Champaign, IL: Human Kinetics.

Sage, G.H. (1986b). Social development. In V.S. Seefeldt (Ed.), *Physical activity and well-being* (pp. 343-371). Reston, VA: American Alliance for Health, Physical Education, Recreation and Dance.

Salke, R.C., Rowland, T.W., & Burke, E.J. (1985). Left ventricular size and function in body builders using anabolic steroids. *Medicine and Science in Sports and Exercise*, **17**, 701-704.

Sallis, J.F. (1987). A commentary on children and fitness: A public health perspective. *Research Quarterly for Exercise and Sport*, **58**, 326-330.

Sallis, J.F., Patterson, T.L., McKenzie, T.L., & Nader, P.R. (1988). Family variables and physical activity in preschool children. *Developmental and Behavioral Pediatrics*, **9**, 57-61.

Saltin, B., Houston, M., & Nygaard, E. (1979). Muscle fiber characteristics in healthy men and patients with juvenile diabetes. *Diabetes, Suppl.* 28, 93-99.

Saris, W.H.M. (1986). Habitual physical activity in children: Methodology and findings in health and disease. *Medicine and Science in Sports and Exercise*, 18, 253-263.

Saris, W.H.M., & Binkhorst, R.A. (1977). The use of pedometer and actometer in studying daily physical activity in man. *European Journal of Applied Physiology*, 37, 219-228.

Saris, W.H.M., Elvers, J.W.H., van't Hof, M.A., & Binkhorst, R.A. (1986). Changes in physical activity of children aged 6 to 12 years. In J. Rutenfranz, R. Mocellin, & F. Klimt (Eds.), *Children and exercise XII* (pp. 121-130). Champaign, IL: Human Kinetics.

Sasaki, J., Shindo, M., Tanaka, H., Ando, M., & Arakawa, K. (1987). A long-term aerobic exercise program decreases the obesity index and increases the high density lipoprotein cholesterol concentration in obese children. *International Journal of Obesity*, 11, 339-345.

Savage, M.P., Petratis, M.M., Thomson, W.H., Berg, K., Smith, J.L., & Sady, S.P. (1986). Exercise training effects on serum lipids of prepubescent boys and adult men. *Medicine and Science in Sports and Exercise*, 18, 197-204.

Scanlan, T.K., & Passer, M.W. (1978). Factors related to competitive stress among male youth sport participants. *Medicine and Science in Sports*, 10, 103-108.

Schaible, T.F., Malhotra, A., Ciambrone, G., & Scheuer, J. (1984). The effects of gonadectomy on left ventricular function and cardiac contractile proteins in male and female rats. *Circulation Research*, 54, 38-49.

Scheuer, J., Malhotra, A., Schaible, T.F., & Capasso, J. (1987). Effects of gonadectomy and hormonal replacement on rat hearts. *Circulation*, 61, 12-19.

Schmidt-Nielsen, K. (1984). *Scaling. Why is animal size so important?* Cambridge: Cambridge University Press.

Schmucker, B., Rigauer, B., Hinrichs, W., & Trawinski, J. (1984). Motor abilities and habitual activity in children. In J. Ilmarinen & I. Valimaki (Eds.), *Children and sport* (pp. 46-52). Berlin: Springer.

Schramm, W., Lyle, J., & Parker, E.B. (1961). *Television in the lives of our children*. Stanford, CA: Stanford University Press.

Scott, E.C., & Johnston, F.E. (1982). Critical fat, menarche, and the maintenance of menstrual cycles. A critical review. *Journal of Adolescent Health Care*, 2, 249-260.

Scrimshaw, N.S., & Guzman, M.A. (1968). Diet and atherosclerosis. *Laboratory Investigation*, 18, 623-628.

Seals, D.R., & Hagberg, J.M. (1984). The effect of exercise training on human hypertension: A review. *Medicine and Science in Sports and Exercise*, 16, 207-215.

Seefeldt, V., & Vogel, P. (1987). Children and fitness: A public health perspective. *Research Quarterly for Exercise and Sport*, **58**, 331-333.

Segal, K.R., & Gutin, B. (1983). Thermic effects of food and exercise in lean and obese women. *Metabolism*, **32**, 581-589.

Segrave, J.O. (1981). *An investigation into the relationship between participation in interscholastic athletics and delinquent behavior*. Unpublished doctoral dissertation, Arizona State University, Tempe.

Segrave, J.O. (1983). Sport and juvenile delinquency. *Exercise and Sport Sciences Reviews*, **11**, 181-209.

Seliger, V., Cermak, V., & Handzo, P. (1971). Physical fitness of the Czechoslovak 12- and 15-year old population. *Acta Paediatrica Scandinavica*, Suppl. 217, 37-41.

Seliger, V., Trefny, Z., Bartunkova, S., & Pauer, M. (1974). The habitual activity and physical fitness of 12 year old boys. *Acta Paediatrica Belgica*, **28**(Suppl.), 54-59.

Seltzer, C.C., & Mayer, J. (1970). An effective weight control program in a public school system. *American Journal of Public Health*, **60**, 679-689.

Servedio, F.J., Bartels, R.L., Hamlin, R.L., Teske, D., Shaffer, T., & Servedio, A. (1985). The effects of weight training, using Olympic style lifts, on various physiological variables in pre-pubescent boys (abstract). *Medicine and Sciences in Sports and Exercise*, **17**, 288.

Sewall, L., & Micheli, L.J. (1986). Strength training for children. *Journal of Pediatric Orthopedics*, **6**, 143-146.

Shaffer, T.E. (1979). The physician and sports medicine. In Ross Roundtable, *Sports medicine for children and youth* (pp. 1-8). Columbus, OH: Ross Laboratories.

Shaffer, T.E. (1983). The physician's role in sports medicine. *Journal of Adolescent Health Care*, **3**, 227-230.

Shangold, M.M. (1986). Gynecological concerns in young and adolescent physically active girls. *Pediatrician*, **13**, 10-13.

Shangold, M., Freeman, R., Thysen, B., & Gatz, M. (1979). The relationship between long-distance running, plasma progesterone, and luteal phase length. *Fertility and Sterility*, **31**, 130-136.

Sharp, M.W., & Reilley, R.R. (1975). The relationship of aerobic physical fitness to selected personality traits. *Journal of Clinical Psychology*, **31**, 428-432.

Shaver, L.G. (1972). Comparison of physical fitness scores of high school girl smokers and non-smokers. *American Corrective Therapy Journal*, **26**, 174-177.

Shaw, K.R., Sheehan, K.H., & Fernandez, R.C. (1987). Suicide in children and adolescents. *Advances in Pediatrics*, **34**, 313-334.

Shaywitz, B.A., Gordon, J.W., Klopper, J.H., & Zelterman, D.A. (1977). The effect of 6-hydroxydopamine on habituation of activity in the developing rat pup. *Pharmacology, Biochemistry, & Behavior*, **6**, 391-396.

Sheehan, G. (1983). Life-styleosis. *The Physician and Sportsmedicine*, **11**, 53.

Sheldahl, L.M. (1986). Special ergometric techniques and weight reduction. *Medicine and Science in Sports and Exercise*, **18**, 25-30.

Shephard, R.J. (1982). *Physical activity and growth*. Chicago: Year Book Medical Publishers.

Shephard, R.J. (1983). Physical activity and the healthy mind. *Canadian Medical Association Journal*, **128**, 525-530.

Shephard, R.J. (1985). Exercise regimens after myocardial infarction: Rationale and results. *Cardiovascular Clinics*, **15**, 145-157.

Shephard, R.J. (1988). Does cardiac rehabilitation after myocardial infarction favorably affect prognosis? *The Physician and Sportsmedicine*, **16**, 116-129.

Shephard, R.J., Allen, C., Bar-Or, O., Davies, C.T.M., Degre, S., Hedman, R., Ishii, K., Kaneko, M., LaCour, J.R., diPrampero, P.E., & Seliger, V. (1969). The working capacity of Toronto schoolchildren. *Canadian Medical Association Journal*, **100**, 560-566.

Shetty, P.S., Jung, R.T., James, W.P.T., Barrand, M.D., & Callingham, B.A. (1981). Postprandial thermogenesis in obesity. *Clinical Science*, **60**, 519-525.

Shively, R.A., Grana, S.W., & Ellis, D. (1981). High school sports injuries. *The Physician and Sportsmedicine*, **9**, 46-50.

Silverman, S., & Anderson, S.D. (1972). Standardization of exercise tests in asthmatic children. *Archives of Disease of Childhood*, **47**, 882-889.

Sim, F.H., & Simonet, W.T. (1988). Ice hockey injuries. *The Physician and Sportsmedicine*, **16**, 92-105.

Simic, B.S. (1980). Childhood obesity as a risk factor in adulthood. In P.J. Collipp (Ed.), *Childhood obesity* (2nd ed., pp. 3-23). Littleton, MA: PSG Publishing.

Simmons, K. (1986). Back to school for youth fitness tests. *The Physician and Sportsmedicine*, **14**, 155-160.

Simon, J.A., & Martens, R. (1979). Children's anxiety in sport and non-sport evaluative activities. *Journal of Sport Psychology*, **1**, 160-169.

Simons-Morton, B.G., O'Hara, N.M., Simons-Morton, D.G., & Parcel, G.S. (1987). Children and fitness: A public health perspective. *Research Quarterly for Exercise and Sport*, **58**, 295-302.

Simonson, M. (1982). Advances in research and treatment of obesity. *Food and Nutrition News*, **53**, 1-4.

Skeie, B., Askanazi, J., Rothkopf, M.M., Rosenbaum, S.H., Kvetan, V., & Ross, E. (1987). Improved exercise tolerance with long-term parenteral nutrition in cystic fibrosis. *Critical Care Medicine*, **15**, 960-962.

Skrobac-Kaczynski, J., & Vavik, T. (1980). Physical fitness and trainability of young male patients with Down syndrome. In K. Berg & B.O. Eriksson (Eds.), *Children and exercise IX* (pp. 300-316). Baltimore: University Park Press.

Sloan, W. (1951). Motor proficiency and intelligence. *American Journal of Mental Deficiency*, **55**, 394-406.

Slusher, H.S. (1964). Personality and intelligence characteristics of selected high school athletes and non-athletes. *Research Quarterly*, **35**, 539-545.

Smilkstein, G. (1980). Psychological trauma in children and youth in competitive sports. *The Journal of Family Practice*, **10**, 737-739.

Smith, B.W., Metheny, W.P., Van Huss, W.D., Seefeldt, V.D., & Sparrow, A.W. (1983). Serum lipids and lipoprotein profiles in elite age-group endurance runners (abstract). *Circulation*, **68**, 191.

Smith, N.J. (1980). Excessive weight loss and food aversion in athletes simulating anorexia nervosa. *Pediatrics*, **66**, 139-142.

Smith, N.J., Smith, R.E., & Smoll, F.L. (1983). *Kidsports. A survival guide for parents*. Reading, MA: Addison-Wesley.

Snell, P.G., & Mitchell, J.H. (1984). The role of maximum oxygen uptake in exercise performance. *Clinics in Chest Medicine*, **5**, 51-62.

Solomon, A.H. & Pangle, R. (1966). *The effects of a structured physical education program on physical, intellectual, and self-concept development of educable retarded boys* (Monograph No. 4). Institute on Mental Retardation and Intellectual Development Behavioral Science.

Sonstroem, R.J. (1978). Physical estimation and attraction scales: Rationale and research. *Medicine and Science in Sports*, **10**, 97-102.

Sonstroem, R.J. (1984). Exercise and self-esteem. *Exercise and Sports Sciences Reviews*, **12**, 123-155.

Spirduso, W.W. (1986). Physical activity and the prevention of premature aging. In V. Seefeldt (Ed.), *Physical activity and well-being* (pp. 141-160). Reston, VA: American Alliance for Health, Physical Education, Recreation and Dance.

Sprynarova, S., & Parizkova, J. (1965). Changes in the aerobic capacity and body composition in obese boys after reduction. *Journal of Applied Physiology*, **20**, 934-937.

Stager, J.M., Robertshaw, D., & Miescher, E. (1984). Delayed menarche in swimmers in relation to age at onset of training and athletic performance. *Medicine and Science in Sports and Exercise*, **16**, 550-555.

Stahl, W.R. (1965). Organ weights in primates and other mammals. *Science*, **150**, 1039-1042.

Stamler, J. (1980). Hypertension: Aspects of risk. In J.C. Hunt, T. Cooper, E.D. Frohlich, R.W. Gifford, N.M. Kaplan, J.H. Laragh, M.H. Maxwell, & C.G. Strong (Eds.), *Hypertension update: Mechanisms, epidemiology, evaluation, management* (pp. 22-37). Bloomfield, NJ: Health Learning Systems.

Stanghelle, J.K. (1988). Physical exercise for patients with cystic fibrosis: A review. *International Journal of Sports Medicine*, **9**(Suppl.), 6-18.

Stanghelle, J.K., Hjeltnes, N., Bangstad, H.J., & Michalsen, H. (1988). Effect of daily short bursts of trampoline exercise during 8 weeks on the pulmonary function and maximal oxygen uptake of children with cystic fibrosis. *International Journal of Sports Medicine*, 9(Suppl.), 32-36.

Stanghelle, J.K., & Skyberg, D. (1983). The successful completion of the Oslo marathon by a patient with cystic fibrosis. *Acta Paediatrica Scandinavica*, **72**, 935-938.

Stark, O., Atkins, E., Wolff, O., & Douglas, J. (1981). Longitudinal study of obesity in the National Survey of Health and Development. *British Medical Journal*, **283**, 13-17.

Stefanik, P.A., Heald, F.P., & Mayer, J. (1959). Caloric intake in relation to energy output of non-obese adolescent boys. *American Journal of Clinical Nutrition*, **7**, 55-62.

Stephens, K.E., Van Huss, W.D., Olson, H.W., & Montoye, H.J. (1984). The longevity, morbidity, and physical fitness of former athletes— an update. In H.M. Eckert & H.J. Montoye (Eds.), *Exercise and health* (pp. 101-119). Champaign, IL: Human Kinetics.

Sterky, G. (1963). Physical work capacity in diabetic school children. *Acta Paediatrica Scandinavica*, **52**, 1-10.

Sterky, G. (1970). *Physical fitness and training in juvenile diabetics*. Leiden: A. Laron.

Sterky, G., Larsson, Y., & Persson, B. (1963). Blood lipids in diabetic and non-diabetic school children. *Acta Paediatrica Scandinavica*, **52**, 11-21.

Stratton, R., Wilson, D.P., Endres, R.K., & Goldstein, D.E. (1987). Improved glycemic control after a supervised 8-week exercise program in insulin-dependent diabetic adolescents. *Diabetes Care*, **10**, 589-593.

Strong, W.B. (1978). *Atherosclerosis: Its pediatric aspects*. New York: Grune & Stratton.

Strong, W.B. (1987). Physical fitness of children: *Mens sana in corpore sano*. *American Journal of Diseases of Children*, **141**, 488.

Strong, W.B., & Alpert, B.S. (1982). The child with heart disease: Play, recreation, and sports. *Current Problems in Pediatrics*, **13**, 1-34.

Strong, W.B., Miller, M.D., Striplin, M., & Salehbhai, M. (1978). Blood pressure response to isometric and dynamic exercise in healthy black children. *American Journal of Diseases of Children*, **132**, 587-591.

Stunkard, A.J., Foch, T.T., & Hrubec, Z. (1986). A twin study of human obesity. *Journal of the American Medical Association*, **256**, 51-54.

Stunkard, A.J., & Pestka, J. (1962). The physical activity of obese girls. *American Journal of Diseases of Children*, **103**, 812-817.

Sullenger, T.E., Parke, L.H., & Wallin, W.K. (1953). The leisure time activities of elementary school children. *Journal of Educational Research*, **46**, 551-554.

Sunderland, G.W. (1976). Fire on ice. *The American Journal of Sports Medicine*, **4**, 264-269.

Sunnegardh, J., Bratteby, L.E., Hagman, U., Samuelson, G., & Sjolin, S. (1986). Physical activity in relation to energy intake and body fat in 8- and 13-year old children in Sweden. *Acta Paediatrica Scandinavica*, **75**, 955-963.

Sunnegardh, J., Bratteby, L., Sjolin, S., Hagman, V., & Hoffstedt, A. (1985). The relationship between physical activity and energy intake of 8- and 13-year old children in Sweden. In R.A. Binkhorst, H.C.G. Kemper, & W.H.M. Saris (Eds.), *Children and exercise XI* (pp. 183-193). Champaign, IL: Human Kinetics.

Svenonius, E., Kautto, R., & Arborelius, M. (1983). Improvement after training of children with exercise-induced asthma. *Acta Paediatrica Scandinavica*, **72**, 23-30.

Sweetgall, R., & Neeves, R. (1987). *Walking for little children*. Newark, DE: Creative Walking.

Tanner, J.M., & Whitehouse, R.H. (1975). Revised standards for triceps and subscapular skinfolds in British children. *Archives of Disease in Childhood*, **50**, 142-145.

Taylor, C.B., Sallis, J.F., & Needle, R. (1985). The relationship of physical activity and exercise to mental health. *Public Health Reports*, **100**, 195-202.

Taylor, C.R., Heglund, N.C., McMahon, T.A., & Looney, T.R. (1980). Energetic cost of generating muscular force during running: A comparison of large and small animals. *Journal of Experimental Biology*, **86**, 9-18.

Thomas, A.E., McKay, D.A., & Cutlip, M.B. (1976). A nomograph method for assessing body weight. *American Journal of Clinical Nutrition*, **29**, 302-304.

Thompson, J.K., Jarvie, G.J., Lahey, B.B., & Cureton, K.J. (1982). Exercise and obesity: Etiology, physiology, and intervention. *Psychological Bulletin*, **91**, 55-79.

Thorland, W.G., & Gilliam, T.B. (1981). Comparison of serum lipids between habitually high and low active preadolescent males. *Medicine and Science in Sports and Exercise*, **13**, 316-321.

Tipton, C.M. (1984). Exercise and resting blood pressure. In H.M. Eckert & H.J. Montoye (Eds.), *Exercise and health* (pp. 32-41). Champaign, IL: Human Kinetics.

Tomassoni, T.L., Galioto, F.M., Vaccaro, P., Vaccaro, J., & Howard, R.P. (1987). The pediatric cardiac rehabilitation program at Children's Hospital National Medical Center, Washington, D.C. *Journal of Cardiopulmonary Rehabilitation*, **7**, 259-262.

Tran, Z.V., Weltman, A., Glass, G.V., & Mood, D.P. (1983). The effects of exercise on blood lipids and lipoproteins: A meta-analysis of studies. *Medicine and Science in Sports and Exercise*, **15**, 393-402.

Treacy, J. & Cunningham, L. (1986, July). Training for high school cross country. *Boston Running News*, 36-40.

Tyroler, H.A., Heyden, S., & Hames, C.G. (1975). Weight and hypertension: Evans County study of blacks and whites. In O. Paul (Ed.),

Epidemiology and control of hypertension (pp. 173-191). New York: Stratton Intercontinental.

Vaccaro, P., Galioto, F.M., Bradley, L.M., & Vaccaro, J. (1987). Effect of physical training on exercise tolerance of children following surgical repair of D-transposition of the great arteries. *Journal of Sports Medicine, 27*, 443-448.

Vaccaro, P., & Mahon, A. (1987). Cardiorespiratory responses to endurance training in children. *Sports Medicine, 4*, 352-363.

Valimaki, I., Hursti, M.L., Pihlakoski, L., & Viikari, J. (1980). Exercise performance and serum lipids in relation to physical activity in school children. *International Journal of Sports Medicine, 1*, 132-136.

Van Camp, S.P., & Choi, J.H. (1988). Exercise and sudden death. *The Physician and Sportsmedicine, 16*, 49-52.

Vandenbroucke, N.P., van Laar, A., & Valkenburg, H.A. (1983). Synergy between thinness and intensive sport activity in delaying menarche. *British Medical Journal, 284*, 1907-1908.

Van Huss, W., Evans, S.A., Kurowski, T., Anderson, D.J., Allen, R., & Stephens, K. (1988). Physiologic characteristics of male and female age-group runners. In E.W. Brown & C.F. Branta (Eds.), *Competitive sports for children and youth* (pp. 143-158). Champaign, IL: Human Kinetics.

Verschuur, R., & Kemper, H.C.G. (1985). Habitual physical activity in Dutch teenagers measured by heart rate. In R.A. Binkhorst, H.C.G. Kemper, & W.H.M. Saris (Eds.), *Children and exercise XI* (pp. 194-202). Champaign, IL: Human Kinetics.

Verschuur, R., Kemper, H.C.G., & Besseling, C.W.M. (1984). Habitual physical activity and health in 13- and 14-year old teenagers. In J. Ilmarinen & I. Valimaki (Eds.), *Children and sport* (pp. 255-261). Berlin: Springer.

Viikari, J., Valimaki, I., Telama, R., Siren-Tiusanen, H., Akerblom, H.K., Dahl, M., Lahde, P.L., Pesonen, E., Pietikainen, M., Suoninen, P., & Uhari, M. (1984). Atherosclerosis precursors in Finnish children: Physical activity and plasma lipids in 3- and 12-year old children. In J. Ilmarinen & I. Valimaki (Eds.), *Children and sport* (pp. 231-240). Berlin: Springer.

Viteri, F., & Torun, B. (1974). Anemia and physical work capacity. *Clinics in Haematology, 3*, 609-626.

Von Dobeln, W. & Eriksson, B.O. (1972). Physical training, maximal oxygen consumption, and dimensions of the oxygen transporting and metabolizing organs in boys 11-13 years of age. *Acta Paediatrica Scandinavica, 61*, 653-660.

Voy, R.O. (1986). The U.S. Olympic Committee experience with exercise-induced bronchospasm, 1984. *Medicine and Science in Sports and Exercise, 18*, 328-330.

Vranic, M., & Berger, M. (1979). Exercise and diabetes mellitus. *Diabetes*, 28, 147-163.

Vrijens, J. (1978). Muscle strength development in the pre- and post-pubescent age. *Medicine and Sport*, 11, 152-158.

Walberg, J., & Ward, D. (1983). Role of physical activity in the etiology and treatment of childhood obesity. *Pediatrician*, 12, 82-88.

Wallberg-Henriksson, H., Gunnarsson, R., Henriksson, J., DeFronzo, R., Felig, P., Ostman, J., & Wahren, J. (1982). Increased peripheral insulin sensitivity and muscle mitochondrial enzymes but unchanged blood glucose control in type I diabetics after physical training. *Diabetes*, 31, 1044-1050.

Wanne, O., Viikari, J., & Valimaki, I. (1984). Physical performance and serum lipids in 14-16 year old trained, normally active, and inactive children. In J. Ilmarinen & I. Valimaki (Eds.), *Children and Sport* (pp. 241-246). Berlin: Springer.

Ward, A. (1987). Soccer: Safe kicks for kids. *The Physician and Sports-medicine*, 15, 150-156.

Ward, D.S., & Bar-Or, O. (1986). Role of the physician and physical education teacher in the treatment of obesity at school. *Pediatrician*, 13, 44-51.

Warren, M.P. (1980). The effects of exercise on pubertal progression and reproductive function in girls. *Journal of Clinical Endocrinology and Metabolism*, 51, 1150-1157.

Washington, R.L., van Gundy, J.C., Cohen, C., Sondheimer, H.M., & Wolfe, R.R. (1988). Normal aerobic and anaerobic exercise data for North American school-age children. *Journal of Pediatrics*, 112, 223-233.

Wasserman, K., Beaver, W.L., & Whipp, B.J. (1985). Mechanisms and patterns of blood lactate increase during exercise in man. *Medicine and Science in Sports and Exercise*, 18, 344-352.

Watkins, L.O., & Strong, W.B. (1984). The child: When to begin preventive cardiology. *Current Problems in Pediatrics*, 14, 1-63.

Watters, R.G., & Watters, W.E. (1980). Decreasing self-stimulatory behavior with physical exercise in a group of autistic boys. *Journal of Autism and Developmental Disorder*, 10, 379-383.

Waxman, M., & Stunkard, A.J. (1980). Caloric intake and expenditure of boys. *Journal of Pediatrics*, 96, 187-193.

Webber, L., Byrnes, W., Rowland, T., & Foster, V. (in press). Serum CK activity and delayed onset of muscle soreness in prepubescent children. *Pediatric Exercise Science*.

Webber, L.S., & Freedman, D.S. (1986). Interrelationships of coronary heart disease risk factors in children. In G.S. Berenson (Ed.), *Causation of cardiovascular risk factors in children* (pp. 65-81). New York: Raven.

Webber, L.S., Freedman, D.S., & Cresanta, J.L. (1986). Tracking of cardiovascular risk factor variables in school-age children. In G.S. Berenson (Ed.), *Causation of cardiovascular risk factors in children* (pp. 42-64). New York: Raven.

Weinhaus, R. (1969). The management of obesity: Some recent concepts. *Missouri Medicine, 66,* 719-730.

Wells, C.L. (1985). *Women, sport, & performance. A physiological perspective.* Champaign, IL: Human Kinetics.

Wells, C.L. (1986a). The effects of physical activity on cardiorespiratory fitness in children. In G.A. Stull & H.M. Eckert (Eds.), *Effects of physical activity on children* (pp. 114-126). Champaign, IL: Human Kinetics.

Wells, C.L. (1986b). Menstruation, pregnancy, and menopause. In V. Seefeldt (Ed.), *Physical activity and well-being* (pp. 211-234). Reston, VA: American Alliance for Health, Physical Education, Recreation and Dance.

Wells, C.L., & Plowman, S.A. (1988). Relationship between training, menarche, and amenorrhea. In E.W. Brown & C.F. Branta (Eds.), *Competitive sports for children and youth* (pp. 195-211). Champaign, IL: Human Kinetics.

Weltman, A., Janney, C., Rians, C.B., Strand, K., Berg, B., Tippitt, S., Wise, J., Cahill, B.R., & Katch, F.I. (1986). The effects of hydraulic resistance strength training in pre-pubertal males. *Medicine and Science in Sports and Exercise, 18,* 629-638.

Weltman, A., Janney, C., Rians, C.B., Strand, K., & Katch, F.I. (1987). The effects of hydraulic resistance strength training on serum lipid levels in prepubertal boys. *American Journal of Diseases of Children, 41,* 777-780.

Weymans, M., Reybrouck, T., Stijns, H.J., & Knops, J. (1985). Influence of age and sex on the ventilatory anaerobic threshold in children. In R.A. Binkhorst, H.C.G. Kemper, & W.H.M. Saris (Eds.), *Children and exercise XI* (pp. 114-118). Champaign, IL: Human Kinetics.

Weymans, M.L., Reybrouck, T.M., Stijns, H.J., & Knops, J. (1986). Influence of habitual levels of physical activity on the cardiorespiratory endurance capacity of children. In J. Rutenfranz, R. Mocellin, & F. Klimt (Eds.), *Children and exercise XII* (pp. 149-156). Champaign, IL: Human Kinetics.

Wheeler, G.D., Wall, S.R., Belcastro, A.N., & Cumming, D.C. (1984). Reduced serum testosterone and prolactin levels in male distance runners. *Journal of the American Medical Association, 252,* 514-516.

Whitehead, R.G., Paul, A.A., & Cole, T.J. (1982). Trends in food energy intakes throughout childhood from one to 18 years. *Human Applied Nutrition, 36,* 57-62.

Wickstrom, R.L. (1983). *Fundamental motor patterns.* Philadelphia: Lea & Febiger.

Widhalm, K., Maxa, E., & Zyman, H. (1978). Effect of diet and exercise upon the cholesterol and triglyceride content of plasma lipoproteins in overweight children. *European Journal of Pediatrics, 127,* 121-126.

Wilkie, D.R. (1950). The relation between force and velocity in human muscle. *Journal of Physiology, 110*, 249-280.

Wilkinson, P.W., Parkin, J.M., Pearlson, G., Strong, H., & Sykes, P. (1977). Energy intake and physical activity in obese children. *British Medical Journal, 1*, 756.

Williams, K.R. (1985). Biomechanics of running. *Exercise and Sport Science Reviews, 13*, 389-441.

Williams, M.H. (1986). Weight control through exercise and diet for children and young athletes. In G.A. Stull & H.M. Eckert (Eds.), *Effects of physical activity on children* (pp. 88-113). Champaign, IL: Human Kinetics.

Williams, R.S. (1985). Exercise training of patients with ventricular dysfunction and heart failure. *Cardiovascular Clinics, 15*, 219-231.

Williams, R.S., Logue, E.E., Lewis, J.L., Barton, T., Stead, N.W., Wallace, A.G., & Pizzo, S.V. (1980). Physical conditioning augments the fibrinolytic response to venous occlusion in healthy adults. *New England Journal of Medicine, 302*, 987-991.

Willman, H.C., & Chun, R.Y.F. (1973). Homeward Bound: An alternative to the institutionalization of adjudicated juvenile offenders. *Federal Probation Quarterly, 37*, 52-58.

Wilmore, J.H. (1983). Body composition in sport and exercise: Directions for future research. *Medicine and Science in Sports and Exercise, 15*, 21-31.

Wilmore, J.H., & McNamara, J.J. (1974). Prevalence of coronary heart disease risk factors in boys 8-12 years of age. *Journal of Pediatrics, 84*, 527-533.

Wilson, V.E., Berger, B.G., & Bird, E.I. (1981). Effects of running and of an exercise class on anxiety. *Perceptual and Motor Skills, 53*, 472-474.

Wolinsky, H., Goldfischer, & Katz, D. (1979). Hydrolase activity in the rat aorta. III. Effects of regular swimming activity and its cessation. *Circulation Research, 45*, 546-553.

Wolman, P. (1984). Feeding practices in infancy and prevalence of obesity in preschool children. *Journal of the American Dietetic Association, 84*, 436-438.

Wong, H.Y.C., David, S.N., & Orimilikwe, S.O. (1974). Effect of exercise on collagen and elastin in cockerels with induced atherosclerosis. In G. Weizel & G. Schettler (Eds.), *Atherosclerosis III* (pp. 362-365). New York: Springer.

Woo, R., Garrow, J., & Pi-Sunyer, F.X. (1982). Effect of exercise on spontaneous caloric intake in obesity. *American Journal of Clinical Nutrition, 36*, 470-477.

Wood, R.E., Boat, T.F., & Doershuk, C.F. (1976). Cystic fibrosis. *American Review of Respiratory Disease, 113*, 833-878.

Yamaji, K., & Miyashita, M. (1977). Oxygen transport systems during exhaustive exercise in Japanese boys. *European Journal of Applied Physiology, 36*, 93-99.

Ylitalo, V.M. (1981). Treatment of obese school children. *Acta Paediatrica Scandinavica*, Suppl. 290, 7-108.

Ylitalo, V.M. (1984). Exercise performance and serum lipids in obese school children before and after a reconditioning program. In J. Ilmarinen & I. Valimaki (Eds.), *Children and sport* (pp. 247-254). Berlin: Springer.

Zach, M.S., Purrer, B., & Oberwalder, B. (1981). Effect of swimming on forced expiration and sputum clearance in cystic fibrosis. *Lancet, 2*, 1201-1203.

Zapletal, A., Misur, M., & Samanek, M. (1971). Static recoil pressure of the lungs in children. *Bulletin Physiopathologie Respiratoire, 7*, 139-143.

Zeidifard, E., Godfrey, S., & Davies, E.E. (1976). Estimation of cardiac output by an N_2O rebreathing method in adults and children. *Journal of Applied Physiology, 41*, 433-438.

Zimmerman, D.R. (1987). Maturation and strenuous training in young female athletes. *The Physician and Sportsmedicine, 15*, 219-222.

Zinman, B., Zuniga-Guajardo, S., & Kelly, D. (1984). Comparison of the acute and long-term effects of exercise on glucose control in type I diabetes. *Diabetes Care, 7*, 515-519.

Zinner, S.H., & Kass, E.H. (1984). Epidemiology of blood pressure in infants and children. In J.M.H. Loggie, M.J. Horan, A.B. Gruskin, A.R. Hohn, J.B. Dunbar, & R.J. Havlik (Eds.), *NHLBI workshop on juvenile hypertension* (pp. 73-92). New York: Biomedical Information Corporation.

Index